ORTHOPEDIC CLINICS OF NORTH AMERICA

www.orthopedic.theclinics.com

Quality, Value, and Patient Safety in Orthopedic Surgery

October 2018 • Volume 49 • Number 4

Editor-in-Chief

FREDERICK M. AZAR

Editorial Board

MICHAEL J. BEEBE
CLAYTON C. BETTIN
JAMES H. CALANDRUCCIO
BENJAMIN J. GREAR
BENJAMIN M. MAUCK
WILLIAM M. MIHALKO
JEFFREY R. SAWYER
THOMAS (QUIN) THROCKMORTON
PATRICK C. TOY
JOHN C. WEINLEIN

ELSEVIER

1600 John F. Kennedy Boulevard • Suite 1800 • Philadelphia, Pennsylvania, 19103-2899.

http://www.orthopedic.theclinics.com

ORTHOPEDIC CLINICS OF NORTH AMERICA Volume 49, Number 4
October 2018 ISSN 0030-5898, ISBN-13: 978-0-323-64093-0

Editor: Lauren Boyle
Developmental Editor: Kristen Helm

Photocopying

Single photocopies of single articles may be made for personal use as allowed by national copyright laws. Permission of the Publisher and payment of a fee is required for all other photocopying, including multiple or systematic copying, copying for advertising or promotional purposes, resale, and all forms of document delivery. Special rates are available for educational institutions that wish to make photocopies for non-profit educational classroom use. For information on how to seek permission visit www.elsevier.com/permissions or call: (+44) 1865 843830 (UK)/(+1) 215 239 3804 (USA).

Derivative Works

Subscribers may reproduce tables of contents or prepare lists of articles including abstracts for internal circulation within their institutions. Permission of the Publisher is required for resale or distribution outside the institution. Permission of the Publisher is required for all other derivative works, including compilations and translations (please consult www.elsevier.com/permissions).

Electronic Storage or Usage

Permission of the Publisher is required to store or use electronically any material contained in this periodical, including any article or part of an article (please consult www.elsevier.com/permissions). Except as outlined above, no part of this publication may be reproduced, stored in a retrieval system or transmitted in any form or by any means, electronic, mechanical, photocopying, recording or otherwise, without prior written permission of the Publisher.

Notice

No responsibility is assumed by the Publisher for any injury and/or damage to persons or property as a matter of products liability, negligence or otherwise, or from any use or operation of any methods, products, instructions or ideas contained in the material herein. Because of rapid advances in the medical sciences, in particular, independent verification of diagnoses and drug dosages should be made.

Although all advertising material is expected to conform to ethical (medical) standards, inclusion in this publication does not constitute a guarantee or endorsement of the quality or value of such product or of the claims made of it by its manufacturer.

Orthopedic Clinics of North America (ISSN 0030-5898) is published quarterly by Elsevier Inc., 360 Park Avenue South, New York, NY 10010-1710. Months of issue are January, April, July, and October. Business and Editorial Offices: 1600 John F. Kennedy Blvd., Suite 1800, Philadelphia, PA 19103-2899. Customer Service Office: 3251 Riverport Lane, Maryland Heights, MO 63043. Periodicals postage paid at New York, NY and additional mailing offices. Subscription prices are $332.00 per year for (US individuals), $713.00 per year for (US institutions), $391.00 per year (Canadian individuals), $870.00 per year (Canadian institutions), $464.00 per year (international individuals), $870.00 per year (international institutions), $100.00 per year (US students), $220.00 per year (Canadian and international students). Foreign air speed delivery is included in all *Clinics* subscription prices. All prices are subject to change without notice. **POSTMASTER:** Send change of address to *Orthopedic Clinics of North America*, **Elsevier Health Sciences Division, Subscription Customer Service, 3251 Riverport Lane, Maryland Heights, MO 63043. Customer Service (orders, claims, online, change of address): Elsevier Health Sciences Division, Subscription Customer Service, 3251 Riverport Lane, Maryland Heights, MO 63043. Tel: 1-800-654-2452 (U.S. and Canada); 314-447-8871 (outside U.S. and Canada). Fax: 314-447-8029. E-mail:** journalscustomerservice-usa@elsevier.com **(for print support);** journalsonlinesupport-usa@elsevier.com **(for online support).**

Reprints. For copies of 100 or more, of articles in this publication, please contact the Commercial Reprints Department, Elsevier Inc., 360 Park Avenue South, New York, NY 10010-1710. Tel.: 212-633-3874; Fax: 212-633-3820; E-mail: reprints@elsevier.com.

Orthopedic Clinics of North America is covered in *MEDLINE/PubMed* (*Index Medicus*), *Cinahl, Excerpta Medica,* and *Cumulative Index to Nursing and Allied Health Literature.*

PROGRAM OBJECTIVE
Orthopedic Clinics of North America offers clinical review articles on the most cutting-edge technologies and techniques in the field, including knee and hip reconstruction, hand and wrist, paediatrics, trauma, shoulder and elbow, and foot and ankle.

TARGET AUDIENCE
Practicing orthopedic surgeons, orthopedic residents, and other healthcare professionals who specialize in orthopedic technologies and techniques for knee and hip reconstruction, hand and wrist, paediatrics, trauma, shoulder and elbow, and foot and ankle.

LEARNING OBJECTIVES
Upon completion of this activity, participants will be able to:
1. Review perioperative safety in the pediatric operating room
2. Discuss continuous quality improvement methods and tools for total joint replacement
3. Recognize the role of business education in the orthopaedic curriculum

ACCREDITATION
The Elsevier Office of Continuing Medical Education (EOCME) is accredited by the Accreditation Council for Continuing Medical Education (ACCME) to provide continuing medical education for physicians.

The EOCME designates this enduring material for a maximum of 15 *AMA PRA Category 1 Credit*(s)™. Physicians should claim only the credit commensurate with the extent of their participation in the activity.

All other healthcare professionals requesting continuing education credit for this enduring material will be issued a certificate of participation.

DISCLOSURE OF CONFLICTS OF INTEREST
The EOCME assesses conflict of interest with its instructors, faculty, planners, and other individuals who are in a position to control the content of CME activities. All relevant conflicts of interest that are identified are thoroughly vetted by EOCME for fair balance, scientific objectivity, and patient care recommendations. EOCME is committed to providing its learners with CME activities that promote improvements or quality in healthcare and not a specific proprietary business or a commercial interest.

The planning committee, staff, authors and editors listed below have identified no financial relationships or relationships to products or devices they or their spouse/life partner have with commercial interest related to the content of this CME activity:
Peter L. Althausen, MD, MBA; Karun Amar, MD; Afshin A. Anoushiravani, MD; Philip Band, PhD; Michael J. Beebe, MD; Clayton C.Bettin, MD; Eric K. Bonness, MD; Lauren Boyle; James H. Calandruccio, MD; Bayard C. Carlson, MD; John J. Carroll, MD; Brett Chamernik, MD; Alberto Criado, MD; Kay Daugherty; Hussein F. Dawiche, MD; Jaime Rice Denning, MD, MS; Thomas C. Dowd, MD; Thomas A. Einhorn, MD; Eric W. Guo; Heather S. Haeberle, BS; Laurence D. Higgins, MD; Joseph P. Iannotti, MD, PhD; Joseph Ingram, MD; Richard Iorio, MD; Kerwyn C. Jones, MD; Raj Karia, MS; Derek M. Kelly, MD; Alison Kemp; Brian Kurcz, MD; Kevin J. Little, MD; Kyle E. Lybrand, MD; Joseph Lyons, BSc; Benjamin M. Mauck, MD; William D. McClain, MD; Anthony J. Mells, BS; Zachary A. Mosher, MD; Feroz A. Osmani, MD; Muhammad T. Padela, MD, MSc; Mohsin Qazi, MD; Prem N. Ramkumar, MD, MBA; Eric T. Ricchetti, MD; Todd Ritzman, MD; Jeffrey R. Sawyer, MD; Yousuf Sayeed, MS; Zain Sayeed, MD, MHA; Patrick Schaefer, MD; Siddartha Simha, BSc; Bilal Sleiman, BS; Jeyanthi Surendrakumar; Michel A. Taylor, MD, MSc, FRCSC; Norfleet B. Thompson, MD; Walid Yassir, MD, MHCM; Bradley J. Zarling, MD; Mark Zekaj, MD.

The planning committee, staff, authors and editors listed below have identified financial relationships or relationships to products or devices they or their spouse/life partner have with commercial interest related to the content of this CME activity:
Benjamin J. Grear, MD: receives royalties from Elsevier, Inc.
A. Noelle Larson, MD: is a consultant/advisor for and receives research support from OrthoPediatrics Corp and K2M, Inc.
William M. Mihalko, MD: participates in a speakers' bureau for Aesculap, Inc. - a B. Braun company and CeramTec GmbH; receives research support from the United States Department of Defense and Stryker; serves as a consultant/advisor for Zimmer Biomet; and receives royalties from Elsevier, Inc.
Todd A. Milbrandt, MD, MS: is a consultant/advisor for and receives research support from OrthoPediatrics Corp.
Selene G. Parekh, MD, MBA: is a consultant/advisor to Baxter, receives royalties and/or owns patents with Wright Medical Group N.V., and is a consultant/advisor to and receives royalties and/or owns patents with Integra LifeSciences and Nextrimity Solutions, Inc.
Thomas (Quin) Throckmorton, MD: participates in a speakers' bureau for Zimmer Biomet, owns stock in Gilead, and receives royalties from Elsevier, Inc.
Patrick C. Toy, MD: has been a consultant/advisor for Zimmer Biomet, Medtronic, and Smith & Nephew. He also receives royalties and/or holds patents with Innomed, Inc.
John C. Weinlein, MD: receives royalties/holds patents with Elsevier, Inc.

UNAPPROVED/OFF-LABEL USE DISCLOSURE
The EOCME requires CME faculty to disclose to the participants:

1. When products or procedures being discussed are off-label, unlabelled, experimental, and/or investigational (not US Food and Drug Administration [FDA] approved); and
2. Any limitations on the information presented, such as data that are preliminary or that represent ongoing research, interim analyses, and/or unsupported opinions. Faculty may discuss information about pharmaceutical agents that is outside of FDA-approved labelling. This information is intended solely for CME and is not intended to promote off-label use of these medications. If you have any questions, contact the medical affairs department of the manufacturer for the most recent prescribing information.

TO ENROLL
To enroll in the *Orthopedic Clinics of North America* Continuing Medical Education program, call customer service at 1-800-654-2452 or sign up online at http://www.theclinics.com/home/cme. The CME program is available to subscribers for an additional annual fee of USD 215.

METHOD OF PARTICIPATION
In order to claim credit, participants must complete the following:
1. Complete enrolment as indicated above.
2. Read the activity.
3. Complete the CME Test and Evaluation. Participants must achieve a score of 70% on the test. All CME Tests and Evaluations must be completed online.

CME INQUIRIES/SPECIAL NEEDS
For all CME inquiries or special needs, please contact elsevierCME@elsevier.com.

EDITORIAL BOARD

FREDERICK M. AZAR, MD – EDITOR-IN-CHIEF
Professor, Department of Orthopaedic Surgery & Biomedical Engineering,
University of Tennessee-Campbell Clinic; Chief-of-Staff, Campbell Clinic, Inc,
Memphis, Tennessee

PATRICK C. TOY, MD – KNEE AND HIP RECONSTRUCTION
Assistant Professor, Department of Orthopaedic Surgery & Biomedical
Engineering, University of Tennessee-Campbell Clinic, Memphis, Tennessee

WILLIAM M. MIHALKO, MD, PhD – KNEE AND HIP RECONSTRUCTION
Professor & J.R. Hyde Chair of Excellence, Chair Joint Graduate Program
in Biomedical Engineering, Department of Orthopaedic Surgery &
Biomedical Engineering, The University of Tennessee Health Science
Center (UTHSC) - Campbell Clinic, Memphis, Tennessee

JOHN C. WEINLEIN, MD – TRAUMA
Assistant Professor, University of Tennessee-Campbell Clinic, Elvis Presley
Memorial Trauma Center, Regional One Health, Memphis, Tennessee

MICHAEL J. BEEBE, MD – TRAUMA
Assistant Professor, Department of Orthopaedic Surgery & Biomedical
Engineering, The University of Tennessee Health Science Center (UTHSC) -
Campbell Clinic, Memphis, Tennessee

JEFFREY R. SAWYER, MD – PEDIATRICS
Professor of Orthopaedic Surgery; Director, Pediatric Orthopaedic Fellowship,
University of Tennessee-Campbell Clinic, Memphis, Tennessee

CONTRIBUTORS

AUTHORS

PETER L. ALTHAUSEN, MD, MBA
Reno Orthopaedic Clinic, Reno, Nevada, USA

KARUN AMAR, MD
Department of Orthopaedics and Sports
Medicine, Detroit Medical Center, Detroit,
Michigan, USA

AFSHIN A. ANOUSHIRAVANI, MD
Department of Orthopaedic Surgery, NYU
Langone Health, New York, New York, USA

PHILIP BAND, PhD
Clinical Researcher, Department of
Orthopaedic Surgery, NYU Langone Medical
Center, Hospital for Joint Disease, New York,
New York, USA

ERIC K. BONNESS, MD
Clinical Fellow, Shoulder Service, Boston
Shoulder Institute, Boston, Massachusetts,
USA

JAMES H. CALANDRUCCIO, MD
Associate Professor, Department of
Orthopaedic Surgery and Biomedical
Engineering, Campbell Clinic, The University
of Tennessee, Memphis, Tennessee, USA

BAYARD C. CARLSON, MD
Department of Orthopedic Surgery, Mayo
Clinic, Rochester, Minnesota, USA

JOHN J. CARROLL, MD
Resident, Department of Orthopaedic
Surgery, SAUSHEC Orthopaedic Residency
Program Position, Fort Sam Houston, Texas,
USA

BRETT CHAMERNIK, MD
Department of Orthopaedics and Sports
Medicine, Detroit Medical Center, Detroit,
Michigan, USA

ALBERTO CRIADO, MD
Department of Orthopaedics and Sports
Medicine, Detroit Medical Center, Detroit,
Michigan, USA

HUSSEIN F. DARWICHE, MD
Department of Orthopaedics and Sports
Medicine, Musculoskeletal Institute of Surgical
Excellence, Detroit Medical Center, Detroit,
Michigan, USA

JAIME RICE DENNING, MD, MS
Assistant Professor, Orthopaedic Surgery,
Cincinnati Children's Hospital Medical Center,
Cincinnati, Ohio, USA

THOMAS C. DOWD, MD
Associate Program Director, Department of
Orthopaedic Surgery, SAUSHEC Orthopaedic
Residency Program Position, Fort Sam
Houston, Texas, USA

THOMAS A. EINHORN, MD
Director of Clinical, Translational Research,
Department of Orthopaedic Surgery,
NYU Langone Medical Center, Hospital
for Joint Disease, New York, New York,
USA

ERIC W. GUO, MD
Wayne State University School of Medicine,
Detroit Medical Center, Detroit, Michigan,
USA

HEATHER S. HAEBERLE, BS
Department of Orthopaedic Surgery, Baylor
College of Medicine, Houston, Texas, USA

LAURENCE D. HIGGINS, MD, MBA
Department of Orthopaedics, King Edward VII
Memorial Hospital, Paget, Bermuda

JOSEPH P. IANNOTTI, MD, PhD
Department of Orthopedic Surgery, Cleveland
Clinic, Cleveland, Ohio, USA

JOSEPH INGRAM, MD
Hand Surgery Fellow, Department
of Orthopaedic Surgery and Biomedical
Engineering, Campbell Clinic, The
University of Tennessee, Memphis,
Tennessee, USA

RICHARD IORIO, MD
Chief of Adult Reconstruction, Department of
Orthopaedic Surgery, NYU Langone Medical
Center, Hospital for Joint Disease, New York,
New York, USA

KERWYN C. JONES, MD
Chair, Department of Orthopedic Surgery,
Akron Children's Hospital, Akron, Ohio, USA;
Associate Clinical Professor, Northeast Ohio
Medical University, Rootstown, Ohio, USA

RAJ KARIA, MS
Research Assistant Professor, Department of
Orthopaedic Surgery, NYU Langone Medical
Center, Hospital for Joint Disease, New York,
New York, USA

DEREK M. KELLY, MD
Associate Professor, Department of
Orthopaedic Surgery and Biomedical
Engineering, The University of Tennessee,
Campbell Clinic, Memphis, Tennessee, USA

BRIAN KURCZ, MD
Department of Surgery, Division of
Orthopaedic Surgery, Southern Illinois
University, Springfield, Illinois, USA

A. NOELLE LARSON, MD
Department of Orthopedic Surgery, Mayo
Clinic, Rochester, Minnesota, USA

KEVIN J. LITTLE, MD
Associate Professor, Orthopaedic Surgery,
Cincinnati Children's Hospital Medical Center,
Cincinnati, Ohio, USA

KYLE E. LYBRAND, MD
Reno Orthopaedic Clinic, Reno, Nevada, USA

JOSEPH LYONS, BSc
Department of Surgery, Chicago Medical
School, North Chicago, Illinois, USA

BENJAMIN M. MAUCK, MD
Instructor, Department of Orthopaedic
Surgery and Biomedical Engineering,
Campbell Clinic, The University of Tennessee,
Memphis, Tennessee, USA

WILLIAM D. McCLAIN, MD
Resident, Department of Orthopaedic
Surgery, SAUSHEC Orthopaedic Residency
Program Position, Fort Sam Houston, Texas,
USA

ANTHONY J. MELLS, BS
Oakland University William Beaumont
School of Medicine, Rochester, Michigan, USA

TODD A. MILBRANDT, MD, MS
Department of Orthopedic Surgery,
Mayo Clinic, Rochester, Minnesota, USA

ZACHARY A. MOSHER, MD
Department of Orthopaedic Surgery and
Biomedical Engineering, The University of
Tennessee, Campbell Clinic, Memphis,
Tennessee, USA

FEROZ A. OSMANI, MD
Clinical Research Fellow, Department
of Orthopaedic Surgery, University of
Illinois at Chicago, Chicago, Illinois,
USA

MUHAMMAD T. PADELA, MD, MSc
Resident, Research Partnership, Department
of Orthopaedics and Sports Medicine,
Detroit Medical Center, Detroit, Michigan,
USA; Rosalind Franklin University of
Medicine and Science, Chicago Medical
School, North Chicago, Illinois,
USA

SELENE G. PAREKH, MD, MBA
Professor, Department of Orthopaedic
Surgery, Duke University Medical Center,
Duke Fuqua School of Business, North
Carolina Orthopedic Clinic, Durham, North
Carolina, USA

MOHSIN QAZI, MD
Department of Orthopaedics and Sports
Medicine, Musculoskeletal Institute of Surgical
Excellence, Detroit Medical Center, Detroit,
Michigan, USA

PREM N. RAMKUMAR, MD, MBA
Department of Orthopedic Surgery, Cleveland
Clinic, Cleveland, Ohio, USA

ERIC T. RICCHETTI, MD
Department of Orthopedic Surgery, Cleveland
Clinic, Cleveland, Ohio, USA

TODD RITZMAN, MD
Director of Education, Department of
Orthopedic Surgery, Akron Children's
Hospital, Akron, Ohio, USA; Associate Clinical
Professor, Northeast Ohio Medical University,
Rootstown, Ohio, USA

JEFFREY R. SAWYER, MD
Professor, Department of Orthopaedic
Surgery and Biomedical Engineering,
The University of Tennessee, Campbell
Clinic, Memphis, Tennessee, USA

YOUSUF SAYEED, MD
Clinical Research Fellow, Department of
Orthopaedic Surgery, NYU Langone Medical
Center, Hospital for Joint Disease, New York,
New York, USA

ZAIN SAYEED, MD, MHA
Resident, Research Partnership,
Department of Orthopaedics and Sports
Medicine, Musculoskeletal Institute of
Surgical Excellence, Detroit Medical Center,
Detroit, Michigan,
USA

PATRICK SCHAEFER, MD
Department of Orthopaedics and Sports
Medicine, Musculoskeletal Institute of Surgical
Excellence, Detroit Medical Center, Detroit,
Michigan, USA

SIDDARTHA SIMHA, BSc
Department of Orthopaedics and Sports
Medicine, Detroit Medical Center, Detroit,
Michigan, USA

BILAL SLEIMAN, BS
Resident, Research Partnership, Department
of Orthopaedics and Sports Medicine, Detroit
Medical Center, Detroit, Michigan, USA

MICHEL A. TAYLOR, MD, MSc, FRCSC
Department of Orthopaedic Surgery, Duke
University Medical Center, Durham, North
Carolina, USA

NORFLEET B. THOMPSON, MD
Instructor, Department of Orthopaedic
Surgery and Biomedical Engineering,
Campbell Clinic, The University of
Tennessee, Memphis, Tennessee, USA

WALID YASSIR, MD, MHCM
Department of Orthopaedics and Sports
Medicine, Detroit Medical Center, Detroit,
Michigan, USA

BRADLEY J. ZARLING, MD
Rosalind Franklin University of Medicine
and Science, Chicago Medical School, North
Chicago, Illinois, USA; Department
of Orthopaedics and Sports Medicine, Detroit
Medical Center, Detroit, Michigan, USA

MARK ZEKAJ, MD
Department of Orthopaedics and Sports
Medicine, Musculoskeletal Institute of Surgical
Excellence, Detroit Medical Center, Detroit,
Michigan, USA

CONTENTS

Knee and Hip Reconstruction
Patrick C. Toy and William M. Mihalko

Technologies continue to shape the path of medical treatment. Orthopedic surgeons benefit from becoming more aware of how twenty-first century information technology (IT) can benefit patients. The percentage of orthopedic patients utilizing IT resources is increasing, and new IT tools are becoming utilized. These include disease-specific applications. This article highlights the opportunity for developing IT tools applicable to the growing population of patients with osteoarthritis (OA) and presents a potential solution that can facilitate the way OA education and treatment are delivered and thereby maximize efficiency for the health care system, the physician, and the patient.

Faced with increasing pressure to reduce costs, hospitals must find new ways to eliminate waste while simultaneously maintaining the highest quality of care. For any institution, these types of changes can be complex and burdensome. This article outlines several methods that have been successful in reducing costs while maintaining high quality and highlights feasible methodologies that can help health care providers implement new quality improvement protocols.

As the Accreditation Council for Graduate Medical Education (ACGME) and National Academy of Medicine (NAM) increase emphasis on quality improvement (QI), continuing medical education must also adapt to meet these increasing demands. In fellowship programs and for attending physicians, QI initiatives exist but are rarer compared with initiatives during residency programs and they are even rarer for orthopedic surgery residents, fellows, and attending physicians. A QI curriculum should be in place at all stages of continuing medical education, as they help meet the criteria of the ACGME and NAM and promote better clinical practice and minimize errors.

Trauma
John C. Weinlein and Michael J. Beebe

Pediatrics
Jeffrey R. Sawyer

The literature within the last 10 years on MRI use in patients with orthopedic implants is reviewed. A literature search returned 15 relevant articles. Only 2 discussed pediatric patients. Overall, significant displacement of implants was infrequent. Radiofrequency-induced heating of implants differed among the studies, but most reported increases of less than 1°C. The authors conclude MRI is safe in patients with orthopedic implants because implant displacement and heating pose little risk to patients. A risk to benefit ratio is warranted, however, to assess the clinical utility and necessity of the study. Further research and individual assessment of implant properties and MRI-related interactions are warranted.

The entire operating room team is responsible for the safety of children in the operating room. As a leader in the operating room, the surgeon is impactful in ensuring that all team members are committed to providing this safe environment, which is achieved by the use of perioperative huddles or briefings, the use of appropriate surgical checklists, operating room standardization, surgeons proficient in the care they provide, and team members who embrace Just Culture.

Distal radius fractures are the most common site of fracture in the pediatric population. Supracondylar humerus fractures are the most common pediatric elbow fracture. Although there is an abundant literature discussing treatment and outcomes of these fractures, there is only an emerging literature specifically discussing the variation in care among surgeons. There is need for standardization of these types of injuries to optimize the quality, safety, and value for patients. Quality improvement methodology differs from traditional research and is meant to be shared and used to implement changes quickly. This article discusses basic quality improvement methodology.

The article addresses patient safety topics in spine surgery, including infection, length of stay, instrumentation strategies, pedicle screw malposition, radiation exposure, and neurologic events. Quality, safety, and value are concepts that are practical, are easy to understand, and can be implemented on any scale and may be matched to individual practices. Furthermore, with quality improvement, there is a culture shift to openly share information, protocols, and strategies so that more patients can rapidly benefit.

Outpatient total ankle arthroplasty (TAA) represents a potential significant source of healthcare cost savings. The ability to institute an effective outpatient TAA program depends on appropriate patient selection, effective management of patient and family expectations, surgeon experience, active involvement and coordination of an experienced multidisciplinary care team which includes anesthesiologists, nurse navigators, recovery room nursing staff, physical and occupational therapists and outpatient clinic personnel. Such a program also requires complete institutional logistical support.

QUALITY, VALUE, AND PATIENT SAFETY IN ORTHOPEDIC SURGERY

FORTHCOMING ISSUES

January 2019
New Technologies
Michael J. Beebe, Clayton C. Bettin,
Tyler J. Brolin, James H. Calandruccio,
Benjamin J. Grear, Benjamin M. Mauck,
William M. Mihalko, Jeffrey R. Sawyer,
Patrick C. Toy, and John C. Weinlein, *Editors*

April 2019
Surgical Considerations for Osteoporosis,
Osteopenia, and Vitamin D Deficiency
Michael J. Beebe, Clayton C. Bettin,
Tyler J. Brolin, James H. Calandruccio,
Benjamin J. Grear, Benjamin M. Mauck,
William M. Mihalko, Jeffrey R. Sawyer,
Patrick C. Toy, and John C. Weinlein, *Editors*

July 2019
Unique or Select Procedures
Michael J. Beebe, Clayton C. Bettin,
Tyler J. Brolin, James H. Calandruccio,
Benjamin J. Grear, Benjamin M. Mauck,
William M. Mihalko, Jeffrey R. Sawyer,
Patrick C. Toy, and John C. Weinlein, *Editors*

RECENT ISSUES

July 2018
Obesity
Michael J. Beebe, Clayton C. Bettin,
James H. Calandruccio, Benjamin J. Grear,
Benjamin M. Mauck, William M. Mihalko,
Jeffrey R. Sawyer, Thomas (Quin) Throckmorton,
Patrick C. Toy, and John C. Weinlein, *Editors*

April 2018
Evidence-Based Medicine
Michael J. Beebe, Clayton C. Bettin,
James H. Calandruccio, Benjamin J. Grear,
Benjamin M. Mauck, William M. Mihalko,
Jeffrey R. Sawyer, Thomas (Quin) Throckmorton,
Patrick C. Toy, and John C. Weinlein, *Editors*

January 2018
Outpatient Surgery
Michael J. Beebe, Clayton C. Bettin,
James H. Calandruccio, Benjamin J. Grear,
Benjamin M. Mauck, William M. Mihalko,
Jeffrey R. Sawyer, Thomas (Quin) Throckmorton,
Patrick C. Toy, and John C. Weinlein, *Editors*

SERIES OF RELATED INTEREST

Clinics in Podiatric Medicine and Surgery
Clinics in Sports Medicine
Foot and Ankle Clinics
Hand Clinics
Physical Medicine and Rehabilitation Clinics

PREFACE

Quality, Value, and Patient Safety in Orthopedic Surgery

Although the goals of medical treatment may seem deceptively simple quality, value, and safety for the patient—the means of attaining these goals are many, varied, and complex. The authors of this issue of *Orthopedic Clinics of North America* have discussed, explained, and proposed methods for improving quality, value, and patient safety in orthopedic procedures ranging from adult reconstructive surgery to pediatric surgery.

Dr Einhorn and colleagues, recognizing the ubiquitous nature of information technology (IT), highlight how IT tools can be developed to disseminate information to patients with osteoarthritis and improve patient-physician communication. Feasible methods for reducing costs and improving quality of care are the focus of the discussion by Dr Guo and colleagues. Dr Simha and colleagues and Dr Mells and colleagues emphasize that quality improvement (QI) needs to be a focus of both resident education and of health care leaders and provide information about QI methods that can promote better, more efficient orthopedic care. The avoidance and treatment of complications are large parts of total joint arthroplasty quality and value. Dr Kurcz and colleagues discuss the role of bearing surface wear in osteolysis after total hip arthroplasty.

As US healthcare costs continue to rise, developing a value-based practice is vital. Drs Lybrand and Althausen make a case for choosing orthopedic trauma implants based on cost savings to the patient, without financial incentive or fear of loss of consulting fees or research support. These two authors further elucidate the complex nature of current medical practice, provide methods for achieving practice stability, and encourage the addition of business education to residency curricula.

In no orthopedic subspecialty is the issue of patient safety such an emotional topic as in pediatric orthopedic surgery. In this section, Drs Mosher, Sawyer, and Kelly encourage physicians to consider the risk-to-benefit ratio when considering MRI evaluation of a child with orthopedic implants, even though their literature review suggested that MRI is safe in these patients. Drs Jones and Ritzman offer a number of suggestions for increasing safety in the operating room; Drs Denning and Little share examples of programs that standardized the surgical care of two common childhood fractures, which resulted in quality improvements in their orthopedic clinics. Finally, Drs Carlson, Milbrandt, and Larson address the topic of safety in spine surgery in children, with discussions of reductions in unplanned returns to the operating room, surgical site infections, and neurologic events.

Reducing costs of orthopedic surgeries is the emphasis of the three upper-extremity articles. Dr Ingram and colleagues discuss reducing the costs of treating carpal tunnel syndrome; Drs Bonness and Higgins provide information for reducing costs of shoulder surgery, and Dr Ramkumar and colleagues investigate the effect of surgical volume on costs in shoulder arthroplasty. The two lower-extremity articles focus on patient safety in foot and ankle surgery. Drs Carroll, McClain, and Dowd review the literature regarding driving limitations in patients with foot or ankle surgery, and Drs Taylor and Parekh highlight the significant cost savings that can be obtained with an effective outpatient total ankle program.

Overall, this issue of *Orthopedic Clinics of North America* brings to the forefront three essential elements of orthopedic treatment—quality, value, and safety—that are becoming more and more important as the health care system continues to evolve, and we appreciate the time and effort these experts have expended to assist us in navigating these often difficult situations.

Frederick M. Azar, MD
University of Tennessee–Campbell Clinic
Department of Orthopaedic Surgery
1211 Union Avenue, Suite 510
Memphis, TN 38104, USA

E-mail address:
fazar@campbellclinic.com

Orthop Clin N Am 49 (2018) xvii
https://doi.org/10.1016/j.ocl.2018.07.001
0030-5898/18/© 2018 Published by Elsevier Inc.

Knee and Hip Reconstruction

The Role of Patient Education in Arthritis Management

The Utility of Technology

Thomas A. Einhorn, MD[a], Feroz A. Osmani, MD[b,*],
Yousuf Sayeed, MD[a], Raj Karia, MS[a], Philip Band, PhD[a],
Richard Iorio, MD[a]

KEYWORDS

- Osteoarthritis • Education • Technology • Arthroplasty • Hip • Knee • Telemedicine

KEY POINTS

- With increasing prevalence, new arthritis management strategies must be developed to curtail its pathologic prognosis.
- The use of information technology (IT) resources, including Web-based platforms and telemedicine, has demonstrated positive results and a growing demand.
- Emerging IT platforms can be used to optimize communication between patients and caregivers in novel ways that can improve outcomes.
- Patients may be able to identify their symptoms early on, and through self-help and exercise programs, gain control over their disease process.
- The Lifetime Initiative for the Management of Arthritis program is an innovative tool that provides a structured exercise regimen, and an easy-access, trusted information source.

INTRODUCTION

Arthritis is a chronic illness that negatively impacts the lives of millions of Americans. It is prevalent in approximately 23% of the US population and was recently reported to affect over 54 million US adults.[1] Per the US Centers for Disease Control and Prevention (CDC), by 2040, this number will increase to a staggering 78 million people, over a quarter of the nation's population.[1]

Osteoarthritis (OA), also known as degenerative arthritis, is the most common form of arthritis and is commonly considered to be associated with aging and obesity. The health and economic burden of OA continue to increase as the US population ages and life expectancy increases. To meet this growing need, the authors have considered how newly available information technology (IT) tools could be used for patient education and disease management. Specifically, the article discusses how IT-based patient education and intervention tools can address gaps in the management of OA. The objective is to modernize treatment, control costs, and improve overall patient outcomes. In the context of this literature review, the authors describe current concepts regarding the diagnosis and treatment of OA, and present a novel IT-based approach that they have developed for OA patients, which

Disclosure Statement: myarthritisrx.com, PCORI Tier III (3411628-003) award funding for Lifetime Initiative for the Management of Arthritis studies.
[a] Department of Orthopaedic Surgery, New York University Langone Medical Center, Hospital for Joint Disease, 380 2nd Avenue, New York, NY 10010, USA; [b] Department of Orthopaedic Surgery, University of Illinois at Chicago, 1740 West Taylor Street, Chicago IL 60612, USA
* Corresponding author.
E-mail address: fosman3@uic.edu

is referred to as the Lifetime Initiative for the Management of Arthritis (LIMA).

LIMA is designed to educate patients about OA, to differentiate diverse OA phenotypes using fingerprints of arthritic disease. The objective of the LIMA project is to identify patients for whom nonoperative management strategies are appropriate, to conserve health care resources, to improve the health status of individuals and populations, and to optimize surgical outcomes when arthroplasty is indicated.

DIAGNOSIS

A diagnosis of OA typically occurs after a positive physical examination indicates degenerative joint disease and is often confirmed by imaging. During examination, the physician may ask the patient to describe his or her symptoms, when the symptoms typically occur, what can make the symptoms better or worse, and inquire about what types of medications the patient is taking. The physical examination reports on gait, deformity, alignment, range of motion, locking, clicking, crepitus, pain, effusion, swelling, and ligamentous stability. At the authors' institution, an IT system has been developed that enables patients to complete validated questionnaires prior to seeing their physician, as part of standard care.[2] The system sends the questionnaires to patients via email prior to their visit, collects data in the waiting room if the questionnaire has not been filled out in advance, and makes this aspect of the patient's history available for review during the office visit. The authors use a measure of joint-specific symptomology (eg, the Knee Injury and Osteoarthritis Outcome Score, KOOS, or the Hip Injury and Osteoarthritis Outcome Score, HOOS), and a preference-based quality of life measure (EQ-5D). Sometimes advanced imaging modalities are prescribed, such as MRI or ultrasound. When patients present with a tense effusion, the joint may be aspirated and synovial fluid analysis performed.

Radiologic assessment of a joint remains the primary factor determining the diagnosis of OA. Paradoxically, radiographic OA in often observed in asymptomatic or minimally involved individuals.[3] The Kellgren and Lawrence (KL) grading scale has been employed to stratify disease severity based on radiologic imaging, dividing patients into 5 groups- Grades 1 through 5.[4] Because symptomatic OA does not always align with the radiographic images, the KL grades must only be used as an adjunct to patient reported pain in order to confirm the diagnosis.

RISK OF OSTEOARTHRITIS INCIDENCE AND PROGRESSION

The incidence and progression of osteoarthritis vary between patients based on several factors. Generally, OA prevalence increases with age.[5] Female gender carries increased risk of OA; the CDC found that OA prevalence was 18% in men and 24% in women.[1] Obesity can cause higher levels of strain on joints, increasing weight-bearing load and the rate of cartilage loss.[6] Obesity was linked to an increase in OA of the hand, hip, and most strongly, the knee.[6] Occupations that were more physically demanding, such as carpenters or dockworkers, were reported to have higher rates of OA.[6]

THE IMPORTANCE OF BIOMARKERS

Joint pain, the cardinal symptom of osteoarthritis, can be periodic or chronic, stable or worsening, disabling or manageable with activity limitation. However, symptoms often do not correlate with radiologic measures of the disease. Inflammation is sometimes clinically evident, but often OA patients experience joint pain with no overt signs of inflammation. OA is a disease with multiple phenotypes that can be clinically distinguished, and it is clinically important to consider phenotype when making treatment decisions.[7]

Although much information about patient OA phenotype can be based on clinical presentation, ongoing work is developing the use of biomarkers in blood and synovial fluid to more precisely inform phenotype-based treatment decisions.[8,9] The most extensively studied biomarkers are measures of cartilage degradation, and of synovial inflammation.[8,9] Cartilage degradation can be monitored via measures of matrix turnover, including type II collagen fragments and propeptide, collagen-associated matrix protein (COMP) and proteoglycan fragments (REFS).[8,9] The inflammatory status of a joint can be determined by measurement of synovial fluid biomarkers, and more precisely defined in terms of the activity of the local innate immune system, including the level of cytokines, chemokines, and protease activity (aggrecanase and metalloprotease forms).[8,9] TSG-6 activity in synovial fluid has been recently identified as a highly significant predictor of the risk for rapid radiologic progression and joint replacement, and is suggested to be useful to inform the timing of arthroplasty.[8,9] Measuring the TSG-6 activity may be important to identify patients at low risk for progression, who should not be rushed into arthroplasty. Joint pain and disability, the primary indications for arthroplasty, are subjective symptoms that are judged by patients and their physicians when making decisions about surgery. The relationship between pain and biomarkers remains an important area of study.[9]

PATIENT-REPORTED OUTCOME MEASURES

There are currently several methods for quantifying the pain and symptomology experienced by patients with OA. Patient-reported outcomes measures (PROMs) focus on the patient's impression of his or her level of pain, quality of life, health status, functionality, symptoms, and overall subjective rating of care. Some commonly used PROMs include the KOOS, HOOS, and the Western Ontario and McMaster University Osteoarthritis Index (WOMAC).[10] The level of impairment from OA has been described through the scope of functional limitations, as patients can be categorized by their abilities (eg, the level of pain they experience when walking or climbing stairs).[11] Physicians must take into account a patient's required activities of daily living (ADLs) when determining a treatment program for OA. It is well-documented that patients with OA can have substantial impairments of their function caused by higher levels of pain associated with specific activities.[11]

INCREASING COMMUNICATION WITH PATIENTS USING INFORMATION TECHNOLOGY

The Internet and personal computing devices create an opportunity to provide patients with a reliable, evidence-based source of knowledge they can use for self-managing their disease. Per the US Census Bureau, in 2013, 83.8% of US households reported computer ownership, and 73.4% had high-speed Internet connections.[12] Smartphone usage rates have increased in recent years, as 68% of US adults reported owning a smartphone in 2015, up from 35% in 2011.[13] With accessibility reaching high levels, there is more opportunity for innovation in the health care industry that may provide a wider audience for IT-driven, customizable, value-based treatment options.

The field of telehealth has expanded medical access to patients throughout the United States.[14] Telehealth gives patients the opportunity to utilize video-conferencing and data storage, and to forward information in the form of text, images, or videos to health care providers. Physicians can now monitor patients remotely, allowing more immediate care delivery. Rural communities have begun to explore telehealth through teleradiology, telepsychiatry, teleopthalmology, teledermatology, and teledentistry. Patients who that do not live near hospitals can now receive care more easily without the need to travel long distances.[15] Telehealth has already been of benefit in several scenarios. One study found that telehealth services utilizing scheduled phone calls from nonclinically trained health advisers for patients with depression resulted in decreased levels of anxiety, greater satisfaction with the care received, and improved self-management and health literacy compared with than standard of care treatment.[16] A Massachusetts General Hospital telemedicine service utilized to manage pain of patients living in rural areas of Massachusetts reported an overall positive response, especially when friendly rapport was established with their health care provider.[17]

For patients who do not speak English, online education now enables text to be translated more easily, and access can occur at the patient's convenience. One study examining patient education for the Latin-American community receiving dialysis found that Web-based education tailored to Hispanic culture led to improved levels of education retention when compared with in-person information given to patients on the same day and 3 weeks after exposure to the Web site.[18] With digital translating services and videoconferencing, translators can also be made available throughout hospitals where interpreters are not physically present.

The quality of materials available to both patients and physicians in the digital world is of variable quality and reliability. Wiechmann and colleagues[19] examined the quality of smartphone applications available in the iTunes App Store being marketed to health care professionals. With over 20,000 applications in the medical category, the search was narrowed to 7699 applications based on appropriate search criteria (using phrases such as critical care, orthopedics, procedures, and emergency medicine). After reviewing the categories, 64.9% of the applications were not relevant to medical professionals who were investigating referring patients to these applications.[19] It is critical to understand and evaluate specific technologies before employing them in one's practice, and especially before recommending them to other physicians or patients.

THE VALUE OF WEB-BASED PATIENT EDUCATION IN ORTHOPEDICS

Patient education plays a critical role in care perception and expectations for treatment effectiveness. Newer therapies, risks for treatment, and even basic prognostic information may be interpreted more keenly by a patient who better educated and knowledgeable about his or her disease. Information that is up-to-date, evidence-based, easily understandable, and in a format that is easy and efficient for a patient is becoming available. Health care provider-to-patient/in-person information transmission is highly inefficient and may not be the best method to educate the population effectively. Heikkinen and colleagues[20] compared the knowledge level improvement of Web-based education of patients undergoing total hip or knee arthroplasty versus those educated face-to-face by a nurse practitioner. They found that individuals receiving Web-based education retained a higher level of useful information than those given face-to-face education from the nurse practitioner.

In another study, Heikkinen and colleagues[21] sought to understand the differences between patients receiving ambulatory orthopedic surgery who were educated about their surgery using 2 different methodologies. Patients receiving Web-based education had higher levels of knowledge retention compared with those patients who communicated with nurses in person to receive information. These studies demonstrate that Web-based education for patients receiving medical care can be superior to in-person education. Web-based education is available whenever and wherever the patient seeks it, and the patient is free to review it at his or her convenience without being subject to the time constraints of health care professionals. Online education should be formatted so that it is accessible to patients of all backgrounds. It can generally be made available in several languages, and should be designed to be understandable and concise, to provide reproducible and consistent outcomes.

GROWING INTEREST IN SELF-MANAGED AND ASSISTED EXERCISE PROGRAMS

Exercise regimens have been well-documented to provide osteoarthritic patients with symptomatic benefits. Jørgensen and colleagues[22] documented the benefits of home-based exercise therapy 7 days a week following unicompartmental knee arthroplasty, versus home-based therapy 5 days a week alongside resistance training 2 days a week, demonstrating that there was no difference in pain scores between the 2 groups after a 1-year follow-up. This suggests that home-based therapies are comparable to supervised

therapies. Group exercise and self-management were found to benefit patients with osteoarthritis, noting the benefit of group interactions to increase sociability, motivation from others, and a sense of cohesion and camaraderie between individuals who were initially strangers.[23]

Wilcox and colleagues[24] compared the effect of the First Step to Active Health self-directed exercise program with a well-balanced Steps to Healthy Eating nutrition control program, finding that those in the exercise group had a greater increase in overall physical activity, although both groups had gained functionality and reported increased psychosocial benefit.

Lee and colleagues[25] found that participation in a structured exercise program resulted not only in significantly decreased pain scores, but also in high patient satisfaction and adherence. Although recent studies have consistently demonstrated the benefits of exercise in the osteoarthritic population, compliance has been the recurring obstacle to improving patient wellness. Unfortunately, it has been well-documented that the effects of exercise eventually disappear with discontinuation. This identifies long-term compliance as an important metric to consider when designing IT-based programs for orthopedic care.

It is important to recognize that there is not a one size fits all self-managed and assisted exercise program. Each individual must have a plan that has been catered to his or her specific needs, goals, and expectations. The personalization of exercise programs is the next step in the development of OA therapy, slowing its progression, and addressing the patient more so than solely the disease.

BENEFITS OF WEARABLE DEVICE APPLICATION

Wearable devices can record and analyze qualities of a patient's daily activities such as distance traveled or number of steps taken in a given timeframe or biometrics like blood pressure or heart rate. One study evaluated the impact of wearable technology on the psychosocial factors of OA management. After interviewing 21 patients with OA in focus groups, researchers found that most patients, 11 out of 21, were not aware of these devices. However, upon learning about them, patients felt that wearable devices can accurately communicate patient functionality to physicians, provide a deeper understanding of shared decision making, increase the potential for customized treatments, and provide a stronger level of clarity for a management plan.[26]

Examining another attribute of wearable devices, Tadano and colleagues[27] also conducted research focused on evaluating patient gait. In their study, 10 subjects with knee OA and 8 healthy volunteers were equipped with H-Gait wearable sensors. The study demonstrated that OA progression led to a more acute angle between the right and left knee and ankle joints on the horizontal plane, and that ankle joints abduct less and less to avoid adduction at the knee in patients as their osteoarthritis increased in severity. These findings can aid in making the diagnosis of symptomatic OA and monitor the progression of the disease in a novel manner. Physicians may be able to monitor patients' gait to stratify patient disease level and suggest treatments.

PATIENT PERSPECTIVE

The authors hosted several focus groups consisting of 10 patients with a diagnosis of OA, the aim of which was to understand patient goals and perspectives. Inclusion criteria included male and female participants ages 18 and older. Questionnaires were distributed asking patients concerning comorbidities, surgical procedures related to OA, medical management of OA, and satisfaction with current management. In addition, patients were asked to describe their current level of OA understanding, the resources that they use to educate themselves regarding their disease process, and which educational modality (in-person, books, Internet, television) they prefer. A brief question-and-answer session was included at the end of all sessions. Reviewing their results, the authors found that most patients do not currently use online or Internet-based information technology programs to help cope with their OA (Fig. 1). The authors' findings also revealed that most patients are more interested in a community program for

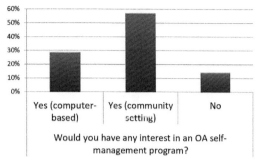

Fig. 2. Interest in osteoarthritis self-management program. N = 7.

managing their osteoarthritis than in a computer-based program, but most were interested in some type of self-management program as part of their therapy (Fig. 2). Most patients were interested in a social framework where they could discuss their disease and treatment options with health care professionals and other patients to tailor treatment to their specific needs and lifestyles. Furthermore, there was a sense of dissatisfaction with the current treatment options available to patients; most the patients interviewed were either neutral or not satisfied with the quality of the treatment they were currently receiving within the health care system (Fig. 3). Lastly, the authors found patients rely on both themselves and their physician equally when planning their treatment for OA (Fig. 4). Taking these results into consideration, it is clear that patients desire to be part of a larger community of OA patients, and many feel that they can guide their own treatment regimens with some direction from a reliable source. The patients felt that the current resources available to them were inadequate for their individual needs. The need for shared decision-making tools was obvious to the patients and the caregivers who participated in the focus groups.

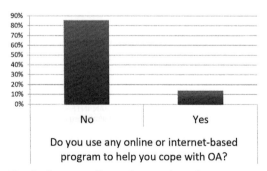

Fig. 1. Current online or Internet-based program usage. N = 7.

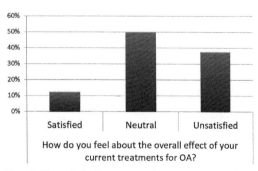

Fig. 3. Overall feelings toward current osteoarthritis treatments. N = 8.

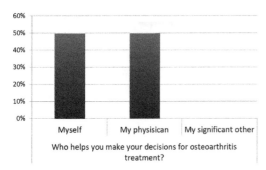

Fig. 4. Responsibility of osteoarthritis treatment. N = 10.

THE DEVELOPMENT OF LIFETIME INITIATIVE FOR THE MANAGEMENT OF ARTHRITIS

The Lifetime Initiative for the Management of Arthritis (LIMA) has been designed to help patients with OA manage their disease process, taking into consideration all that has been highlighted in this review. LIMA is a patient-facing digital platform designed for evidence-based patient education, and the evaluation and symptomatic management of OA. Utilizing bioinformatics tools, patients are stratified by disease severity and risk of progression and provided a treatment regimen that is customized to their individual needs. Self-evaluation and staging algorithms are unique elements that form the therapeutic foundation of LIMA.

Through focus group sessions, the authors determined that there is demand for an all-encompassing evidence-based resource that patients can use to learn more about their disease and how to manage symptoms. Participation in LIMA provides patients with access to evidence-based information that is relevant to their individual problem, along with treatment-appropriate options.

Upon initial presentation, participants with a joint complaint will engage the LIMA platform, prior to or after the initial doctor visit. Through a series of interactive questionnaires, a unique algorithm scores the patient based on severity and risk of progression. The LIMA algorithm metrics include participant demographics, pain measurements, participant-reported outcomes scores, activity, health status, and participant expectations. These variables are used to calculate the likelihood of meeting expectations based on the selected intervention, providing a probability of treatment success.

Based on the participant's severity and risk score, a recommendation is made for either self-management, assisted self-management, or physician intervention. Assisted self-management includes an arthritis coach, over-the-counter medications, wellness, health assessments, physical therapy, and a customized exercise regimen. The purpose of this management plan is essentially for early identification, symptom and disability

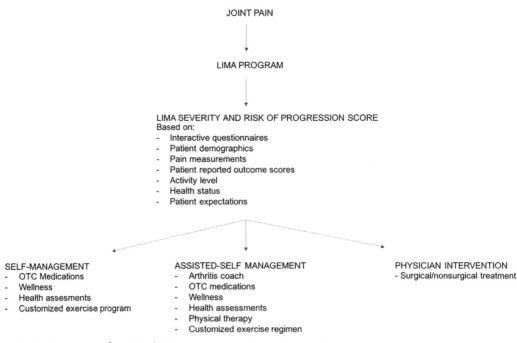

Fig. 5. LIMA program: from initial joint pain presentation to intervention.

improvement, and minimization of the risk of OA progression.

The LIMA program will provide a structured exercise program, and an easy-access, trusted information source. The technology platform includes progress tracking, self-monitoring and coaching as required, and a social media component. Participants are encouraged to take responsibility for those behavioral patterns that influence the OA disease process. The objective of the tools that LIMA provides is to engage participants in a social platform and improve compliance with their recommended intervention regimens, increasing mobility, satisfaction, and adherence, while decreasing pain scores (Fig. 5).

SUMMARY

Emerging IT platforms can be used to optimize communication between patients and caregivers in novel ways that can improve outcomes. The LIMA platform is designed to engage patients, and help patients understand the value of conservative measures to relieve pain and improve health status. Future patients are expected to be better equipped to adapt to a changing health care landscape that will utilize newer IT resources for self-managed therapies. Properly curated, Web-based education platforms can provide a useful source of evidence-based, standardized patient education. Physicians who treat arthritis should consider how the availability of these IT tools can help provide the best management strategies for their patients, but it is important that all new platforms be properly evaluated before introducing them to patients.

REFERENCES

1. At a glance — arthritis. Atlanta (GA): US Department of H.ealth and Human Services, Centers for Disease Control and Prevention; 2016.
2. Karia RJ, Zhou X, Slover JD, et al. Patient specific variables influence patient reported outcome scores in TKA population. Osteoarthritis and Cartilage. 23. A350. 10.1016/j.joca.2015.02.643.
3. Bedson J, Croft PR. The discordance between clinical and radiographic knee osteoarthritis: a systematic search and summary of the literature. BMC Musculoskelet Disord 2008;9:116.
4. Petersson IF, Boegård T, Saxne T, et al. Radiographic osteoarthritis of the knee classified by the Ahlbäck and Kellgren & Lawrence systems for the tibiofemoral joint in people aged 35-54 years with chronic knee pain. Ann Rheum Dis 1997;56(8): 493–6.
5. Dibonaventura MD, Gupta S, McDonald M, et al. Impact of self-rated osteoarthritis severity in an employed population: cross-sectional analysis of data from the national health and wellness survey. Health Qual Life Outcomes 2012;10:30.
6. Zhang Y, Jordan JM. Epidemiology of osteoarthritis. Clin Geriatr Med 2010;26(3):355–69.
7. Van der Esch M, Knoop J, Van der Leeden M, et al. Clinical phenotypes in patients with knee osteoarthritis: a study in the Amsterdam osteoarthritis cohort. Osteoarthr Cartil 2015;23(4):544–9.
8. Wisniewski HG, Colón E, Liublinska V, et al. TSG-6 activity as a novel biomarker of progression in knee osteoarthritis. Osteoarthritis Cartilage 2014;22(2):235–41.
9. Band PA, Heeter J, Wisniewski HG, et al. Hyaluronan molecular weight distribution is associated with the risk of knee osteoarthritis progression. Osteoarthritis Cartilage 2015;23(1):70–6.
10. Ramkumar PN, Harris JD, Noble PC. Patient-reported outcome measures after total knee arthroplasty: a systematic review. Bone Joint Res 2015;4(7):120–7.
11. Mcdonough CM, Jette AM. The contribution of osteoarthritis to functional limitations and disability. Clin Geriatr Med 2010;26(3):387–99.
12. File T, Ryan C. "Computer and internet use in the United States: 2013," American community survey reports, ACS-28. Washington, DC: U.S. Census Bureau; 2014.
13. Anderson M. "Technology device ownership: 2015." Pew Research Center Internet Science Tech RSS. Washington DC: The Pew Charitable Trusts; 2015. Available at: http://www.pewinternet.org/2015/10/29/technology-device-ownership-2015/. Accessed May 3, 2016.
14. What is telehealth? Center for Connected Health Policy. Available at: http://www.cchpca.org/what-is-telehealth. Accessed May 7, 2017.
15. Rural Health Information Hub. Telehealth use in rural healthcare introduction. Grand Forks (ND): RHIHub; 2014. Available at: https://www.rural-healthinfo.org/topics/telehealth. Accessed May 3, 2016.
16. Salisbury C, O'cathain A, Edwards L, et al. Effectiveness of an integrated telehealth service for patients with depression: a pragmatic randomised controlled trial of a complex intervention. Lancet Psychiatry 2016;3(6):515–25.
17. Hanna GM, Fishman I, Edwards DA, et al. Development and patient satisfaction of a new telemedicine service for pain management at Massachusetts General Hospital to the Island of Martha's Vineyard. Pain Med 2016;17(9):1658–63.
18. Gordon EJ, Feinglass J, Carney P, et al. A Website intervention to increase knowledge about living kidney donation and transplantation among Hispanic/Latino dialysis patients. Prog Transplant 2016;26(1):82–91.

19. Wiechmann W, Kwan D, Bokarius A, et al. There's an app for that? Highlighting the difficulty in finding clinically relevant smartphone applications. West J Emerg Med 2016;17(2):191–4.

20. Heikkinen K, Helena LK, Taina N, et al. A comparison of two educational interventions for the cognitive empowerment of ambulatory orthopaedic surgery patients. Patient Educ Couns 2008; 73(2):272–9.

21. Heikkinen K, Leino-kilpi H, Salanterä S. Ambulatory orthopaedic surgery patients' knowledge with Internet-based education. Methods Inf Med 2012; 51(4):295–300.

22. Jørgensen PB, Bogh SB, Kierkegaard S, et al. The efficacy of early initiated, supervised, progressive resistance training compared to unsupervised, home-based exercise after unicompartmental knee arthroplasty: a single-blinded randomized controlled trial. Clin Rehabil 2017;31(1):61–70.

23. Ettinger WH, Burns R, Messier SP, et al. A randomized trial comparing aerobic exercise and resistance exercise with a health education program in older adults with knee osteoarthritis. The Fitness Arthritis and Seniors Trial (FAST). JAMA 1997;277(1):25–31.

24. Wilcox S, Mcclenaghan B, Sharpe PA, et al. The steps to health randomized trial for arthritis: a self-directed exercise versus nutrition control program. Am J Prev Med 2015;48(1):1–12.

25. Lee FI, Lee TD, So WK. Effects of a tailor-made exercise program on exercise adherence and health outcomes in patients with knee osteoarthritis: a mixed-methods pilot study. Clin Interv Aging 2016;11:1391–402.

26. Belsi A, Papi E, Mcgregor AH. Impact of wearable technology on psychosocial factors of osteoarthritis management: a qualitative study. BMJ Open 2016; 6(2):e010064.

27. Tadano S, Takeda R, Sasaki K, et al. Gait characterization for osteoarthritis patients using wearable gait sensors (H-Gait systems). J Biomech 2016; 49(5):684–90.

Improving Total Joint Replacement with Continuous Quality Improvement Methods and Tools

Eric W. Guo, MD[a], Zain Sayeed, MD, MHA[b,c,d,*],
Muhammad T. Padela, MD, MSc[b,c,d], Mohsin Qazi, MD[c,d],
Mark Zekaj, MD[c,d], Patrick Schaefer, MD[c,d],
Hussein F. Darwiche, MD[c,d]

KEYWORDS

- Total joint arthroplasty • Total knee arthroplasty • Total hip arthroplasty • Quality improvement
- Lean six sigma • Clinical pathways • BPCI

KEY POINTS

- Applying quality improvement techniques from other industries can provide a legitimate template for improving the health care system.
- Standardization and simplification are feasible adjustments that can drastically improve outcomes for patients.
- Eliminating inefficiencies in the delivery of total joint arthroplasty in the context of novel compensation models can decrease cost and increase value for all stakeholders while maintaining quality for patients.
- There are multiple studies that have established a foundation for less-experienced health care institutions to draw upon to aid the transition to high-quality, economically efficient protocols.

INTRODUCTION

Total joint arthroplasty (TJA) is frequently indicated in patients with severe degenerative osteoarthritis. As the population continues to age, the demand for these surgeries will continue to rise. It is estimated that by 2030, the number of annual total hip arthroplasties (THAs) and total knee arthroplasties (TKAs) in the United States could reach 572,000 and 3.48 million, respectively.[1]

Studies have reported that joint arthroplasty surgeries are cost-effective. Cost-effectiveness can be portrayed as a comparison of the cost of a surgical or medical intervention with the gain of quality-adjusted life years (QALYS). The threshold value for cost-effectiveness has not been standardized on a large scale, but there have been recommendations for thresholds of $50,000 to $200,000 per QALY, or 2 to 3 times the per capita gross income.[2] There have been several studies on TJA that report cost-effectiveness well below these numbers. For example, Chang and colleagues[3] reported a $4600 cost per QALY gained in THAs. Similarly, for TKA, Losina and colleagues[4] found a cost-effectiveness to QALY ratio ranging from

[a] Wayne State University School of Medicine, Detroit Medical Center, 4707 St Antoine Street, Detroit, MI 48201, USA; [b] Chicago Medical School at Rosalind Franklin University, 3333 Greenbay Road, North Chicago, IL 60064, USA; [c] Department of Orthopaedic Surgery, Detroit Medical Center, 4201 St Antoine Street, Suite 9B, Detroit, MI 48201, USA; [d] Resident Research Partnership, 233 Fielding Street, Suite B, Ferndale, MI 48220, USA
* Corresponding author.
E-mail address: zainsayeed@gmail.com

Orthop Clin N Am 49 (2018) 397–403
https://doi.org/10.1016/j.ocl.2018.05.002
0030-5898/18/© 2018 Elsevier Inc. All rights reserved.

$9700 to $21,700 for low- and high-risk patients, respectively. The cost per QALY for TJA is well below the previously mentioned thresholds, suggesting that TJA is an economically efficient way to improve a patient's quality of life.

Although cost-effective, TJA is highly variable in its delivery, which presents many opportunities for quality improvement. Tomek and colleagues[5] collected data from several health care systems to identify differences in TKA delivery. They found variations in each system and identified characteristics such as having a dedicated TKA operating team and multispecialty involvement in perioperative care as factors associated with improved patient and hospital outcomes. Studies have shown there are also fluctuating costs for TKA and THA within and between hospitals. Bozic and colleagues[6] compiled data on patients admitted for TKA or THA from 61 hospitals. They noted that the cost of a knee and hip implant displayed high degrees of variability, ranging from $1797 to $12,093 USD and $2392 to $12,651 USD respectively. Even including this wide range of implant costs, there was still a significant portion of variability unaccounted for. As economic pressures to decrease cost continue to rise, standardization of TJA delivery will become increasingly critical to reduce waste, eliminate inefficiencies, and ultimately improve the quality of TJA.

Lean six sigma (LSS) and the use of standard clinical pathways are quality improvement methodologies that have shown promise. LSS is a quality improvement system that was originally implemented in manufacturing industries, but has been applied to the health care field over the past 20 years.[7,8] The purpose of LSS is to use systematic and analytical approaches to identify inefficiencies and improve them. Clinical pathways, on the other hand, are evidence-based changes to homogenize perioperative protocols to minimize variation with the goal of improving efficiency and quality.

As the population in the United States continues to age, the demand for these TJA will only continue to rise. Evaluating and implementing novel cost-cutting procedures can be difficult for any organization. The purpose of this article is to analyze current quality improvement techniques and provide a framework of feasible changes that institutions can draw from to facilitate the transition to value-based health care.

BENCHMARKING

Setting internal benchmarks that are in accordance to external benchmarks set by national regulatory committees can lead to direct improvements on quality. Benditz and colleagues[9] demonstrated that using a system of benchmarking with feedback mechanisms led to a decrease in pain after THA, increase in patient satisfaction, and an improvement of quality. Benditz and colleagues assembled a multidisciplinary team to establish and implement a regular system of data analysis and internal benchmarking. Some of the parameters that were benchmarked included mean numerical rating score (NRS), maximum pain, minimum pain, and patient satisfaction. The health care team was then informed of the data and feedback reported from patients. Constant communication and suggestions for improvement among patient, nurses, and physicians were encouraged. After implementation of the continuous benchmarking and feedback program, patients reported decreased mean maximal pain scores and increased satisfaction scores. Through consistent benchmarking, feedback, and communication, the researchers were able to improve the quality of THA. Benditz and colleagues[10] then applied this benchmarking with a direct feedback process to TKA and noted similar improvements in pain score and patient satisfaction. In larger health care systems where implementation of any standard protocol can be complex and difficult, benchmarking can be a simple yet effective technique to improve patient outcomes.

In addition to internal benchmarks, hospitals must ensure that the benchmarks they set either meet or exceed the standards set by the Agency for Healthcare Research and Quality and other national health care quality evaluators.

LEAN SIX SIGMA

LSS is similar to benchmarking, but there are some differences. LSS is a methodology originally implemented in manufacturing industries to use systematic and reproducible approaches to improve quality. There are several management techniques described as LSS tools that may aid in effective quality improvement implementation. Perhaps the most fundamental roadmap in LSS methodology is the DMAIC process. In practice, this means defining a goal, measuring current performance, analyzing the root of the defect, improving and/or eliminating the defect, and controlling future process performance. During the measure phase, a SIPOC (suppliers, inputs, process, outputs, customer) diagram is frequently used it help identify waste (**Box 1**) in a process.

Box 1
Sources of waste identified
1. Defects
2. Overproduction
3. Waiting
4. Nonutilized talent
5. Transportation
6. Inventory
7. Motion
8. Extra processing
With respect to orthopedic surgery and joint replacement, nonutilized talent, waiting, defects, and overproduction are the most relevant.

Improta and colleagues[11] used this DMAIC roadmap to systematically analyze and identify critical processes for improvement in THA. The team set a goal of reducing hospital length of stay (LOS) to less than 14 days. LOS data were then measured and analyzed. The authors found a major source of increased LOS was excessive and unnecessary delays in the preoperative phase during surgery risk assessment and preparation. For the improve phase, the authors implemented many changes. First, the hospital implemented a prehospitalization service in which all tests and examinations were done without hospitalization. Second, they standardized the discharge process. Third, they simplified bureaucratic procedures such as reserving operating rooms to decrease communication errors. Finally, they held regular meetings with health care managers and clinical staff to discuss the negative economic impacts of noncompliance with the new changes in protocol. During the control phase, the new processes were frequently checked and reviewed to ensure the new clinical pathway was being implemented properly and effectively. After incorporating these changes, the authors reported a reduced length of stay from 18.9 days to 10.6 days. The authors were able to effectively identify inefficiencies in their system and improve them by following the core tenets of the LSS methodology.

Similarly, stakeholders in the joint replacement process at the Richard L. Roudebush VA Medical Center (RLR VAMC) used different LSS techniques to improve efficiency for TJA. Gayed and colleagues[12] focused on implementing single-piece flow, a Lean principle focused on interconnecting various steps of a process. The stakeholders in this situation wanted to take the disconnected processes of the preoperative clinic, hospital admission, and postoperative

care and make them a more connected process. They identified barriers that would prevent them from implementing the appropriate changes and their associated waste before enacting changes to overcome the barriers. For example, the team identified surgeon-specific barriers including inadequate operating room (OR) time, unclear expectations for discharge, and the extra work required for patients with delayed discharges. These concerns were addressed by adding additional OR time, shifting the OR case load to earlier in the week to compensate for lack of social work support on weekends, hiring an additional surgeon, and securing administrative support to be able to discharge patients as soon as they were medically cleared. Another interesting finding from this study was that a lack of standardization was a common cause of inefficiencies. After the team addressed and overcame these obstacles, they experienced improvements in LOS, non-VA care, cost savings, and return on investment (ROI). LOS decreased from 5.3 days to 3.4 days. Non-VA care was reduced, resulting in cost savings of $1.02 million when comparing the preproject period to the postproject period. The ROI was estimated at $1 million annually after accounting for an implementation cost of $25,000. This provides another example of how applying LSS methods was an effective way to improve total joint replacement quality. Hospitals seeking to decrease costs and improve quality of TJA should strongly consider using LSS methods.

STANDARDIZING CLINICAL PATHWAYS

Developing and implementing standard clinical pathways can improve total joint replacement quality. Clinical pathways are multidisciplinary processes that are intended to deliver standardized, evidence-based care to patients with minimal variability. Duncan and colleagues[13] examined a cohort of consecutive patients having primary TKA with traditional perioperative techniques, followed by a primary TKA on the contralateral knee using a newly implemented clinical pathway. The researchers measured and compared patient clinical and hospital economic outcomes of the standardized clinical pathway with the traditional pathway. They found that patients undergoing TKA after implementation of the clinical pathway had a shorter LOS, lower visual analog scale (VAS) pain scores, decreased opioid requirements, and decreased frequency of urinary retention. Additionally, more patients could independently transfer from bed to chair on the day of surgery compared with before implementation of the standardized clinical pathway. There was also a reduced direct hospital cost by an estimated mean of $956 per surgical episode of care. The new, standardized pathway was superior for 2 reasons. There were improved patient outcomes and decreased costs for the hospital.

Although standardization in TJA has been shown to effectively improve quality, the complex nature of the many perioperative variables involved in TJA can make it difficult for hospitals to develop and implement their own pathways. Van Citters and colleagues[14] developed a novel TJA clinical pathway that focused on standardization, communication across interdisciplinary care teams, patient-centeredness, and patient and family engagement designed to serve as a guideline for TJA programs to implement their own care pathways. The researchers identified several high-performing hospitals, conducted interviews with interdisciplinary care teams from these hospitals, and drafted a care pathway via collaboration with a multistakeholder panel. The interviews focused on care processes that could promote safe, effective, efficient, and patient-centered care. The proposed pathway was organized into 4 care periods: preoperative surgical visit, preoperative preparation and planning for surgery, hospital admission for surgery through hospital discharge, and postdischarge care. After conducting the interviews, Van Citters and colleagues identified 17 proposed system- and patient-level suggestions that applied across all 4 care periods. These 17 suggestions were further organized into 3 categories: standardization and process improvement, communication and collaboration, and patient and family engagement and education. Developing a standardized pathway is a difficult task, and there is a lack of step-by-step instructions for pathway implementation. The proposed pathway and suggestions from Van Citters and colleagues can serve as a reference for other institutions to implement their own quality improvement measures (Table 1).

SIMPLIFICATION

As previously stated, implementing care pathways for total joint replacement can be difficult because of the complexity and variability of multistep pathways, and stakeholders may be reluctant to buy in. Simplification can help institutions apply system-wide clinical pathways in an efficient and sustainable manner. Loftus and colleagues[15] sought to rapidly deploy a standardized TKA care pathway in a large health

care system. To do this, researchers focused on just 2 key aspects: early activity and avoidance of a continuous urinary catheter for all TKA patients. After enacting the changes, there was a 10.5% reduction in overall complications, fewer readmissions, and a reduction of $1040 cost per case. Loftus and colleagues showed that adapting a new clinical pathway in a large health care system does not have to be complicated or cumbersome. They focused on just 2 areas of improvement and decreased the costs, complications and readmissions associated with TKA. Barber and colleagues[16] implemented the same pathway for THA (integrating early activity after surgery and avoidance of a continuous urinary catheter) that Loftus and colleagues used for TKA at the same institution and reported similar improvements.

STANDARDIZATION IN THE CONTEXT OF BUNDLED PAYMENTS

In addition to improved quality to patients, there are also economic incentives for stakeholders to adopt standardized TJA clinical pathways. In 2011, the US Centers for Medicare and Medicaid Services (CMS) initiated the Bundled Payment for Care Improvement (BPCI) initiative. The goal of this new payment model was to innovate higher quality and more coordinated care while decreasing the cost to Medicare. Iorio and colleagues[17] began participation in the BPCI model 2, which includes services provided 72 hours before hospital admission, the inpatient stay, and 90-day postdischarge. They developed and implemented a standardized clinical pathway for TJA that helped coordinate the tasks of attending physicians, residents, nurses, nurse practitioners, and social workers. After 1 year of using the standard care pathway, Iorio and colleagues reported decreased LOS and increased discharge to home with stable readmission rates. They were able to decrease LOS without compromising quality to the patients, which can lead to decreased costs to the hospital. The subsequent increase in value for hospitals and physicians provides further reason for stakeholders to develop and implement standardized care pathways for TJA. Dundon and colleagues[18] performed an analysis at the same institution as Iorio and colleagues and compared data from year 3 after enrolling in the BPCI initiative to year 1. They found increased reduction in LOS, increased home self-care discharges, and a 6% reduction of total allows claims per case. This suggests that continued improvement over initial gains reported in year 1 is possible.

Table 1
Standardization of clinical pathways

Study	Purpose	Conclusions/Outcomes
Duncan et al,[13] 2013	1. Develop a standardized pathway for TKA 2. Analyze the effects of the standardized primary TKA protocol on patients who previously had a primary TKA on the contralateral knee with an unstandardized protocol	1. Decreased LOS, decreased VAS pain score, decreased opioid requirements, decreased urinary retention, and increased number of patients who could move from bed to chair the day of surgery 2. Decreased cost of $956 per episode of care
Van Citters et al,[14] 2014	1. Develop a novel TJA pathway that could serve as a guideline for institutions	1. Numerous improvement suggestions were collected from multiple disciplines 2. Several suggestions applicable to all periods of care were identified
Loftus et al,[15] 2014	1. Develop and analyze a simplified TKA pathway that could be easily implemented in health care institutions	1. The pathway focused on emphasizing early activity after surgery and discontinued use of continuous urinary catheters 2. Reported reduced costs, readmissions, and complications 3. This pathway changed only 2 aspects of a pathway and had significant improvements in quality and efficiency
Barber et al,[16] 2017	1. Apply the same pathway that Loftus et al used to THA	1. Researchers reported similar improvements in quality and efficiency that Loftus et al noted.

In a recent report, Kim and colleagues identified 5 key factors to their success in the context of BPCI.[19] They (1) implemented improved screening of patients and comorbidities before surgery to decrease readmission rates, (2) optimized care coordination and patient education, (3) minimized narcotic, (4) optimized blood management, (5) and minimized postacute facility and resource utilization.

Developing and implementing clinical pathways can be complicated and costly, making stakeholders reluctant to buy in. However, the previously mentioned studies show that there

simple and effective pathways that can be implemented, and that there are significant improvements in patient and hospital economic outcomes (**Fig. 1**).

DISCUSSION

Despite increasing pressure to decrease costs, the patient-centered perspective must be maintained. Some cost-saving pathways can be detrimental to the patient. Lovecchio and colleagues[20] compared patient outcomes for those who underwent outpatient THA and TKA

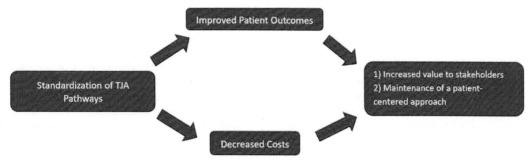

Fig. 1. Why should stakeholders buy in?

pathways and those who underwent fast-track inpatient TKA and THA pathways. They found that outpatients had higher rates of medical complications, including bleeding requiring transfusion, deep venous thromboembolism requiring treatment, and increased rates of reoperation compared with fast-track inpatients. In addition to negative patient outcomes, outpatient TJA can negate the potential cost savings and decrease value to stakeholders, since complications and reoperations will increase costs to the hospital.

As economic pressure increases to reduce costs, it is still of utmost importance to provide high-quality health care to patients. The number of TJAs performed will continue to increase as the population ages. Some methods to decrease costs may do harm to patients, but there are many other methods that can effectively decrease costs while maintaining or improving quality.

It is difficult to standardize and implement clinical pathways, but the improvements in quality and increased value to stakeholders justify the cost. LSS and associated quality improvement methodologies from other industries have shown promise in TJA. This systematic approach of analyzing, reviewing, and improving processes has led to improved outcomes for patients and health care providers. Health care institutions could further benefit from continuing to borrow quality improvement techniques from other industries. Standardization promotes collaboration between multiple disciplines to develop the best pathway. Furthermore, it is much easier to analyze the efficacy of a standard pathway. Identifying 1 or 2 components of a pathway for improvement can lead to drastic increases in quality. In addition to providing higher-quality TJA to patients, pathway standardization provides the added incentive of increased value to stakeholders. Reducing costs while maintaining or improving quality can lead to improved outcomes and increased value for patients and stake holders alike, especially in the context of new reimbursement models such as the BPCI.

REFERENCES

1. Kurtz S, Ong K, Lau E, et al. Projections of primary and revision hip and knee arthroplasty in the United States from 2005 to 2030. J Bone Joint Surg Am 2007;89(4):780–5.
2. Neumann PJ, Cohen JT, Weinstein MC. Updating cost-effectiveness — the curious resilience of the $50,000-per-QALY threshold. N Engl J Med 2014; 371(9):796–7.
3. Chang RW, Pellisier JM, Hazen GB. A cost-effectiveness analysis of total hip arthroplasty for osteoarthritis of the hip. JAMA 1996;275(11):858–65.
4. Losina E, Walensky RP, Kessler CL, et al. Cost-effectiveness of total knee arthroplasty in the United States: patient risk and hospital volume. Arch Intern Med 2009;169(12):1113–21 [discussion: 1121–12].
5. Tomek IM, Sabel AL, Froimson MI, et al. A collaborative of leading health systems finds wide variations in total knee replacement delivery and takes steps to improve value. Health Aff (Millwood) 2012;31(6):1329–38.
6. Bozic KJ, Ward L, Vail TP, et al. Bundled payments in total joint arthroplasty: targeting opportunities for quality improvement and cost reduction. Clin Orthop Relat Res 2014;472(1):188–93.
7. Mason SE, Nicolay CR, Darzi A. The use of Lean and six sigma methodologies in surgery: a systematic review. Surgeon 2015;13(2):91–100.
8. de Koning H, Verver JP, van den Heuvel J, et al. Lean six sigma in healthcare. J Healthc Qual 2006;28(2):4–11.
9. Benditz A, Greimel F, Auer P, et al. Can consistent benchmarking within a standardized pain management concept decrease postoperative pain after total hip arthroplasty? A prospective cohort study including 367 patients. J Pain Res 2016;9:1205–13.
10. Benditz A, Drescher J, Greimel F, et al. Implementing a benchmarking and feedback concept decreases postoperative pain after total knee arthroplasty: a prospective study including 256 patients. Sci Rep 2016;6:38218.
11. Improta G, Balato G, Romano M, et al. Lean Six Sigma: a new approach to the management of patients undergoing prosthetic hip replacement surgery. J Eval Clin Pract 2015;21(4):662–72.
12. Gayed B, Black S, Daggy J, et al. Redesigning a joint replacement program using Lean Six Sigma in a Veterans Affairs hospital. JAMA Surg 2013; 148(11):1050–6.
13. Duncan CM, Moeschler SM, Horlocker TT, et al. A self-paired comparison of perioperative outcomes before and after implementation of a clinical pathway in patients undergoing total knee arthroplasty. Reg Anesth Pain Med 2013;38(6):533–8.
14. Van Citters AD, Fahlman C, Goldmann DA, et al. Developing a pathway for high-value, patient-centered total joint arthroplasty. Clin Orthop Relat Res 2014;472(5):1619–35.
15. Loftus T, Agee C, Jaffe R, et al. A simplified pathway for total knee arthroplasty improves outcomes. J Knee Surg 2014;27(3):221–8.
16. Barber C, Fraser JF, Mendez GG, et al. The halo effect: an unintended benefit of care pathways. J Knee Surg 2017;30(3):264–8.
17. Iorio R, Clair AJ, Inneh IA, et al. Early results of medicare's bundled payment initiative for a 90-

day total joint arthroplasty episode of care. J Arthroplasty 2016;31(2):343–50.

18. Dundon JM, Bosco J, Slover J, et al. Improvement in total joint replacement quality metrics: year one versus year three of the bundled payments for care improvement initiative. J Bone Joint Surg Am 2016; 98(23):1949–53.

19. Kim K, Iorio R. The 5 clinical pillars of value for total joint arthroplasty in a bundled payment paradigm. J Arthroplasty 2017;32(6):1712–6.

20. Lovecchio F, Alvi H, Sahota S, et al. Is outpatient arthroplasty as safe as fast-track inpatient arthroplasty? A propensity score matched analysis. J Arthroplasty 2016;31(9 Suppl):197–201.

Professional Formation of Physicians Focused on Improving Care
How Do We Get There?

Siddartha Simha, BSc[a,b], Zain Sayeed, MD, MHA[a,b,*],
Muhammad T. Padela, MD, MSc[a,b], Alberto Criado, MD[a,b],
Karun Amar, MD[a,b], Walid Yassir, MD, MHCM[a,b]

KEYWORDS

- Quality improvement • Orthopedic surgery • Quality improvement initiatives
- Quality improvement measures • Quality improvement benefits

KEY POINTS

- Quality improvement (QI) is being emphasized heavily by the Accreditation Council for Graduate Medical Education and National Academy of Medicine.
- QI training begins strong in residency, but wavers through continuing medical education such as fellowship programs and finally as an attending physician.
- QI measures are limited in all stages of continuing medical education for orthopedic surgery.

INTRODUCTION

In recent years, there has been an increasing emphasis by both the National Academy of Medicine (NAM) and the Accreditation Council for Graduate Medical Education (ACGME) to integrate quality improvement (QI) initiatives into the residency curriculums. Quality improvement (QI) is defined by Batalden & Davidoff as "the combined and unceasing efforts of everyone—healthcare professionals, patients and their families, researchers, payers, planners and educators—to make the changes that will lead to better patient outcomes (health), better system performance (care) and better professional development".[1] QI has been receiving emphasis after the NAM, formerly named the Institute of Medicine (IOM), aimed to recognize the drawbacks of healthcare. In efforts to improve the field positively, the NAM released two publications, *To Err Is Human: Building a Safer Health System*, and *Crossing the Quality Chasm: A New Health System for the 21st Century*. Both publications highlight the prevalence of preventable mistakes in the field of medicine. In the latter publication, released in 2001, the NAM provided six aims for improvement which were general and far reaching: the six aims were built around health care being "safe, effective, patient-centered, timely, efficient, [and] equitable".[2] Subsequently, in 2003, the NAM released another publication titled, *Health Professions Education: A Bridge to Quality*, in which five competencies were clearly highlighted that were far more specific and direct: "Provide patient-centered care, work in interdisciplinary teams, employ evidence-based practice, apply quality improvement, [and] utilize informatics".[3]

Additionally, the ACGME, a non-profit council responsible for accrediting residency programs

---

Funding Sources: No additional funding sources were used for this article.

Conflicts of Interest: No conflicts of interest are evident for authors of this article.

[a] Children's Hospital of Michigan, Department of Pediatric Orthopaedics, 1st Floor Main, 3901 Beaubien Street, Detroit, MI 48201, USA; [b] Resident Research Partnership, 233 Fielding Street, Suite B, Ferndale, MI 48220, USA

* Corresponding author. Children's Hospital of Michigan, Department of Pediatric Orthopaedics, 1st Floor Main, 3901 Beaubien Street, Detroit, MI 48201, USA

E-mail address: zainsayeed@gmail.com

throughout the United States, released their own set of competencies for graduate medical education in 2002. These competencies are skills that the ACGME holds residents accountable for developing and are as follows: Patient care, medical knowledge, practice-based learning and environment, interpersonal and communication skills, professionalism, and systems based practice. To no surprise there is a clear emphasis on quality improvement in the competencies put forth by the ACGME. More specifically, this emphasis is highlighted in two of the competencies – Practice-based learning and systems-based practice.

Practice-based learning and improvement emphasizes residents investigating and evaluating their practices, and eventually using their evaluations to reflect and improve their practice. The ACGME commonly assesses this competency through "audit of clinical practice (quality performance measures), evidence-based medicine logs, case logs, [and] rating scales/evaluation forms".[4] Systems-based practice focuses on residents being able to call upon resources to provide optimal and efficient care. The ACGME commonly assesses this competency through "audit of clinical practice (quality performance measures), multi-source feedback (MSF), [and] rating scales/evaluation forms".[4] By obtaining proficiency in these competencies, the ACGME hopes for residents to be able to reflect upon their practices and find methods to improve the quality of care they are delivering to patients. These competencies put forth by the NAM and ACGME are summarized in **Table 1**. Though the ACGME and the NAM emphasize the importance of QI, there may not be enough focus on QI throughout the training of medical professionals, especially orthopedic surgeons. Within our review, we aim to investigate the extent of QI measures throughout the various steps of medical education en route to becoming an orthopedic surgery attending – orthopedic residency, fellowships, and finally, as an attending. Through this assessment, it will become clear that though QI is

beginning to be preached extensively in different residency programs to meet the demands of the ACGME and NAM, further QI measures need to be implemented in orthopedics. Additionally, we will see that the emphasis on QI training begins strong and is prominent in residency programs, but wavers through fellowship programs and finally as an attending physician.

ORTHOPEDIC RESIDENCY

Having QI initiatives in orthopedic residency is crucial to the education of the resident. Residency is the first legitimate exposure many physicians have to independently manage and care for patients. Thus, emphasizing QI at an early stage in medical education allows residents to develop the proper foundation in order to provide care to their patients that is, not only efficient, but also continuously improving in quality.

The Surgical Council on Resident Education (SCORE) has made a national curriculum available for residency programs to incorporate. This curriculum contains a significant amount of skills that surgical residents are responsible for developing throughout the course of their residency. As suggested by ACGME, this curriculum contains a specific category titled as "Practice-Based Learning & Improvement"; all four of the requirements residents are responsible for achieving for this category correlate with QI. The fact that the SCORE emphasizes QI throughout their surgical education curriculum, although not as prominently as other competencies, highlights the increasing importance of QI in residency programs. Specific to orthopedic surgery, the American Board of Orthopedic Surgery (ABOS) and the ACGME both released milestones intended for residency programs to use when reporting performance of their residents to the ACGME. In these milestones, there is a specific requirement by ABOS and ACGME for residents to be able to "work in interprofessional teams to enhance patient safety and quality

Table 1 Summary of NAM and ACGME competencies		
Organization	**National Academy of Medicine (NAM)**	**Accreditation Council for Graduate Medical Education (ACGME)**
Emphasized competencies	1. Provide patient centered care 2. Work in interdisciplinary teams 3. Employ evidence-based practice 4. Apply quality improvement[a] 5. Utilize informatics	1. Patient care 2. Medical knowledge 3. Practice-based learning and improvement[a] 4. Interpersonal and communication skills 5. Professionalism 6. Systems-based practice[a]

[a] Indicates important competency for QI.

care".[5] In order for a resident to achieve full marks in this category, they must "develop and publish quality improvement project results [and/or] lead a local or regional quality improvement project".[5] With this increasing stress on QI by various organizations such as SCORE, ACGME, and ABOS, studies are being conducted to assess correlations between emphasizing QI in residency and improved clinical outcomes; and, after investigation of the literature, there does seem to be beneficial results from the incorporation of QI measures into various residency curriculums.[6–8]

For example, A systematic review conducted by Medbery and colleagues[6] delved into the present literature and investigated the availability of a QI curriculum. Medbery and colleagues[6] found that though difficult to implement, the foundation for a surgical QI curriculum does in fact exist. However, implementing these particular curriculums poses significant issues. A few of the issues that Medbery and co. addressed were lack of formal training in QI, a low level of confidence in teaching QI, and lack of integration of the QI curriculum. Finally, they noted a deficit in consistency between different institutions as differences in size and resource availability pose barriers to QI curriculum implementation.

Hall Barber and colleagues[7] investigated an experimental approach to teaching QI – Barber and co. research a graduate medical education curriculum held at the Department of Family Medicine (DFM) at Queen's University aiming to create an Innovative and broad QI curriculum. The DFM's program combines an experimental team project with numerous didactics and hopes to educate residents on QI. The residents are paired into teams and select a topic in the field of QI to investigate; they then research the topic, and provide possible improvement ideas.

Finally, a study conducted at Henry Ford Hospital investigated the effect of training their residents in QI in response to the ACGME's implementation of QI as a core competency. In this study, a QI process, more specifically a modified Plan-Do-Study-Act (PDSA), was implemented at the medical intensive care unit (MICU) of Henry Ford Hospital to further improve not only the residency curriculum's educational effectiveness, but also the clinical results. The PDSA activities "focused on improving clinical outcomes, but also outlined educational goals for residents and fellows, defined teaching methods, and determined assessment methods for ACGME curricula".[8] The study investigated clinical outcomes pre- and post- QI education and recognized improvement in two areas that

were previously lacking – iatrogenic pneumothorax rate and sepsis-specific mortality. The authors highlight that after the QI curriculum implementation, clinical outcomes in these two areas improved dramatically.[8]

Though literature shows that measures are being implemented to avoid errors and increase quality of care in orthopedic practice, a lack of evidence exists assessing QI curriculums in orthopedic residency programs.[9] However, the benefits QI curriculums provide, such as allowing residents to navigate real-world issues, like "securing project buy-in, negotiating with peers, and developing solutions to problems" is sufficient enough to advocate for implementation of these initiatives into orthopedic residency programs.[7] Additionally, residents that participated in the experimental study conducted at DFM were able to use the QI principles they learned and lead QI initiatives. Thus, QI curriculums may help residents perform better in the operating rooms and with their patients, and may allow residents to pass their knowledge to future generations.

ORTHOPEDIC FELLOWSHIP

Though there is a fair amount of literature regarding QI measures being implemented into residency programs, the amount of literature decreases drastically when investigating QI in fellowship programs, especially orthopedic fellowships. A potential etiology may be due to the assumption that QI is being heavily emphasized in residency programs and by the time residents complete their training they are already well versed in QI methodology. However, as earlier stated, though residency programs do stress QI measures, there is no gold standard curriculum throughout all residency programs. Thus, the emphasis on QI should be maintained in fellowship programs especially with the difficulty in establishing a universal QI curriculum in residencies.

One effective QI measure in literature was implemented at Mayo Clinic. Mayo Clinic, in the 2010 to 2011 curriculum year, implemented a QI education program into the curriculum of the Mayo Clinic Combined Critical Care Fellowship (CCF) – the goal of this implementation was to deliver QI training that could be applied to enhance patient care "as an integral part of the demanding CCF curriculum, and as a model for other fellowship programs to follow".[10] The program consisted of two Mayo Quality Academy instructors and five additional physicians who were experts in the QI content. The seven instructors would then work with the fellows to assess them on "satisfaction, knowledge, and skill transfer".[10] Not only was the program a success, with all 20 fellows becoming Bronze certified and 14 even becoming Silver certified, but the fellows were demonstrated improvement in patient safety and care. The program has been successfully implemented in the CCF curriculum and is currently in the fourth year. A program such as this would cement QI practices in physicians' clinical practice and would teach both the principles required for QI, and would allow for these fellows to pass on their knowledge to faculty, as they would have become either Bronze or Silver certified. Furthermore, implementation of these methods in orthopedic surgery may be especially beneficial. It may assist both the fellow in future board recertification exams, and also has the potential to decrease readmission rates, improve clinical outcomes, and decrease rate of surgical site infections.[11]

Another study, also conducted at Mayo Clinic, taught QI to both neurology residents and fellows, and then had these physicians work on a project regarding QI. The QI project was approached using DMAIC: Define, measure, analyze, improve, control. DMAIC is the methodology employed by Lean Six Sigma (LSS)for effective problem-solving; however, DMAIC is not solely used by LSS managers, but is employed by other organizations for a variety of purposes. In this study, the residents and fellows first addressed a deficit in quality, which was the abundant number of delayed muscle biopsies. Then, they measured the baseline data for 1 year. Next, the data was analyzed to identify reasons as to why muscle biopsies were being delayed or canceled. After these reasons were acknowledged, interventions were implemented to address them and improve the problem. Finally, the last part of DMAIC can only be addressed over time to see if the implementations were maintained and controlled[12] (this information is summarized in **Table 2**). Integrating this type of QI instruction in an orthopedic fellowship curriculum, and also a residency curriculum, is not only feasible but may provide a framework for addressing various gaps in quality. For example, there is a high prevalence of postoperative DVT/PE in orthopedic patients. Performing a DMAIC QI improvement project on this would allow for addressing the problem, creating a solution, and potentially maintaining this solution.

ORTHOPEDIC ATTENDINGS

QI knowledge and implementation, along with evidence of implementation of QI in clinical practice, is a vital part of being a physician.

Table 2
DMAIC improvement cycle

DMAIC	Step	Example in Literature
D	Define	Gap in quality regarding canceled muscle biopsies
M	Measure	Baseline data was taken for 1 y regarding if and why muscle biopsy was canceled
A	Analyze	Data was analyzed for common reasons for cancellation
I	Improve	Interventions were implemented such as changing time of biopsy to afternoon, creating patient informational handout, etc.
C	Control	Will be addressed in time

Data from Kassardjian CD, Williamson ML, van Buskirk DJ, et al. Residency training: quality improvement projects in neurology residency and fellowship: applying DMAIC methodology. Neurology 2015;85(2):e7–10.

Not only may it assist with clinical outcomes and improved patient care, but demonstration of QI implementation in clinical practice is necessary for board recertification; for example, the American Board of Orthopedic Surgery (ABOS) evaluates candidates available for recertification on their "focus on quality improvement [via] a stringent peer review process and submission of case lists".[13] Thus, knowledge and demonstration of QI is likely beneficial to the hospital, the patient, and the physician themselves.

However, when reviewing the literature regarding QI measures in continuing medical education for physicians, it is evident that there is a wide array of research being done in order to assess gaps or deficits in surgical procedures and treatments. However, it is harder to find literature on the importance of continued QI training for physicians – this is especially important with attendings as it is vital to ensure that physicians are up to date with the most recent methods in QI. This is not to say that QI curriculums are not being implemented, as seen in the following example.

A model initiative, known as the Physician Quality Improvement Initiative (PQII), has been implemented by The Council of Academic Hospitals of Ontario. This initiative uses "a well-established multi-source feedback program" to collaborate with chiefs in a hospital and provide feedback to current physicians.[14] The program consists of a facilitated feedback review with the chief and allows for an open dialogue in which QI is emphasized on the agenda. When this program was being evaluated for its effectiveness, 90% of the participants believed that the feedback provided by the chief promoted QI.[14] Additionally, communication was enhanced and relationships were fostered. A model such as this may be very simple to implement in orthopedic surgery. Through feedback and enhanced communication, physicians and chiefs can partake in a conversation focused on methods that the physician can improve quality of care. By opening communication lines potential deficits in care can be addressed and improved.

RECOMMENDATION

We propose, as a possible initiative that could be incorporated into orthopedic surgery residency or fellowship programs, a hospital-specific database where residents are able to log difficult situations that they face – whether it is procedural, such as placing a traction pin in the ER, or simply difficulty finding sterile equipment. Then, at the end of the month in each rotation, the staff would gather and discuss how to prevent these problems or find methods to ease these problems, if possible. Another initiative would be having attendings track down resident errors and logging these errors. Then, at the end of the month, the attending can meet with each resident and discuss methods in order to reduce the frequency of these mistakes, or even eliminate them altogether. Initiatives such as the aforementioned would minimize mistakes and increase efficiency, thus reducing-costs and improving patient care.

SUMMARY

Through the literature, it is clear to see that QI measures are being implemented in various institutions in order to meet the ACGME and NAM criteria to emphasize the impact patient-centered care. However, the existence of these programs in orthopedics is not as well outlined or even researched thoroughly. Though the benefits of incorporating a QI curriculum in the training of residents, fellows, and attendings, are well defined through numerous publications across various residencies, there still is not one universal curriculum regarding the topic, in orthopedics or other residency programs. Nonetheless, with the increasing

requirement of the ACGME and NAM, we may soon see the implementation of a general curriculum across residencies to ensure that QI and patient-centered care are both central and fundamental parts of continuing medical education.

REFERENCES

1. Batalden PB, Davidoff F. What is "quality improvement" and how can it transform healthcare? Quall Saf Health Care 2007;16(1):2–3.
2. Crossing the quality chasm: a new health system for the 21st century. Institute of Medicine. 2001. Crossing the Quality Chasm: A New Health System for the 21st Century. Washington, DC: The National Academies Press. Available at: https://doi.org/10.17226/10027.
3. In: Greiner AC, Knebel E, editors. Health professions education: a bridge to quality. Washington, DC: 2003.
4. Holmboe ES, Edgar L, Hamstra S. The milestones guidebook. ACGME; 2016. Available at: https://www.acgme.org/Portals/0/MilestonesGuidebook.pdf. Accessed December 15, 2016.
5. ACGME, ABOS. The orthopaedic surgery milestones project. 2015. Available at: https://www.acgme.org/Portals/0/PDFs/Milestones/OrthopaedicSurgeryMilestones.pdf. Accessed December 15, 2016.
6. Medbery RL, Sellers MM, Ko CY, et al. The unmet need for a national surgical quality improvement curriculum: a systematic review. J Surg Educ 2014;71(4):613–31.
7. Hall Barber K, Schultz K, Scott A, et al. Teaching quality improvement in graduate medical education: an experiential and team-based approach to the acquisition of quality improvement competencies. Acad Med 2015;90(10):1363–7.
8. Buckley JD, Joyce B, Garcia AJ, et al. Linking residency training effectiveness to clinical outcomes: a quality improvement approach. Jt Comm J Qual Patient Saf 2010;36(5):203–8.
9. Anoushiravani AA, Sayeed Z, El-Othmani MM, et al. High reliability of care in orthopedic surgery: are we there yet? Orthop Clin North Am 2016;47(4):689–95.
10. Kashani KB, Ramar K, Farmer JC, et al. Quality improvement education incorporated as an integral part of critical care fellows training at the Mayo Clinic. Acad Med 2014;89(10):1362–5.
11. Surgery UDoO, Children Olf. 2015 quality & outcomes report. 2015. UCLA Department of Orthopaedic Surgery. 2015 Quality Outcomes Report. Available at: http://ortho.ucla.edu/workfiles/About_

Us/Quality/Ortho%20QB%202015%20%20%282%29.pdf. Accessed March 27, 2017.

12. Kassardjian CD, Williamson ML, van Buskirk DJ, et al. Residency training: quality improvement projects in neurology residency and fellowship: applying DMAIC methodology. Neurology 2015; 85(2):e7–10.

13. (ABOS) ABoOS. Maintenance of certification. Available at: https://www.abos.org/moc.aspx. Accessed March 27, 2017.

14. Wentlandt K, Bracaglia A, Drummond J, et al. Evaluation of the physician quality improvement initiative: the expected and unexpected opportunities. BMC Med Educ 2015;15:230.

Walk a Mile in the Leadership's Shoes
Why Focus on Quality Improvement?

Anthony J. Mells, BS[a],
Muhammad T. Padela, MD, MSc[b,c,d],
Bilal Sleiman, BS[b,c,d], Brett Chamernik, MD[b,c,d],
Bradley J. Zarling, MD[b,c,d], Zain Sayeed, MD, MHA[b,c,d],*

KEYWORDS

- Quality improvement • Michigan Arthroplasty Registry Collaborative Quality Initiative
- Value-based care • Pay for performance
- Medicare Access and CHIP Reauthorization Act of 2015 (MACRA)

KEY POINTS

- Lack of quality health care results in avoidable medical errors, cost inefficiencies, and poorer clinical outcomes.
- Physician and hospital reimbursements are closely tied to meeting QI standards.
- As QI initiatives are implemented by leaders in health care, strict adherence to QI standards by all members of the health care team is essential to their success.

INTRODUCTION

In order to maximize quality improvement (QI) in medicine, the health care system must find ways to harness value-based care.[1] To accomplish this, quality measures such as improved outcomes, shorter length of stays (LOS), and reduced complications must coincide with lower expenses.

It has been estimated that between 98,000 and 210,000 people die annually as a result of preventable harm in hospitals, making medical errors the leading cause of preventable death in the United States.[2,3] Preventable death is an extreme result of poor quality and medical errors. However, other examples such as wrong site surgeries, postoperative infections, and lack of operating room (OR) efficiency all contribute to lower quality and increased expenses that burden the health care system.

In addition to the devastating complications that can result from preventable mistakes, medical errors are estimated to cost the United States health care system $29 billion annually.[4] To combat this, recent changes in health care reimbursement are emphasizing the importance QI. The Medicare Access and CHIP (Children's Health Insurance Program) Reauthorization Act reimburses physicians.[5] Merit-based incentives payment systems and advanced alternative payment models will encourage physicians and health care systems to meet certain quality benchmarks in order to receive full reimbursement. Medicare is also transitioning the

---

Funding Sources: No additional funding sources were used for this article.
Conflicts of Interest: No conflicts of interest are evident for authors of this article.

[a] Oakland University William Beaumont School of Medicine, 586 Pioneer Drive, Rochester, MI 48309, USA; [b] Chicago Medical School at Rosalind Franklin University, 3333 Greenbay Road, North Chicago, IL 60064, USA; [c] Department of Orthopaedic Surgery, Detroit Medical Center, 4201 St Antoine Street, Suite 9B, Detroit, MI 48201, USA; [d] Resident Research Partnership, 233 Fielding Street, Suite B, Ferndale, MI 48220, USA
* Corresponding author. Department of Orthopaedic Surgery, Detroit Medical Center, 4201 St Antoine Street, Suite 9B, Detroit, MI 48201, USA
E-mail address: zainsayeed@gmail.com

physician reimbursement system from a pay-for-service to a pay-for-performance based system.[6]

The need to improve clinical outcomes, patient safety, and satisfaction, alongside the financial incentives that payors are placing on improved quality, has forced leaders in the health care field to place increased emphasis on the QI process.[7] This article aims to assess the history and background of quality improvement, while analyzing QI activities among various stakeholders such as physicians, nurses, hospitals, patients, and payors.

History and Background of Quality Improvement

Dr. Ernest Codman was the first physician to emphasize the importance of quality measures for physicians and hospitals.[8] In the early twentieth century, other surgeons refused to measure outcomes evaluations, while Codman continually documented all errors with the hopes of making improvements to patient care.[9] Today's emphasis on QI initiatives has continually grown over the past 100 years as a direct result of Codman's insights and teachings of the importance of QI.[8–10]

More recently, nationally quantified surgical QI was first made possible by The American College of Surgeons National Surgical Quality Improvement Program (ACS NSQIP). Founded in the mid-1980s by the Veterans Health Administration, ACS NSQIP was the first and only physician validated nationwide quality improvement program.[11] It has since been expanded to include hundreds of surgical hospitals and provides a risk-adjusted database of outcomes of all noncardiac surgeries.[12]

Health care systems began to take further action in the 1990s. The first QI initiative of the American Academy of Orthopedic Surgeons (AAOS) was in 1998, as AAOS instituted the Sign Your Site initiative.[2,4,13] From 1995 to 2006 a total of 279 cases of wrong-site surgery were identified, 86 of which were orthopedic procedures.[2] It has also been estimated that 25% of surgeons will perform at least 1 wrong site surgery in a 35 -year career.[14] It is difficult to tell how successful the Sign Your Site initiative has been, as data appear to be mixed in reporting a decline in wrong-site surgeries.[2,15,16] QI initiatives such as this one require years of implementation and participation in order to measure a significant improvement in wrong-site surgeries, and continual involvement is recommended.[17]

QI initiatives do not require the backing of a national organization or governmental influence in order to make an impact. Local and regional efforts can have an even bigger impact on QI, as these initiatives can be more targeted and relevant to a specific population. The Michigan Arthroplasty Registry Collaborative Quality Initiative (MARCQI) is a Blue Cross and Blue Shield of Michigan-sponsored registry that tracks total arthroplasties in the state and identifies areas for QI.[18,19] The database provides information on thousands of arthroplasties from hundreds of different surgeons and has helped to improve processes that prevent and minimize complications including deep vein thrombosis (DVT), infections, transfusions, and readmission.[19]

Although improved quality and reduced cost are vitally important to the health care system as a whole, the real beneficiaries of QI are the patients. Reduced complications, fewer repeat surgeries, mitigated pain, and improved function are the quality metrics that matter most to patients. Through an outcome initiative, the AAOS developed a patient-oriented self-report measures questionnaire as part of the Musculoskeletal Outcomes Data Evaluation and Management System (MODEMS).[20] This system allowed patients to self-report their improved function and quality following a hip or knee arthroplasty. Although MODEMS as described no longer exists, other self-reported measures have evolved to be important instruments in accurately and precisely measuring patient's pain and satisfaction. An example of this is the Patient Reported Outcomes Measurement Information System (PROMIS) developed by the National Institutes of Health (NIH), which has allowed for a more standardized and validated tool to measure outcomes in clinical research.[20,21] Other studies have solicited participation by requesting that the patient write his or her own initials on the area that needs the surgery.[22] Despite the limited efficacy of patients marking their own surgical site, the benefits of enlisting patients to aid in the QI process should not be overlooked.

LEADERSHIP'S ROLE IN QUALITY IMPROVEMENT

The entire health care system depends on various types of leaders who all have different but vital roles in helping the system to run effectively. Senior management's involvement on QI teams has shown to positively correlate with quality indicators.[23] Physicians, nurses, hospitals, and payors all stand to benefit from collaborative QI efforts. As a result, quality assurance committees comprised of health care leaders and key stakeholders are essential to a successful QI program.

Physicians

The value of an orthopedic surgeon's time cannot be overstated. With a finite amount of operating time available each day, it is important to maximize the efficiency of the OR. When surgical schedules are delayed, not only is the value of the surgeon's time decreased, but it inconveniences patients and costs the organization money. By examining multiple different orthopedic departments over a 30-day period, it was determined that 15% of overall OR time was lost because of inefficiency, correlating to an average of 79 hours per month.[24] This inefficiency was calculated by adding underuse time (time that the patient was ready for surgery but not yet in the OR) and spill-over time (excess time spent in the OR because of unexpected prolongations).[24] After the implementation of a quality assurance committee that addressed the problem and adjusted the policies and guidelines, time waste was reduced by 35%.[24] Eliminating time waste in the OR results in the timely completion of more cases, ultimately improving the surgeon's overall efficiency.

As efficiency and quantity increase, it is important to acknowledge the trend away from payments based on quantity alone. The unsustainable rising cost of health care makes QI imperative, and the Centers for Medicare & Medicaid Services (CMS) have implemented regulations to facilitate this. The shift from pay for service to pay for performance is an evolving dynamic that impacts the reimbursement of surgeons.[25] Under the pay-for-service model, physicians get paid an equivalent amount for each patient, incentivizing quantity alone. Alternatively, pay for performance rewards physicians based upon successfully meeting specific quality metrics. Reimbursement is deducted for underperformance, measured by readmissions, surgical complications, or lack of correct diagnostic testing. This emphasizes objective measurements in order to quantify the quality of health care that is delivered to patients. For example, the Physician Quality Reporting System (PQRS) requires physicians to report certain quality measures to CMS and calculates physician reimbursement based upon successful fulfillment (or failure) of the required metrics.[25,26] Ultimately, surgeons' level of reimbursement is now more strongly correlated to the level of quality they are able to provide.

Another CMS initiative that has dramatically changed orthopedic surgery reimbursement is the Bundled Payments for Care Improvement (BPCI) for total joint arthroplasty.[27] BPCI is composed of 4 different models that provide physicians with fixed payments irrespective of all other factors. One orthopedic department that studied its implementation of BPCI found that the average cost of an arthroplasty surgery decreased by 20% from year 1 to year 3 of BPCI.[28] These cost savings were largely the result of shorter LOS, fewer discharges to inpatient facilities, and lower readmission rates.[28] The substantial cost savings and higher-quality health care that BPCI provides for total joint arthroplasty patients demonstrate the value of initiatives such as these to physicians and patients alike.

With regards to health care economics, competition among orthopedic surgeons should have the potential to produce lower costs and better results However, this surgeon mentality also fosters a cut-throat environment that discourages collaborative efforts that can ultimately improve an orthopedic surgery department. An example of a hybrid medical directorship at a St. Louis Hospital showed that when 3 previous competing surgeons joined forces, the infection and readmission rates declined while their Press-Ganey patient satisfaction scores increased to the 95th percentile.[29] Collaboration among professionals has the potential for cost savings and a higher level of care for patients.

Other Health Care Providers

Nonphysician health care providers play an integral role In a successful surgery. Nurses are critical for the early physical, emotional, and psychosocial preparations for surgery.[30] Although certain questions regarding the surgery and preadmission education are ideally directed to the physician, in reality, nurses are often tasked with providing much of this information to the patient and his or her family.[31] Nurses are commonly relied upon to ensure that there is proper understanding of the surgical process.[30] Surgical timeouts are standard practice that undoubtedly improve quality.[32] Nurses play a vital role in ensuring that all systems are go before the actual operation can begin.

In addition to their vital role on the health care team's path toward QI, nurses have a lot to gain from the changing dynamic in the OR. A comparison with the aviation industry demonstrates this philosophic shift. In the 1970s, the airline industry had a poor safety record. The sentinel event demonstrating this was a tragic and deadly crash known as the 1977 Tenerife Airport Disaster, in which 1 plane attempted to take off before another plane had fully cleared the runway.[33] Many factors contributed to this accident, including financial pressures, weather conditions, and poor communication. Importantly, the pilot at fault was one of the airline's most senior and accomplished pilots, and concerned crew members were not comfortable questioning the decision-making of such an esteemed superior. Part of the airline industry's success in turning this around was a QI project that changed the culture in the cockpit. The revamped culture encouraged and empowered anyone in the airplane to question another's decision, even if it was the captain's decision. This fostered the concept of shared decision making, which significantly reduced avoidable aviation errors.[33]

A similar culture shift in the health care industry, and the OR in particular, can provide a safer environment for patients.[34] Establishment of a system of cross checking gives any member of the surgical team the authority to question the surgical process at any time without fear of reprimand.[16] Although physicians may initially feel threatened by such a culture change, the drive toward improved quality must always be the primary goal. An important adjunct to this would also be to foster a culture of education in the OR. Surgeons train their whole lives in order to gain the expertise of performing such invasive and complicated procedures. Surgical technicians and nurses cannot be expected to have the same understanding as a physician, but encouraging education of the rest of the surgical team can greatly improve this dynamic. Team members should be encouraged to ask the surgeon questions, while the surgeon should welcome such inquiries and educate others in order to build team camaraderie and encourage this kind of culture shift.

Hospitals

QI initiatives provide benefit to hospitals from a cost savings, as well as a market share perspective. As health care delivery has evolved, and payments have been reduced, health systems have been incentivized to reduce the amount of time that patients spend in the hospital. Between the years 1993 and 2006, the mean hospital LOS decreased from 8.81 days to 6.33 days.[35] QI in orthopedic surgery strives to continue to decrease LOS. For example, a study involving 182,146 patients undergoing arthroplasty in over 300 hospitals was analyzed. When physicians adhered to evidence-based processes such as antibiotic and DVT prophylaxis, a significant reduction in readmissions and shorter LOS were observed.[36]

One way to facilitate an overall shorter LOS and significant cost savings is by performing simultaneous bilateral total knee arthroplasty (TKA) as opposed to staged TKA, which requires 2 separate operations. If patients have symptomatic bilateral osteoarthritis of the knee, and bilateral TKA is indicated, replacing both knees during the same operation can result in significant cost savings for the hospitals. In 1 nationwide study of over 400,000 TKAs, The estimated cost of simultaneous bilateral TKA was $43,401, while staged bilateral TKA cost a total of $72,233.[37] Importantly, the quality-adjusted life years (QALY) for these procedures was 9.31 and 9.29 respectively.[37] Combining 2 operations into 1 day requires less resources on all levels of care, and results in equal or improved outcomes.

The vast amount of data now available through electronic health records (EHRs), provides a new way to track various metrics that can be integrated into QI processes. Hospitals can more efficiently gather information on their various departments, employees, and patients. For example, using inpatient pharmacy data and diagnosis codes can provide a more accurate determination of surgical site infections, after arthroplasty.[38] Automated surveillance based on EHR data demonstrated that surgical site infections were actually occurring twice as often as previously determined using traditional surveillance methods. Although this more accurate data reflect poorly on the studied hospitals, it shows that leveraging large databases can provide more accurate statistical results. It also substantially reduces the resources necessary for manual chart review, as computer systems allow for a reduction in chart surveillance of up to 90%.[39] Furthermore, large-scale, system-wide data analyses can potentially recognize problems before they occur, predict risks, and ultimately prevent harm to patients.

Payors

The insurance industry is likewise capable of leveraging large databases, but on a much grander scale. Sophisticated analysis of claims data is being used to identify payment irregularities. Cost overruns, abuse, or fraud would go largely undetected without these important computer systems.[40] These capabilities allow for adjustments in reimbursements that result in health care cost savings across the entire system. As previously discussed, MARCQI was started and funded by Blue Cross Blue Shield of Michigan in order to share information and promote the most effective QI initiatives in the state. One important example is an analysis of the root causes of unnecessary use of skilled nursing facilities (SNFs) following total hip arthroplasty (THA) or TKA. MARCQI set a goal of reducing postoperative SNF utilization to 15% of cases and outlines suggestions for accomplishing this.[41]

Payors also stand to benefit from reduction of avoidable errors and poor outcomes. By definition, QI necessitates improved outcomes, resulting in fewer payments for surgical revisions and extended hospitalizations. This cost savings goes directly to the insurance company's bottom line.

As the CMS are often viewed as the implementers and enforcers of QI initiatives, Medicare is deeply dependent on QI for its survival. Cost savings have been discussed previously at every level of leadership; however, the expense grows exponentially when examined on a national scale. For example, THA has been shown to be one of the safer joint replacement procedures, with fewer complications compared with TKA.[42] Complications of THA occur 20.16% of the time, the most common being transfusions (17.9%), acute renal failure (2.3%), and infections (0.3%).[43] In 2013, Medicare spent $2.8 billion on the 174,167 Medicare beneficiaries who had THA.[43] The costs of complication or adverse events were $87.1 million for transfusions, $21.5 million for acute renal failure, and $10.9 million for infections.[43] The hundreds of millions of dollars being spent on complications from 1 relatively safe orthopedic surgery demonstrate the value and reasoning for CMS to heavily rely on QI. It is clear that CMS and other payors play an integral role with an enormous stake in successful QI. However, payors are still only 1 facet of the broad and diverse set of programs and ideas aimed at achieving better outcomes at a reduced cost.

IMPORTANCE OF PHYSICIAN-LED DIRECTIVES

Despite its many benefits, change in the health care industry can be difficult. One can expect resistance to leadership-driven QI from staff members due to the belief that it will be more time consuming. This is why it is essential for QI to be physician driven, in order to gain the acceptance of the medical staff. As the leaders of the health care team, physicians must buy into these initiatives in order for them to be successful. For example, Michigan physicians utilized the MARCQI database to institute data-driven transfusion protocols. This led to

an 80% reduction in the rate of postoperative total joint arthroplasty transfusions.[18] The physicians recognized a problem, identified a potential solution, and were able to get the entire orthopedic service line on board, resulting in a successful QI initiative.[19]

Physician leaders also must engage administrators in the conversation about quality, and convince them that quality drives productivity, efficiency, reputation, and reimbursement. It is crucial that QI initiatives be presented to physicians in a manner that proves that physicians will become more efficient and have better outcomes.[44]

FUTURE DIRECTIONS

Data-driven management and the influence of technology on the health care system will continue to grow with time. The government QI measures that have been put in place are primarily used to assess physicians, and lack a needed focus on improved clinical outcomes. With so much hidden potential in what is termed big data, hospitals will begin extracting and utilizing data from hospital-wide EHR systems in real time.[45] The goal of this is to improve efficiency across the entire hospital, as these advanced analytics allow for action to be taken at the point of care.

As the volume of EHR systems continues to grow, the interoperability of these systems has not kept pace.[46] It is important that EHR systems converge into an information network that can be utilized to extract meaningful data that will influence the direction of QI.[47–49] As previously demonstrated, large orthopedic registries such as MARCQI play a crucial role in identifying areas of potential improvement and then discovering solutions.[19] It is also possible to compare across different regions and hospitals to evaluate discrepancies in postoperative complications and resource use.[50] A related example of this is called The CRIMSON initiative, in which over 200 hospitals were integrated electronically and shared physician performance data, which allowed hospitals to compare themselves with others and work toward optimizing their productivity.[51] Big data applications will need to continue to evolve in order to manage more diverse clinical information.[52]

SUMMARY

The ongoing quest for meaningful QI is a relatively recent phenomenon that is here to stay. The importance of QI to patients, physicians, hospitals, and the longevity of the US health care system has been thoroughly demonstrated. QI has various benefits to all of the leaders in health care, and when properly implemented, results are beneficiary to all parties involved. Successful initiatives are heavily reliant on physician and hospital leadership that have the passion and influence to help change the culture in ORs and hospitals across the country. As QI efforts continue, and reimbursements inevitably become more complex, strong leadership will result in hospitals and physicians being rewarded for their effective health care delivery systems.

REFERENCES

1. Nwachukwu BU, Hamid KS, Bozic KJ. Measuring value in orthopaedic surgery. JBJS Rev 2013; 1(1):e2.

2. Wong DA, Herndon JH, Canale ST, et al. Medical errors in orthopaedics. J Bone Joint Surg Am 2009;91(3):547–57.

3. James JT. A new, evidence-based estimate of patient harms associated with hospital care. J Patient Saf 2013;9(3):122–8.

4. Schweitzer KM, Brimmo O, May R, et al. Incidence of wrong-site surgery among foot and ankle surgeons. Foot Ankle Spec 2011;4(1):10–3.

5. Burgess M. H.R.2-114th Congress (2015-2016): Medicare Access and CHIP Reauthorization Act of 2015. Washington, DC: 114th Congress; 2015.

6. Pierce RG, Bozic KJ, Bradford DS. Pay for performance in orthopaedic surgery. Clin Orthop Relat Res 2007;457(457):87–95.

7. Rosenthal MB, Fernandopulle R, Song HR, et al. Paying for quality: providers' incentives for quality improvement. Health Aff 2004;23(2):127–41.

8. Donabedian A. The end results of health care: Ernest Codman's contribution to quality assessment and beyond. Milbank Q 1989;67(2):233–56.

9. Codman EA. The classic: a study in hospital efficiency: as demonstrated by the case report of first five years of private hospital. Clin Orthop Relat Res 2013;471:1778–83.

10. Neuhauser D. Heroes and martyrs of quality and safety. Qual Saf Health Care 2002;11(1):103.

11. Molina CS, Thakore RV, Blumer A, et al. Use of the national surgical quality improvement program in orthopaedic surgery. Clin Orthop Relat Res 2015; 473:1574–81.

12. Khuri SF, Daley J, Henderson W, et al. The Department of Veterans Affairs' NSQIP: the first national, validated, outcome-based, risk-adjusted, and peer-controlled program for the measurement and enhancement of the quality of surgical care. National VA Surgical Quality Improvement Program. Ann Surg 1998;228(4):491–507.

13. Canale ST. Wrong-site surgery: a preventable complication. Clin Orthop Relat Res 2005;433:26–9.

14. Meinberg EG, Stern PJ. Incidence of wrong-site surgery among hand surgeons. J Bone Joint Surg Am 2003;85-A(2):193–7.

15. Wong DA, Watters WC. To err is human: quality and safety issues in spine care. Spine (Phila Pa 1976) 2007;32(11 Suppl):S2–8.

16. Lee SH, Kim JS, Jeong YC, et al. Patient safety in spine surgery: regarding the wrong-site surgery. Asian Spine J 2013;7(1):63–71.

17. Wong DA, Lewis B, Herndon J, et al. Patient safety in North America: beyond "operate through your initials" and "sign your site." J Bone Joint Surg Am 2009;91-A(6):1534–41.

18. Markel DC, Allen MW, Zappa NM. Can an arthroplasty registry help decrease transfusions in primary total joint replacement? A quality initiative. Clin Orthop Relat Res 2016;474(1):126–31.

19. Hughes R, Hallstrom B, Igrisan R, et al. Michigan Arthroplasty Registry Collaborative Quality Initiative (MARCQI) as a model for regional registries in the United States. Orthop Res Rev 2015;7:47.

20. Saleh KJ, Bershadsky B, Cheng E, et al. Lessons learned from the hip and knee musculoskeletal outcomes data evaluation and management system. Clin Orthop Relat Res 2004;429:272–8.

21. Kashikar-Zuck S, Carle A, Barnett K, et al. Longitudinal evaluation of Patient Reported Outcomes Measurement Information Systems (PROMIS) measures in pediatric chronic pain HHS Public Access. Pain 2016;157(2):339–47.

22. DiGiovanni CW, Kang L, Manuel J. Patient compliance in avoiding wrong-site surgery. J Bone Joint Surg Am 2003;85-A(5):815–9.

23. Weiner BJ, Alexander JA, Shortell SM, et al. Quality improvement implementation and hospital performance on quality indicators. Health Serv Res 2006;41(2):307–34.

24. Weinbroum AA, Ekstein P, Ezri T. Efficiency of the operating room suite. Am J Surg 2003;185(3):244–50.

25. Kamal RN, Ring D, Akelman E, et al. Quality measures in upper limb surgery. J Bone Joint Surg Am 2016;98(6):505–10.

26. Centers for Medicare & Medicaid Services. Physician quality reporting system. 2016. Available at: https://www.cms.gov/Medicare/Quality-Initiatives-Patient-Assessment-Instruments/PQRS/index.html. Accessed February 19, 2017.

27. Center for Medicare & Medicaid Innovation. Bundled payments for care improvement (BPCI) initiative: general information. Available at: https://innovation.cms.gov/initiatives/bundled-payments/. Accessed February 19, 2017.

28. Dundon J, Bosco J, Sayeed Y, et al. Improvement in total joint replacement. J Bone Joint Surg Am 2016; 98(23):1949–53.

29. Mathias J. Hybrid medical leadership turns competitors into collaborators. OR Manager 2014; 30(10):1–5.

30. Geier KA. A practical guide to improving patient outcomes. Orthop Nurs 2000;19(Suppl):22–8.

31. Heikkinen K, Salanterä S, Suomi R, et al. Ambulatory orthopaedic surgery patient education and cost of care. Orthop Nurs 2011;30(1):20–8.

32. Mclaughlin N, Winograd D, Chung HR, et al. Impact of the time-out process on safety attitude in a tertiary neurosurgical department. World Neurosurg 2014;76:2–5.

33. Nance JJ. Why hospitals should fly: the ultimate flight plan to patient safety and quality care. Bozeman (MT): Second River Healthcare Press; 2008.

34. Lingard L, Espin S, Whyte S, et al. Communication failures in the operating room: an observational classification of recurrent types and effects. Qual Saf Health Care 2004;13:330–4.

35. Bueno H, Ross JS, Wang Y, et al. Trends in Length of Stay and Short-Term Outcomes among Medicare Patients Hospitalized for Heart Failure: 1993–2008. JAMA 2010;303(21):2141–7.

36. Bozic KJ, Maselli J, Pekow PS, et al. The influence of procedure volumes and standardization of care on quality and efficiency in total joint replacement surgery. J Bone Joint Surg Am 2010; 92(16):2643–52.

37. Odum SM, Troyer JL, Kelly MP, et al. A Cost-utility analysis comparing the cost-effectiveness of simultaneous and staged bilateral total knee arthroplasty. J Bone Joint Surg Am 2013;95(16):1441–9.

38. Bolon MK, Hooper D, Stevenson KB, et al. Improved surveillance for surgical site infections after orthopedic implantation procedures: extending applications for automated data. Clin Infect Dis 2009;48(9):1223–9.

39. Inacio MCS, Paxton EW, Chen Y, et al. Leveraging electronic medical records for surveillance of surgical site infection in a total joint replacement population. Infect Control Hosp Epidemiol 2011;32(4):351–9.

40. Srinivasan U, Arunasalam B. Leveraging big data analytics to reduce healthcare costs. IT Prof 2013; 15(6):21–8.

41. Nasser S, Steenbergh K. MARCQI joint replacement workgroup toolkit. In: Hallstrom Brian R, editor. Strategies to reduce unnecessary skilled nursing facility admissions. Detroit (MI): Michigan Arthroplasty Registry Collaborative Quality Initiative; 2017. p. 1–17.

42. Choi JK, Geller JA, Yoon RS, et al. Comparison of total hip and knee arthroplasty cohorts and short-term outcomes from a single-center joint registry. J Arthroplasty 2012;27(6):837–41.

43. Culler SD, Jevsevar DS, Shea KG, et al. The incremental hospital cost and length-of-stay associated with treating adverse events among Medicare beneficiaries undergoing THA during fiscal year 2013. J Arthroplasty 2016;31(1):42–8.

44. Bradley EH, Holmboe ES, Mattera JA, et al. Data feedback efforts in quality improvement: lessons learned from US hospitals. Qual Saf Health Care 2004;13. https://doi.org/10.1136/qshc.2002.4408.

45. Elton J, Ural A. Predictive medicine depends on analytics. Harv Bus Rev 2014. Available at: https://hbr.org/2014/10/predictive-medicine-depends-on-analytics. Accessed May 7, 2017.

46. Castillo VH, Martínez-García AI, Pulido J. A knowledge-based taxonomy of critical factors for adopting electronic health record systems by physicians: a systematic literature review. BMC Med Inform Decis Mak 2010;10. https://doi.org/10.1186/1472-6947-10-60.

47. Auerbach A. Healthcare quality measurement in orthopaedic surgery current state of the art. Clin Orthop Relat Res 2009. https://doi.org/10.1007/s11999-009-0840-8.

48. Anoushiravani AA, Patton J, Sayeed Z, et al. Big data, big research implementing population health-based research models and integrating care to reduce cost and improve outcomes. Orthop Clin North Am 2016. https://doi.org/10.1016/j.ocl.2016.05.008.

49. Saleh KJ, Bozic KJ, Graham DB, et al. Quality in orthopaedic surgery–an international perspective: AOA critical issues. J Bone Joint Surg Am 2013; 95(1):e3.

50. Bozic KJ, Kurtz SM, Lau EM, et al. The epidemiology of revision total knee arthroplasty in the United States. Clin Orthop Relat Res 2010;468(1): 45–51.

51. Hardy K. CRIMSON initiative aims at performance transparency and improved care quality. Healthcare IT News 2009. Available at: http://www.healthcareitnews.com/news/crimson-initiative-aims-performance-transparency-and-improved-care-quality. Accessed June 18, 2017.

52. Raghupathi W, Raghupathi V. Big data analytics in healthcare: promise and potential. Health Inf Sci Syst 2014;2:3.

Osteolysis as it Pertains to Total Hip Arthroplasty

Brian Kurcz, MD[a], Joseph Lyons, BSc[b], Zain Sayeed, MD, MHA[c], Afshin A. Anoushiravani, MD[d], Richard Iorio, MD[d,*]

KEYWORDS

- Osteolysis • Total hip arthroplasty • Imaging • Management

KEY POINTS

- Osteolysis is a long-term complication of total hip arthroplasty (THA).
- Because of advancements in prosthesis design, metallurgy, and enhanced bearing surfaces, fewer revision THAs will be linked to osteolysis and aseptic loosening.
- The material properties of bearing surfaces have been enhanced with the goal of reducing the component wear rates and the prevalence of osteolysis.
- Advancements in imaging modalities, including 3-dimensional computer tomography and metal artifact reduction sequence MRI, have made it possible to detect osteolysis earlier in the process, enabling orthopedic surgeons to intervene before widespread bone loss.
- Despite advancements in implant design and diagnostic and treatment modalities, no preventative therapies are currently available for the management of osteolysis other than removing and replacing the source of bearing surface wear.

INTRODUCTION

Total hip arthroplasty (THA) is a successful and cost-effective procedure for the management of debilitating hip arthritis. In 2015, more than 350,000 primary THA procedures were performed in the United States; this number is projected to increase at an annual rate of 6% over the next 5 years.[1] As younger, more active patients seek THA, the number of revision surgeries will theoretically increase.[1] Recent studies have demonstrated that the revision burden associated with THA comprises 15% of all THAs in the United States[2] and is associated with increased cost and patient morbidity.[3–5] Moreover, the burden associated with revision THA (rTHA) continues to decrease as implant failures secondary to polyethylene (PE) and metal wear become less common, with recent studies reporting that osteolysis may account for 9% to 20% of all rTHAs.[6] Although the prevalence of rTHA continues to decrease, managing osteolysis remains challenging and requires a comprehensive evaluation of the patient, prosthesis, and joint biomechanics. The purpose of this article is to review the pathophysiology responsible for osteolysis, discuss available diagnostic and treatment modalities, and explore future interventions for the management of osteolysis following THA.

Historical Background

Osteolysis is the process of progressive destruction of periprosthetic bone, characterized on serial radiographs as progressive radiolucent lines or cavitation at the implant-bone or cement-bone interface.[7] John Charnley first discussed cystic erosions in the femoral diaphysis in association with stem fractures. He found the tissue around the implant contained cement particles, and he equated the erosion to a deficient cement mantle.[8] William Harris and

[a] Division of Orthopaedic Surgery, Southern Illinois University, 701 North 1st Street, Springfield, IL 62781, USA;
[b] Department of Surgery, Chicago Medical School, 3333 Green Bay Road, North Chicago, IL 60064, USA;
[c] Department of Orthopaedic Surgery, Detroit Medical Center, 4201 Saint Antoine, Detroit, MI 48201, USA; [d] Division of Orthopaedic Surgery, Albany Medical Center, 43 New Scotland, Albany, NY, USA
* Corresponding author.
E-mail address: Richard.iorio@nyumc.org

Orthop Clin N Am 49 (2018) 419–435
https://doi.org/10.1016/j.ocl.2018.06.001
0030-5898/18/© 2018 Elsevier Inc. All rights reserved.

colleagues[9] later described localized bone resorption around a loose THA, as evidenced by the large amounts of macrophages containing phagocytosed cement particles. The evidence at the time suggested that bone cement was causing osteolysis, popularizing the term "cement disease."[10] It was not until cementless components were introduced in the 1980s that particulate debris generated from the implant was implicated as the cause of osteolysis.[11–13] It is now recognized that osteolysis is not a "cement disease," but rather a "particle disease" in which debris generated from any component of the prosthesis causes disease.[14–17] PE is considered the primary culprit, being responsible for 90% of the debris.[14–16]

Pathophysiology

The primary mechanism responsible for osteolysis involves an immunologic response to particulate debris, subsequently resulting in progressive bone loss and implant loosening.[18] During this immunologic reaction, particles are phagocytosed by macrophages, activating direct and indirect osteolysis. Direct osteolysis results from bone resorption by macrophages.[19] Indirect osteolysis is more common and results from osteoclast overstimulation and osteoblast inhibition by proinflammatory cytokines such as interleukin 1 beta (IL-1β) released by activated macrophages.[20,21] The end result is progressive bone resorption and possible loosening of the femoral or acetabular component. Presence of wear debris does not always result in osteolysis; however, osteolysis is more likely to occur when production of wear particles exceeds the individual's capacity to remove the debris, usually occurring when wear rates exceed more than or equal to 0.1 mm/y[22,23]

Wear refers to the loss of prosthetic material from the interface of articulating surfaces.[24] As illustrated in Fig. 1, particulate wear debris can be generated through 4 different modes of wear. Although the generation of particulate debris often occurs at several interfaces, most of the wear occurs at the juncture between the femoral and acetabular components. This specific mode of wear produces biologically active particles less than or equal to 1 μm in diameter.[25]

The movement of particulate debris within the joint may further facilitate development of osteolysis. Increased fluid pressure secondary to inflammation can propel synovial fluid through the joint space or along the bone implant interface, spreading debris and potentially initiating an immunologic response in adjacent bone.[26] In addition, prosthesis loading can significantly increase the pressure within the membrane between the implant and bone, disrupting normal perfusion of the bone leading to osteonecrosis.[27,28] Finally, adaptive bone remodeling or stress shielding may alter proximal femoral load distribution increasing the risk for osteolysis.[29]

Early cementless femoral stems such as the Harris-Galante I had patch porous coating on the proximal one-third of the implant. With non-circumferential titanium fiber metal pads on the anterior, posterior, and medial aspects of the stem, it was thought in early studies that this provided fibrous channels that allowed PE liner particulate wear to flow through to the distal aspects of the stem. Through joint position, and muscle contraction, joint fluid pressure can reach up to 198 mm Hg, which can force particulate debris through these fibrous channels.[30] Five-year studies demonstrated that in these early stem designs osteolysis may begin within 12 to 18 months, primarily affecting the distal end of the prosthesis in Gruen zones 3 and 5.[13] In a recent long-term study looking at 21- to 27-year results of Harris-Galante I femoral stems, most cases diagnosed with osteolysis were limited to the proximal areas of the femur in Gruen zones 1 and 7.[31] Thus, the evidence currently available is contradictory and does not fully support the hypothesis that patch porous coating may propagate particle flow to the diaphyseal portion of the stem, promoting osteolysis and loosening.

RISK FACTORS
Patient Related

A patient's activity level following THA plays an important role in the development of osteolysis. A study by Schmalzried and colleagues[32] demonstrated a direct relationship between the volume of particulate debris and patient activity. Younger, more active male patients were found to have increased wear patterns increasing their risk for developing osteolysis.[32] Lubbeke and colleagues[33] reported that 24% of patients who maintained high activity levels after THA developed femoral osteolysis. Similarly, Flugsrad and colleagues[34] demonstrated that patients engaging in intermediate to intense activity were 4 times more likely than less active patients to develop acetabular loosening. Although morbid obesity ($\geq$40 kg/m^2) has historically been considered a relative contraindication for THA,[35] it has not been directly linked to osteolysis.[36,37] However, it is well recognized that

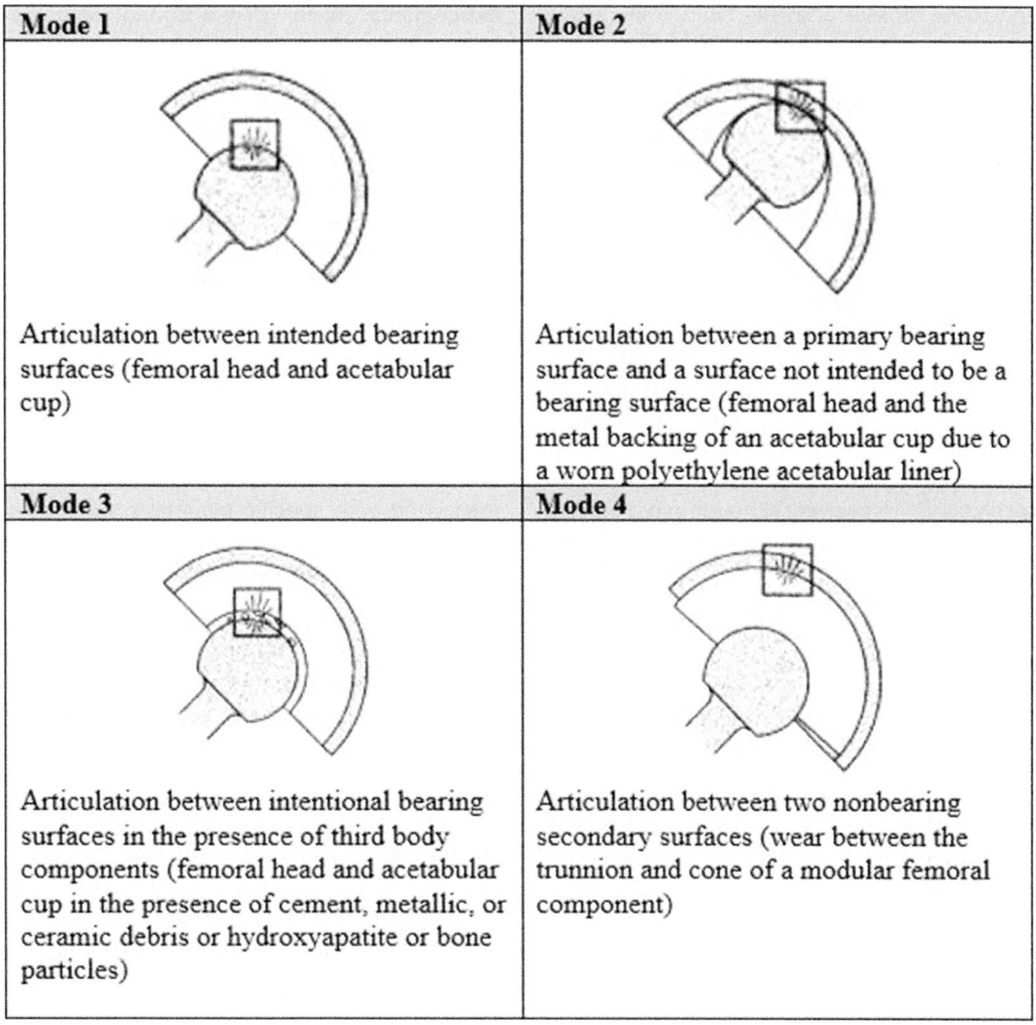

Mode 1	Mode 2
Articulation between intended bearing surfaces (femoral head and acetabular cup)	Articulation between a primary bearing surface and a surface not intended to be a bearing surface (femoral head and the metal backing of an acetabular cup due to a worn polyethylene acetabular liner)
Mode 3	**Mode 4**
Articulation between intentional bearing surfaces in the presence of third body components (femoral head and acetabular cup in the presence of cement, metallic, or ceramic debris or hydroxyapatite or bone particles)	Articulation between two nonbearing secondary surfaces (wear between the trunnion and cone of a modular femoral component)

Fig. 1. Modes of wear in periprosthetic hips. (*Reprinted with permission from* Wright TM, Goodman SB, editors. Implant Wear in Total Joint Replacement. Rosemont (IL): American Academy of Orthopaedic Surgeons; 2001.)

obesity is closely associated with a host of comorbidities drastically increasing the risk for poor outcomes and revision arthroplasty.[38]

MECHANICAL FACTORS
Bearing Surfaces
The rate of wear is influenced by the properties inherent to the bearing surface. A cobalt chromium femoral head articulating with an ultra-high molecular weight PE acetabular component has been shown to be an acceptable bearing surface with excellent long-term results.[39] Conventional PE has excellent mechanical integrity due to its chain entanglements, high molecule density, and moderate crystallinity.[40] Despite this, the wear from the conventional PE

components was a major contributor to osteolysis. To address this issue, orthopedic manufacturers introduced highly cross-linked PE (HXLPE) as a more resilient substitute for conventional PE. In addition, in 1998 manufacturers began treating HXLPE with gamma irradiation in a vacuum, breaking the carbon-hydrogen chains producing free radicals, enhancing wear characteristics.[41,42]

There is conflicting evidence regarding the performance of conventional versus HXLPE in THA. Several biomechanical and clinical studies have shown improved wear patterns with HXLPE when compared with conventional PE.[43–45] Recent studies have reported that HXLPE not only produces less debris, but the particles tend to be smaller and less biologically active compared with conventional PE.[43] Decreased wear rates with HXLPE have been shown with short-, mid-, and long-term follow-up.[46–48] A randomized control trial conducted by Engh and colleagues[46] comparing HXLPE and conventional PE reported a 95% reduction in wear and decreased osteolysis at 5 years with the use of HXLPE. Another study by Hanna and colleagues[48] with a 13-year follow-up showed significantly less osteolysis and lower revision rates with the use of HXLPE liners compared with conventional PE liners. Several meta-analyses have also suggested that HXLPE reduces wear debris compared with conventional PE[49,50] and that these improved wear patterns are associated with a decreased prevalence of osteolysis.[46,49] However, although most studies report favorable short- and mid-term outcomes, longer-term wear rates at 15 years may be inferior with HXLPE (0.883 mm) when compared with conventional PE (0.836 mm).[51]

In an effort to further reduce wear rates, manufacturers have also developed vitamin E-infused HXLPE, which incorporates the ant oxidative properties of vitamin E with the reduced wear rates associated with HXLPE.[52] During the manufacturing of vitamin E-infused HXLPE, PE powder is mixed with vitamin E and then irradiated.[53] The irradiation process cross-links the HXLPE while locking the vitamin E directly within the PE chain, providing long-lasting oxidative stability.[53] Although no long-term studies assessing the effectiveness of vitamin E HXLPE are available, short- and midterm follow-up have suggested improved wear rates.[54] Greene and colleagues[55] recently presented a multicenter prospective study of 977 THA patients in which the vitamin E–infused PE group had no evidence of osteolysis at 5 years.

Advancements in Bearing Surfaces

Because of the complications associated with PE wear, there has been renewed interest in ceramic components. Clinical and laboratory results indicate that wear rates can decrease by 10% to 50% when bearing surfaces are composed of ceramic-on-PE (CoPE) rather than cobalt chromium-on-PE.[56] Particulate debris produced by CoPE bearing surfaces tends to be nanometric in size and less biologically active.[57–59] Clinical results have demonstrated superior wear patterns and reduced osteolysis improving implant survivorship, presenting orthopedic surgeons with an alternative in young active patients.[60] In addition, laboratory experiments have demonstrated improved wear rates and decreased osteolytic potential with ceramic-on-ceramic (CoC) when compared with CoPE bearings.[61] Two recent meta-analyses comparing CoC and CoPE bearings in THA demonstrated lower wear rates in the CoC cohorts; however, this did not affect the rate of osteolysis, implant loosening, and the need for revision surgery.[62,63] Although improved wear rates with ceramic heads provide an attractive alternative to metal components, there currently is no conclusive evidence supporting the use of CoC- or CoPE bearing surfaces in all patients. In addition, CoC components are prone to squeaking, stripe wear, bearing surface fracture, and chipping during insertion. These negative attributes are associated with specific material properties of modular CoC components, including stem metal. Femoral stems made of a β titanium alloy, also called TMZF (Ti-12Mo-6Zr-2Fe [wt.%]) alloy, have been used as part of modular hip replacements since the early 2000s.[64] In 2011, such stems were recalled by the US Food & Drug Administration due to increased production of wear debris.[64] The wear associated with small movement of the stem and neck at the junction where they fit together in the modular CoC hip replacement. In addition, a study by Yoon and colleagues examined the ceramic femoral heads and acetabular components in 10 patients with THA diagnosed with osteolysis. Visible wear and damage to the load bearing surface of ceramic heads were noted. Studies examining the metallic rim around the ceramic acetabular insert may be warranted, although most studies using electron microscopy report ceramic wear debris within phagosomes of macrophages.[65]

Surgeons must also consider whether the increased cost of ceramic provides enough benefit to justify its use. Carnes and colleagues[66] recently performed a cost analysis to determine if the lifetime revision cost savings of CoPE implants offsets the higher initial costs when compared with metal-on-PE implants. The investigators concluded that lower revision rates can make the more expensive implants more cost-effective but this is reliant on the patient's age as well as the implant cost difference. For instance, when the CoPE implant costs $325 more than the metal-on-PE variant, then in order for the procedure to be cost-effective the patient should be younger than 85 years. However, when the cost difference increases to $600, the patient should be younger than 65 years. Thus, in order to comply with value-based care initiatives, surgeons must fully consider the advantages and disadvantages associated with each prosthesis component.

Fixation of Femoral Component

Although the Charnley low-friction arthroplasty developed in 1962 remains the gold standard for cemented fixation due to its excellent survival in long-term follow-up,[67,68] there has been a shift toward the use of uncemented stems in THA in recent years. Both cemented and uncemented femoral stems have demonstrated excellent survival rates, with revisions, when required, usually due to osteolysis and aseptic loosening.[69–72] There has, however, been conflicting evidence regarding the superiority of either cemented or uncemented femoral stems when looking at rates of wear and osteolysis. Wechter and colleagues[73] recently examined a large community joint registry and found that cemented stems were 3.76 times as likely as uncemented stems to be revised for aseptic loosening or loosening related to wear/osteolysis, whereas other studies have demonstrated no difference.[74–76] There is speculation that variability in patient age, sex, weight, comorbidities, and activity level may contribute to these differences. A recent study by Kim and colleagues,[77] in which patients received simultaneous bilateral THA with a cemented stem in one hip and an uncemented stem in the other hip, sought to permit more meaningful comparison of the outcomes by eliminating these variables. The investigators reported no significant difference in wear and osteolysis between the 2 groups at 25- to 27-year follow-up. Each study has its own inherent limitations, and the preference to use cemented or uncemented femoral fixation is multifactorial and depends on the treating physician.

Fixation of Acetabular Component

Although early acetabular components were cemented, the use of cementless acetabular components in THA has gained popularity over the past 4 decades. Today most of the THAs performed in the United States use uncemented acetabular components.[78] Clement and colleagues[79] analyzed 16 comparative studies of cemented and uncemented sockets and found a slightly higher rate of osteolysis in the cemented sockets. However, the extent and severity of osteolysis was greater in the uncemented cohort. The investigators hypothesized that the increased severity of osteolysis was due to accelerated wear in uncemented fixation.[79] It has been suggested that modularity of uncemented acetabular components contributes to

increased backside wear, accelerating the progression of osteolysis.[80–83] As a result, monoblock press-fit acetabular components may reduce PE wear and osteolysis. Monoblock sockets have no liner-shell micromotion, eliminating the risk of backside wear.[84,85] In addition, the absence of dome holes prevents wear debris from directly accessing the subchondral bone, further reducing the risk of acetabular osteolysis.[82] Nevertheless, several studies have reported conflicting results on the advantages and disadvantages associated with monoblock and modular acetabular components.[85–87]

Femoral Head Size

There is a trend toward increasing femoral head size in THA, because a larger femoral head improves range of motion and joint stability, reducing the risk of impingement and dislocation.[88] However, increasing the femoral head size also increases the bearing surface, potentially affecting PE wear rates and osteolysis. A study by Howie and colleagues[89] reported no significant difference in linear and volumetric wear rates between 28-mm and 36-mm femoral heads with 1- to 3-year follow-up. Similarly, Hammerberg and colleagues[90] reported no statistical difference in linear wear rates between smaller (28–32 mm) and larger (38–44 mm) femoral heads. Although the investigators of another study did note an association between larger head size (36–40 mm) and increased volumetric wear rate, the rate increase did not exceed the threshold associated with osteolysis.[91]

Modular Designs

Modular THA designs use a single head-neck taper junction connecting the femoral stem to the prosthesis head allowing for intraoperative adjustments of limb length, femoral offset, and head diameter. Dual modular THA designs have an additional taper junction between an interchangeable neck and stem, permitting further intraoperative flexibility and partial revision of the prosthesis if necessary.[92] The use of these designs, however, introduces additional interfaces from which wear debris can form. Trunnion wear, characterized by corrosion and fretting of the taper, can occur at both the head-neck and the neck-stem taper junctions, producing adverse local tissue reactions, including osteolysis, similar to that seen in resurfacing implants in which there is no taper junction.[93–95]

Retrieval studies of metal-on-metal designs have shown that the taper contributes, on average, 32.9% of the total wear volume and may exceed wear volume generated at the bearing surface. The development and severity of trunnionosis is influenced by several biomechanical, implant design and material-related factors.[96] Tan and colleagues[97] demonstrated an effect of taper design, head length, head size, and implant material composition on tribocorrosion at the modular head-neck taper interface of THA implants, with (1) narrower tapers, (2) longer head lengths, and (3) larger head sizes demonstrating increased fretting damage and corrosion.[98,99] In addition, trunnion wear is considered to be most significant in the setting of metal-on-metal modular THA designs, particularly when using a titanium neck. Although trunnionosis remains an infrequent cause for implant failure, it should be considered in patients with modular head-neck or neck-stem implants who present with unexplained pain or late recurrent instability, possibly due to osteolysis caused by hardware debris.

DIAGNOSIS OF OSTEOLYSIS
Symptoms
Most patients with osteolysis have no clinical symptoms until the implant has loosened or the PE insert has worn considerably.[100] A small subset of patients may present with thigh or groin pain due to femoral or acetabular component loosening, respectively.[101] Pain associated with osteolysis often presents after a pain-free interval following the index procedure. In addition, micromotion and loosening at the bone-prosthesis interface may cause start-up pain and pain that ceases with rest.[102] Because many of the radiographic findings of osteolysis overlap with infection,[103] it is imperative that the surgeon determines the location, severity, and timing of pain as well as the presence or absence of a postoperative pain-free interval during the history and physical examination. Pain that is associated with rest and lack of a pain-free interval after index arthroplasty can suggest periprosthetic joint infection,[102] and diagnosis of mechanical loosening requires a negative infection workup.[104] Loosening and infection can of course present simultaneously in the presence of osteolysis (Fig. 2).

Imaging Studies
It is crucial that orthopedic surgeons diagnose osteolysis as early as possible, because outcomes are best when bone stock is preserved.[100,105–109] rTHA in patients with extensive osteolysis is associated with suboptimal outcomes due to bony

and soft tissue deficiencies that frequently require grafts and restrictive implants.[110] The timely diagnosis and management of osteolysis is essential for optimal outcomes.[111–114]

Subclinical osteolysis should be followed closely. Diagnosis and surveillance of wear-induced osteolysis requires several imaging modalities to be used to assess the extent of particulate wear, location of lesion, and risk of progression. Clinically serial radiographs are most commonly used to identify and estimate acetabular PE wear rates. More advanced imaging including radiostereometric analysis can be used to accurately quantify the magnitude of penetration of the femoral head into the PE bearing surface of the acetabular component.[115] The role of other imaging modalities including 3-dimensional computed tomography (CT) and MRI in the setting of PE wear analysis has not been well defined. Although there is no clear consensus on how to best measure PE wear, radiographs should be obtained anytime a patient has symptomatic THA, and subsequent radiographs should be obtained at follow-up visits to evaluate progression.

When evaluating for osteolysis it is crucial to compare the immediate postoperative radiograph with the most recent radiograph, with views in the anterior, posterior, and iliac oblique planes.[116–118] Plain radiographs may demonstrate progressive and/or extensive gapping at the bone-cement, bone-prosthesis, or cement-prosthesis interface. Although easily obtained, plain radiographic evaluation often substantially underestimates the extent of involvement in the bone and soft tissue and is unlikely to detect small osteolytic lesions.[119] Moreover, plain radiographs may inaccurately portray the location of the lesion.[119–121] 3D CT has proved to be superior to plain radiographs for the detection and monitoring of osteolytic lesions.[122] CT scanning can be used in conjunction with plain radiograph when osteolysis is suspected. Such an approach will identify the extent and location of disease (Fig. 3) permitting adequate management.[119] On CT, well-defined lucencies and the absence of osseous trabeculae in continuity with the prosthesis are characteristic findings associated with osteolysis and are better defined than with plain radiographs.[123] Howie and colleagues[122] demonstrated that the amount of osteolysis found on the initial CT scan and the patient's activity level are strong predictors of disease progression.

MRI is another useful imaging modality to detect and quantify osteolysis. Although the sensitivity for detecting osteolysis with CT

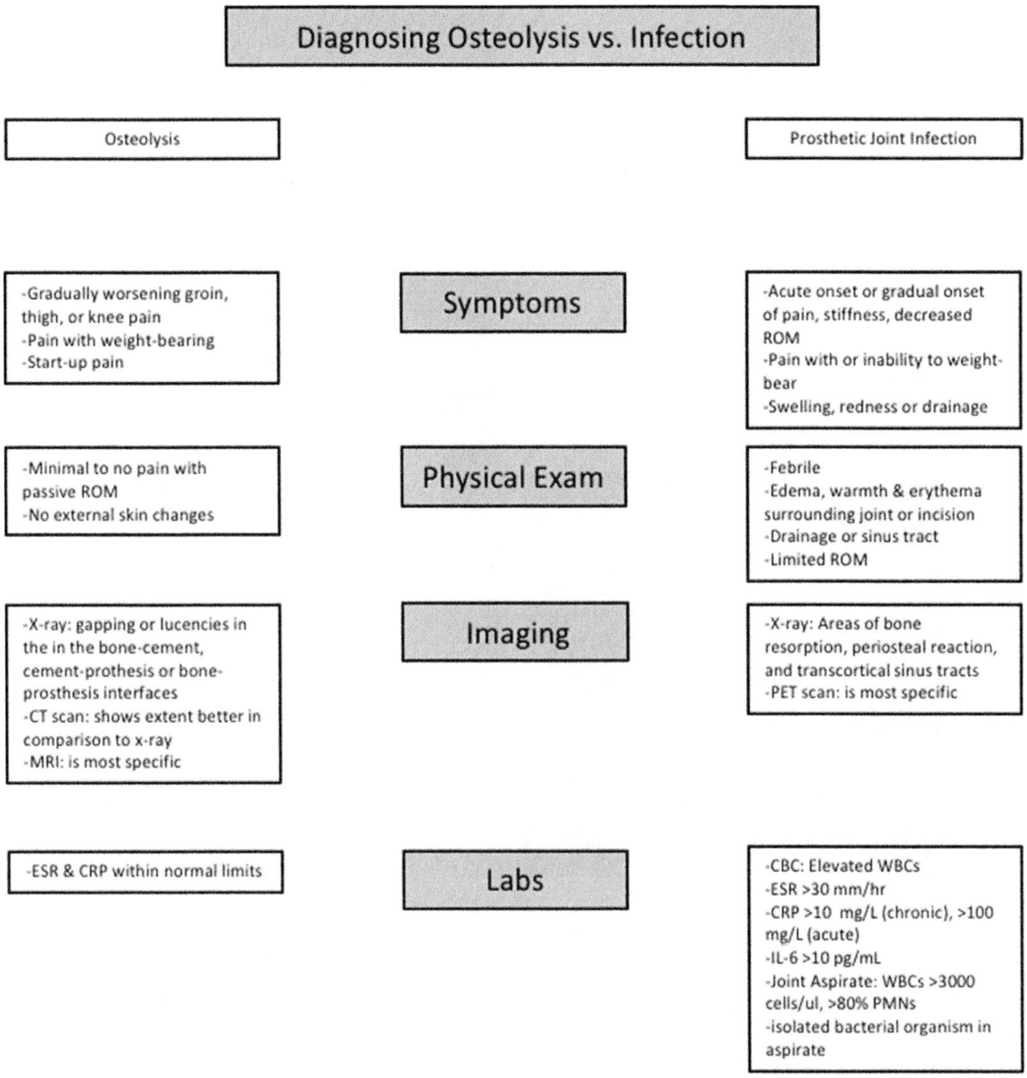

Diagnosing Osteolysis vs. Infection

| Osteolysis | | Prosthetic Joint Infection |

Osteolysis		Prosthetic Joint Infection
-Gradually worsening groin, thigh, or knee pain -Pain with weight-bearing -Start-up pain	**Symptoms**	-Acute onset or gradual onset of pain, stiffness, decreased ROM -Pain with or inability to weight-bear -Swelling, redness or drainage
-Minimal to no pain with passive ROM -No external skin changes	**Physical Exam**	-Febrile -Edema, warmth & erythema surrounding joint or incision -Drainage or sinus tract -Limited ROM
-X-ray: gapping or lucencies in the in the bone-cement, cement-prothesis or bone-prosthesis interfaces -CT scan: shows extent better in comparison to x-ray -MRI: is most specific	**Imaging**	-X-ray: Areas of bone resorption, periosteal reaction, and transcortical sinus tracts -PET scan: is most specific
-ESR & CRP within normal limits	**Labs**	-CBC: Elevated WBCs -ESR >30 mm/hr -CRP >10 mg/L (chronic), >100 mg/L (acute) -IL-6 >10 pg/mL -Joint Aspirate: WBCs >3000 cells/ul, >80% PMNs -isolated bacterial organism in aspirate

Fig. 2. Comparatively evaluating the diagnosis of osteolysis versus infection.

imaging is 75%,[119] MRI is significantly more sensitive at 95%.[119] In addition, MRI is most effective at detecting small lesions less than 3 cm^3.[119] The sensitivity and specificity of different imaging modalities for the detection of osteolysis is summarized in Table 1.

MANAGEMENT

Management of osteolysis following THA relies on the patient's symptoms and disease severity.[13,124,125] The primary aim of surgical intervention in the setting of osteolysis following THA is to identify and remove the origin of the osteolysis, loose hardware and wear debris, and graft osteolytic lesions.[101] rTHA is guided by a set of variables, including patient age, extent of bone loss, rate of disease progression, risk of fracture, activity level, symptomology, component fixation, and general patient health.[101] Patient pain may indicate THA involvement. Although pain symptoms may vary, groin pain is typically associated with the acetabular component, whereas thigh pain is reflective of the femoral component.

Patients diagnosed with asymptomatic osteolysis are typically managed nonsurgically. Current management guidelines are not well established but the authors recommend radiographic surveillance every 12 to 18 months. The goals of nonsurgical management include the stabilization of bone loss and control of symptoms. Patient education, physical therapy, and activity modification may be used to manage symptoms and maintain function. The

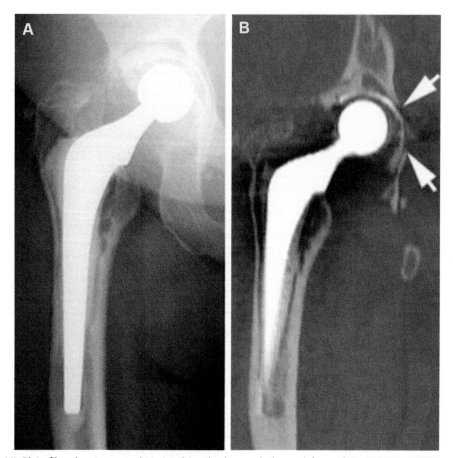

Fig. 3. (A) Plain film showing osteolysis involving both acetabular and femoral components. (B) Coronal CT showing additional findings not revealed on plain radiograph in medial wall of the acetabulum (arrows). (From Cahir JG, Toms AP, Marshall TJ, et al. CT and MRI of hip arthroplasty. Clin Radiol 2007;62(12):1166; with permission.)

decision to revise patients with asymptomatic periacetabular osteolysis is multifactorial. Important variables to consider include impending prosthesis failure due to wear through of the PE liner or large, rapidly progressing osteolytic lesions particularly when fixation of the cup is threatened. Furthermore, the comorbidity profile and life expectancy of the patient and prosthesis track record should also be considered. As the disease progresses, patient symptomology may worsen warranting rTHA.

Table 1		
Sensitivity and specificity of imaging modalities for detection of osteolysis		
Imaging Modality	**Sensitivity**	**Specificity**
Plain radiograph	57.6%–64%[a]	92.9%
CT	75%	95%
MRI	95%	98%

[a] Depend on radiograph orientation anterior-posterior versus oblique views, respectively.
Data from Refs.[119,145,146]

Femoral Component

For asymptomatic osteolysis around a well-fixed cemented femoral component, treatment avoids removal of the stem and focuses on curettage and grafting of the boney defects, as well as exchange of the femoral head and bearing surface.[101] A cemented femoral component that has become loose due to osteolysis must be revised.

Osteolysis around an uncemented femoral component is treated similarly, requiring revision when loose. However, controversy arises when there is osteolysis around a well-fixed uncemented femoral component. In this case, there are 2 surgical options. The first option is to completely revise the implant. The second is to debride and graft the osteolytic lesion and replace the bearing surface.[126] Several factors must be considered including the location of the osteolytic lesions, extent of fixation, and the implant track record. Metaphyseal lesions are often amenable to grafting, whereas diaphyseal lesions are at risk for periprosthetic fracture and should be revised.[126] Moreover, the extent of

Table 2
Classification of osteolysis around uncemented femoral components

Osteolysis Cemented Classification	Suggested Intervention
Type 1	• The stem is well fixed • Metaphyseal osteolysis only • Sufficient ingrowth or ongrowth to provide long-term stability	• Stem retention, debridement, and grafting
Type 2	• The stem is well fixed • Significant diaphyseal or metaphyseal osteolysis • Limited area of osseointegration	• Stem removal, reclassify extent of osteolysis
Type 3	• Implant is loose	• Stem removal and reconstruction

Data from Maloney WJ. The surgical management of femoral osteolysis. J Arthroplasty 2005;20(4 Suppl 2):75–8.

fixation and the quality of remaining bony apposition should also be assessed to ensure long-term implant stability. Lastly, implants with poor clinical track records may be considered for revision.[126] Using the aforementioned criteria, Maloney and colleagues developed a management protocol for patients with uncemented stems and femoral osteolytic disease (Table 2).[126]

The Paprosky classification (Table 3) can be used to classify femoral bone deficits using the location of bone loss and amount of remaining proximal and diaphyseal bone.[127] Paprosky classification Type I and II bone deficits can be revised using extensively porous-coated femoral stems or mid-modular cementless stems.[128]

Types III and IV disease can be managed with impaction grafting or allograft prosthetic composites and cemented stems. **Fig. 4** illustrates the recommended operative algorithm for patients with femoral component osteolysis.

Acetabular Component

Revision of the acetabular component is more complex and is often performed when the prosthesis becomes loose. Cemented cups normally have a linear osteolytic pattern around the cement-bone interface, which can lead to loosening of the acetabular component.[129] When loosening occurs, revision is indicated with a cementless acetabular component. Any bone stock deficiencies must be treated with an appropriate graft.[7] If osteolysis is discovered around a stable cemented component, wear should be assessed intraoperatively. If the wear is minimal, the cup can be retained, but if significant acetabular cup wear is apparent, the component should be replaced and bone deficits grafted.

Uncemented acetabular components often remain well fixed even in the presence of extensive osteolysis because the cementless component has areas of ingrowth.[130] An expansive pattern of osteolysis is usually seen on radiograph and is often illustrated with radiolucent regions at the bone-implant interface expanding away from the implant into the surrounding cancellous bone.[129,131,132] These lesions predominately occur in zones 2 and 3 but may occur in any of the Charnley zones.[129] Patients with well-fixed cups are often asymptomatic,[133] but if the osteolytic process is allowed to progress until symptomatic, revision may be challenging. Loosening of an uncemented acetabular component may signify major structural compromise of the pelvis, stemming from pelvic discontinuity or pelvic column deficiencies.[133–135]

Early reports advocated the removal of a well-fixed cup during revision surgery for osteolysis,

Table 3
Paprosky classification of femoral bone loss

Type	I	II	IIIa	IIIb	IV
Description	Minimal metaphyseal bone loss	Extensive metadiaphyseal bone loss with intact diaphysis	Extensive metadiaphyseal bone loss, minimum of 4 cm of intact cortical bone in the diaphysis	Extensive metadiaphyseal bone loss, less than 4 cm of intact cortical bone in the diaphysis	Extensive metadiaphyseal bone loss and a nonsupportive diaphysis

Data from Paprosky WG, Weeden SH. Extensively porous-coated stems in femoral revision arthroplasty. Orthopedics 2001;24(9):871–2.

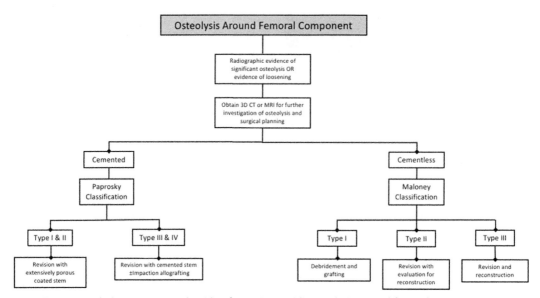

Fig. 4. Recommended management algorithm for patients with osteolysis around femoral component.

allowing the surgeon to accurately assess, debride, and graft osteolytic regions.[130,134,136] However, removing a well-fixed cup can substantially damage the surrounding bone and tissue compromising the integrity of the pelvis.[133–135] In addition, rTHA is associated with significant morbidity and should be avoided if possible. Thus, in the setting of acetabular osteolysis it is crucial that the orthopedic surgeon be cognizant of disease severity and risk for progression, because both premature or delayed interventions may adversely affect outcomes.[137]

In order to assist orthopedic surgeons and guide treatment of acetabular osteolysis, a classification system was proposed by Rubash and colleagues[109] for uncemented cups based on the stability of the shell and exchangeability of the liner. As described in **Table 4**, acetabular components can be classified into 3 categories, which may effectively guide treatment.[109,135,137,138] In patients with more complex disease, the Gross classification system (**Table 5**) may help guide management, particularly in patients with Type IV and V disease. These severe circumstances often require elaborate cage-cup constructs or customized triflange implants. **Fig. 5** illustrates the recommended operative algorithm,

Table 4		
Classification of osteolysis around uncemented acetabular components		
Osteolysis Uncemented Classification		
Type 1	• Focal osteolysis with a well-fixed shell and the PE liner is exchangeable • The cup is stable but is associated with a discrete focal osteolytic lesion, usually located in zones 1 or 3 or both and occasionally adjacent to the screws[7] • An acetabular socket should not be removed if it is well fixed with intraoperative testing and if the following criteria were met: (1) the cup was not malpositioned; (2) the locking mechanism was intact; (3) the metal shell was not damaged; (4) the PE liner was of adequate thickness; (5) the implant had an acceptable track record; and (6) the implant was a modular implant[112]		
Type 2	• Focal osteolysis with a well-fixed shell, but the PE liner is nonexchangeable or the locking mechanism is defective or suboptimal so cup has to be removed • If the components are stable but do not meet the criteria for Type 1, they are classified as Type 2 defects		
Type 3	• Osteolysis with obvious loosening of the cup • The component is unstable and has migrated into the osteolytic lesion, necessitating revision of the components		

Data from Rubash HE, Sinha RK, Paprosky W, et al. A new classification system for the management of acetabular osteolysis after total hip arthroplasty. Instr Course Lect 1999;48:37–42.

Table 5					
Gross classification of acetabular bone loss					
Type	**I**	**II**	**III**	**IV**	**V**
Description	No substantial loss of bone stock	Contained loss of bone stock	Minor column defect: uncontained loss of bone stock involving <50% of acetabulum	Major column defect: uncontained loss of bone stock involving ≥ 50% of acetabulum	Pelvic discontinuity with uncontained loss of bone stock

Data from Garbuz D, Morsi E, Mohamed N, et al. Classification and reconstruction in revision acetabular arthroplasty with bone stock deficiency. Clin Orthop Relat Res 1996(324):98–107; with permission.

in the setting of osteolysis of the acetabular component.

Pharmacologic Management

Physiologic modalities of preventing osteolysis have also been investigated. One of the promising treatments is denosumab, an RANKL antibody.[139–141] Other antiinflammatory immune modulators including IL-1Ra and AM630, a cannabinoid receptor 2, and inhibitor of IL-1b and tumor necrosis factor alpha have reduced particulate debris in early animal studies; however, it will be some time until they are clinically available.[142,143]

Cost

Revision procedures are costly and are associated with increased morbidity and mortality. Further complicating the matter is the extensive societal and economic burden associated with rTHA. The Charlson Comorbidity Index (CCI) may be used to predict patient outcomes during revision surgery. In a study by Nichols and colleagues[144] the highest cost scenarios were observed in patients with a CCI greater than 2, demonstrating the predictive nature of CCI for postoperative complications and resource utilization patterns.[144]

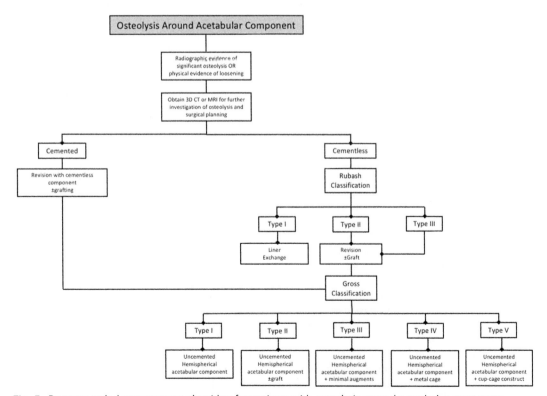

Fig. 5. Recommended management algorithm for patients with osteolysis around acetabular component.

SUMMARY

Although osteolysis was first recognized in the setting of THA many decades ago, it remains a significant challenge affecting the longevity of the implant. Osteolysis is the result of an immunologic reaction against particulate wear debris that arises due to several host, prosthesis, and mechanical factors. When there is significant wear and osteolysis around a THA, surgical intervention is often indicated. Because rTHA is associated with increased cost and patient morbidity, it is crucial that wear rates be kept to a minimum and patients be evaluated for osteolysis regularly. Significant efforts have been made to develop new technologies and materials with enhanced wear properties, thereby reducing the prevalence of osteolysis amongst THA recipients.

REFERENCES

1. Kurtz SM, Ong KL, Lau E, et al. Impact of the economic downturn on total joint replacement demand in the United States: updated projections to 2021. J Bone Joint Surg Am 2014; 96(8):624–30.
2. Bozic KJ, Kamath AF, Ong K, et al. Comparative epidemiology of revision arthroplasty: failed THA poses greater clinical and economic burdens than failed TKA. Clin Orthop Relat Res 2015; 473(6):2131–8.
3. Crowe JF, Sculco TP, Kahn B. Revision total hip arthroplasty: hospital cost and reimbursement analysis. Clin Orthop Relat Res 2003;(413):175–82.
4. Katz RP, Callaghan JJ, Sullivan PM, et al. Long-term results of revision total hip arthroplasty with improved cementing technique. J Bone Joint Surg Br 1997;79(2):322–6.
5. Paprosky WG, Weeden SH, Bowling JW Jr. Component removal in revision total hip arthroplasty. Clin Orthop Relat Res 2001;(393):181–93.
6. Haynes JA, Stambough JB, Sassoon AA, et al. Contemporary surgical indications and referral trends in revision total hip arthroplasty: a 10-year review. J Arthroplasty 2016;31(3):622–5.
7. Saleh KJ, Thongtrangan I, Schwarz EM. Osteolysis: medical and surgical approaches. Clin Orthop Relat Res 2004;(427):138–47.
8. Charnley J. Postoperative infection after total hip replacement with special reference to air contamination in the operating room. Clin Orthop Relat Res 1972;87:167–87.
9. Harris WH, Schiller AL, Scholler JM, et al. Extensive localized bone resorption in the femur following total hip replacement. J Bone Joint Surg Am 1976;58(5):612–8.
10. Jones LC, Hungerford DS. Cement disease. Clin Orthop Relat Res 1987;(225):192–206.
11. Harris WH. Osteolysis and particle disease in hip replacement. A review. Acta Orthop Scand 1994; 65(1):113–23.
12. Harris WH. The problem is osteolysis. Clin Orthop Relat Res 1995;(311):46–53.
13. Tanzer M, Maloney WJ, Jasty M, et al. The progression of femoral cortical osteolysis in association with total hip arthroplasty without cement. J Bone Joint Surg Am 1992;74(3): 404–10.
14. Campbell P, Ma S, Yeom B, et al. Isolation of predominantly submicron-sized UHMWPE wear particles from periprosthetic tissues. J Biomed Mater Res 1995;29(1):127–31.
15. Maloney WJ, Smith RL, Schmalzried TP, et al. Isolation and characterization of wear particles generated in patients who have had failure of a hip arthroplasty without cement. J Bone Joint Surg Am 1995;77(9):1301–10.
16. Margevicius KJ, Bauer TW, McMahon JT, et al. Isolation and characterization of debris in membranes around total joint prostheses. J Bone Joint Surg Am 1994;76(11):1664–75.
17. Jacobs JJ, Roebuck KA, Archibeck M, et al. Osteolysis: basic science. Clin Orthop Relat Res 2001;(393):71–7.
18. Rubash HE, Sinha RK, Shanbhag AS, et al. Pathogenesis of bone loss after total hip arthroplasty. Orthop Clin North Am 1998;29(2):173–86.
19. Athanasou NA, Quinn J, Bulstrode CJ. Resorption of bone by inflammatory cells derived from the joint capsule of hip arthroplasties. J Bone Joint Surg Br 1992;74(1):57–62.
20. Gupta SK, Chu A, Ranawat AS, et al. Osteolysis after total knee arthroplasty. J Arthroplasty 2007; 22(6):787–99.
21. Yao J, Cs-Szabo G, Jacobs JJ, et al. Suppression of osteoblast function by titanium particles. J Bone Joint Surg Am 1997;79(1):107–12.
22. Green TR, Fisher J, Stone M, et al. Polyethylene particles of a 'critical size' are necessary for the induction of cytokines by macrophages in vitro. Biomaterials 1998;19(24):2297–302.
23. Dumbleton JH, Manley MT, Edidin AA. A literature review of the association between wear rate and osteolysis in total hip arthroplasty. J Arthroplasty 2002;17(5):649–61.
24. Kandahari AM, Yang X, Laroche KA, et al. A review of UHMWPE wear-induced osteolysis: the role for early detection of the immune response. Bone Res 2016;4:16014.
25. McKellop HA, Campbell P, Park SH, et al. The origin of submicron polyethylene wear debris in total hip arthroplasty. Clin Orthop Relat Res 1995;(311):3–20.

26. Dalling JG, Math K, Scuderi GR. Evaluating the progression of osteolysis after total knee arthroplasty. J Am Acad Orthop Surg 2015;23(3):173–80.

27. Aspenberg P, Van der Vis H. Migration, particles, and fluid pressure. A discussion of causes of prosthetic loosening. Clin Orthop Relat Res 1998;(352):75–80.

28. Aspenberg P, van der Vis H. Fluid pressure may cause periprosthetic osteolysis. Particles are not the only thing. Acta Orthop Scand 1998;69(1):1–4.

29. Chen HH, Morrey BF, An KN, et al. Bone remodeling characteristics of a short-stemmed total hip replacement. J Arthroplasty 2009;24(6):945–50.

30. Schmalzried TP, Jasty M, Harris WH. Periprosthetic bone loss in total hip arthroplasty. Polyethylene wear debris and the concept of the effective joint space. J Bone Joint Surg Am 1992;74(6):849–63.

31. Kawamura H, Mishima H, Sugaya H, et al. The 21- to 27-year results of the Harris-Galante cementless total hip arthroplasty. J Orthop Sci 2016;21(3):342–7.

32. Schmalzried TP, Szuszczewicz ES, Northfield MR, et al. Quantitative assessment of walking activity after total hip or knee replacement. J Bone Joint Surg Am 1998;80(1):54–9.

33. Lubbeke A, Garavaglia G, Barea C, et al. Influence of patient activity on femoral osteolysis at five and ten years following hybrid total hip replacement. J Bone Joint Surg Br 2011;93(4):456–63.

34. Flugsrud GB, Nordsletten L, Espehaug B, et al. The effect of middle-age body weight and physical activity on the risk of early revision hip arthroplasty: a cohort study of 1,535 individuals. Acta Orthop 2007;78(1):99–107.

35. Charnley J. Long-term results of low-friction arthroplasty. Hip 1982;42–9.

36. Lubbeke A, Garavaglia G, Barea C, et al. Influence of obesity on femoral osteolysis five and ten years following total hip arthroplasty. J Bone Joint Surg Am 2010;92(10):1964–72.

37. Andrew JG, Palan J, Kurup HV, et al. Obesity in total hip replacement. J Bone Joint Surg Br 2008;90(4):424–9.

38. Werner BC, Higgins MD, Pehlivan HC, et al. Super obesity is an independent risk factor for complications after primary total hip arthroplasty. J Arthroplasty 2017;32(2):402–6.

39. Kumar N, Arora GN, Datta B. Bearing surfaces in hip replacement - evolution and likely future. Med J Armed Forces India 2014;70(4):371–6.

40. Li S, Burstein AH. Ultra-high molecular weight polyethylene. The material and its use in total joint implants. J Bone Joint Surg Am 1994;76(7):1080–90.

41. Jacobs CA, Christensen CP, Greenwald AS, et al. Clinical performance of highly cross-linked polyethylenes in total hip arthroplasty. J Bone Joint Surg Am 2007;89(12):2779–86.

42. Ries MD, Pruitt L. Effect of cross-linking on the microstructure and mechanical properties of ultra-high molecular weight polyethylene. Clin Orthop Relat Res 2005;440:149–56.

43. Minoda Y, Kobayashi A, Sakawa A, et al. Wear particle analysis of highly crosslinked polyethylene isolated from a failed total hip arthroplasty. J Biomed Mater Res B Appl Biomater 2008;86(2):501–5.

44. Heiner AD, Galvin AL, Fisher J, et al. Scratching vulnerability of conventional vs highly cross-linked polyethylene liners because of large embedded third-body particles. J Arthroplasty 2012;27(5):742–9.

45. Dorr LD, Wan Z, Shahrdar C, et al. Clinical performance of a Durasul highly cross-linked polyethylene acetabular liner for total hip arthroplasty at five years. J Bone Joint Surg Am 2005;87(8):1816–21.

46. Engh CA Jr, Stepniewski AS, Ginn SD, et al. A randomized prospective evaluation of outcomes after total hip arthroplasty using cross-linked marathon and non-cross-linked Enduron polyethylene liners. J Arthroplasty 2006;21(6 Suppl 2):17–25.

47. Bragdon CR, Doerner M, Martell J, et al. The 2012 John Charnley Award: clinical multicenter studies of the wear performance of highly crosslinked remelted polyethylene in THA. Clin Orthop Relat Res 2013;471(2):393–402.

48. Hanna SA, Somerville L, McCalden RW, et al. Highly cross-linked polyethylene decreases the rate of revision of total hip arthroplasty compared with conventional polyethylene at 13 years' follow-up. Bone Joint J 2016;98-B(1):28–32.

49. Kurtz SM, Gawel HA, Patel JD. History and systematic review of wear and osteolysis outcomes for first-generation highly crosslinked polyethylene. Clin Orthop Relat Res 2011;469(8):2262–77.

50. Mu Z, Tian J, Wu T, et al. A systematic review of radiological outcomes of highly cross-linked polyethylene versus conventional polyethylene in total hip arthroplasty. Int Orthop 2009;33(3):599–604.

51. Tsukamoto M, Ohnishi H, Mori T. Fifteen-year comparison of wear and osteolysis analysis for cross-linked or conventional polyethylene total hip arthroplasty for hip dysplasia - a retrospective cohort study. J Arthroplasty 2017;32(1):161–5.

52. Nebergall AK, Troelsen A, Rubash HE, et al. Five-year experience of vitamin E-diffused highly cross-linked polyethylene wear in total hip arthroplasty assessed by radiostereometric analysis. J Arthroplasty 2016;31(6):1251–5.

53. Inc. Z. Vivacit-E® Vitamin E highly crosslinked polyethylene long-term performance for high demand patients. Available at: http://www.zimmerbiomet.

com/content/dam/zimmer-biomet/medical-professionals/hip/vivacit-e/vivacite-white-paper.pdf. Accessed March 1, 2018.

54. Bladen CL, Teramura S, Russell SL, et al. Analysis of wear, wear particles, and reduced inflammatory potential of vitamin E ultrahigh-molecular-weight polyethylene for use in total joint replacement. J Biomed Mater Res B Appl Biomater 2013;101(3):458–66.

55. Greene M, SN, Nebergall A, et al. 5 year long-term multicenter outcomes with vitamin E polyethylene liners and porous-titanium coated shells. AAHKS 24th Annual Meeting. Dallas, Texas, November 6–9, 2014.

56. Simon JA, Dayan AJ, Ergas E, et al. Catastrophic failure of the acetabular component in a ceramic-polyethylene bearing total hip arthroplasty. J Arthroplasty 1998;13(1):108–13.

57. Lewis PM, Al-Belooshi A, Olsen M, et al. Prospective randomized trial comparing alumina ceramic-on-ceramic with ceramic-on-conventional polyethylene bearings in total hip arthroplasty. J Arthroplasty 2010;25(3):392–7.

58. Choy WS, Kim KJ, Lee SK, et al. Ceramic-on-ceramic total hip arthroplasty: minimum of six-year follow-up study. Clin Orthop Surg 2013;5(3):174–9.

59. Molloy D, Jack C, Esposito C, et al. A mid-term analysis suggests ceramic on ceramic hip arthroplasty is durable with minimal wear and low risk of squeak. HSS J 2012;8(3):291–4.

60. Garino JP. Cermic hip replacement history. Semin Arthroplasty 2011;22(4):214–7.

61. Affatato S, Goldoni M, Testoni M, et al. Mixed oxides prosthetic ceramic ball heads. Part 3: effect of the ZrO2 fraction on the wear of ceramic on ceramic hip joint prostheses. A long-term in vitro wear study. Biomaterials 2001;22(7):717–23.

62. Dong YL, Li T, Xiao K, et al. Ceramic on ceramic or ceramic-on-polyethylene for total hip arthroplasty: a systemic review and meta-analysis of prospective randomized studies. Chin Med J (Engl) 2015; 128(9):1223–31.

63. Si HB, Zeng Y, Cao F, et al. Is a ceramic-on-ceramic bearing really superior to ceramic-on-polyethylene for primary total hip arthroplasty? A systematic review and meta-analysis of randomised controlled trials. Hip Int 2015;25(3):191–8.

64. Yang X, Hutchinson CR. Corrosion-wear of beta-Ti alloy TMZF (Ti-12Mo-6Zr-2Fe) in simulated body fluid. Acta Biomater 2016;42:429–39.

65. Yoon TR, Rowe SM, Jung ST, et al. Osteolysis in association with a total hip arthroplasty with ceramic bearing surfaces. J Bone Joint Surg Am 1998;80(10):1459–68.

66. Carnes KJ, Odum SM, Troyer JL, et al. Cost analysis of ceramic heads in primary total hip arthroplasty. J Bone Joint Surg Am 2016; 98(21):1794–800.

67. Berry DJ, Harmsen WS, Cabanela ME, et al. Twenty-five-year survivorship of two thousand consecutive primary Charnley total hip replacements: factors affecting survivorship of acetabular and femoral components. J Bone Joint Surg Am 2002;84-A(2):171–7.

68. Sochart DH, Porter ML. The long-term results of Charnley low-friction arthroplasty in young patients who have congenital dislocation, degenerative osteoarthrosis, or rheumatoid arthritis. J Bone Joint Surg Am 1997;79(11):1599–617.

69. Collis DK, Mohler CG. Comparison of clinical outcomes in total hip arthroplasty using rough and polished cemented stems with essentially the same geometry. J Bone Joint Surg Am 2002;84-A(4):586–92.

70. de Nies F, Fidler MW. The Harris-Galante cementless femoral component: poor results in 57 hips followed for 3 years. Acta Orthop Scand 1996; 67(2):122–4.

71. Learmonth ID, Grobler GP, Dall DM, et al. Loss of bone stock with cementless hip arthroplasty. J Arthroplasty 1995;10(3):257–63.

72. Ong A, Wong KL, Lai M, et al. Early failure of precoated femoral components in primary total hip arthroplasty. J Bone Joint Surg Am 2002;84-A(5): 786–92.

73. Wechter J, Comfort TK, Tatman P, et al. Improved survival of uncemented versus cemented femoral stems in patients aged < 70 years in a community total joint registry. Clin Orthop Relat Res 2013; 471(11):3588–95.

74. Grant P, Aamodt A, Falch JA, et al. Differences in stability and bone remodeling between a customized uncemented hydroxyapatite coated and a standard cemented femoral stem A randomized study with use of radiostereometry and bone densitometry. J Orthop Res 2005;23(6):1280–5.

75. Karrholm J, Malchau H, Snorrason F, et al. Micromotion of femoral stems in total hip arthroplasty. A randomized study of cemented, hydroxyapatite-coated, and porous-coated stems with roentgen stereophotogrammetric analysis. J Bone Joint Surg Am 1994;76(11):1692–705.

76. Strom H, Kolstad K, Mallmin H, et al. Comparison of the uncemented Cone and the cemented Bimetric hip prosthesis in young patients with osteoarthritis: an RSA, clinical and radiographic study. Acta Orthop 2006;77(1):71–8.

77. Kim YH, Park JW, Kim JS, et al. Twenty-five- to twenty-seven-year results of a cemented vs a cementless stem in the same patients younger than 50 years of age. J Arthroplasty 2016;31(3):662–7.

78. Morshed S, Bozic KJ, Ries MD, et al. Comparison of cemented and uncemented fixation in total hip replacement: a meta-analysis. Acta Orthop 2007; 78(3):315–26.

79. Clement ND, Biant LC, Breusch SJ. Total hip arthroplasty: to cement or not to cement the acetabular socket? A critical review of the literature. Arch Orthop Trauma Surg 2012;132(3):411–27.

80. Chen PC, Mead EH, Pinto JG, et al. Polyethylene wear debris in modular acetabular prostheses. Clin Orthop Relat Res 1995;(317):44–56.

81. Fehring TK, Smith SE, Braun ER, et al. Motion at the modular acetabular shell and liner interface. A comparative study. Clin Orthop Relat Res 1999;(367):306–14.

82. Huk OL, Bansal M, Betts F, et al. Polyethylene and metal debris generated by non-articulating surfaces of modular acetabular components. J Bone Joint Surg Br 1994;76(4):568–74.

83. McCombe P, Williams SA. A comparison of polyethylene wear rates between cemented and cementless cups. A prospective, randomised trial. J Bone Joint Surg Br 2004;86(3):344–9.

84. Baad-Hansen T, Kold S, Nielsen PT, et al. Comparison of trabecular metal cups and titanium fiber-mesh cups in primary hip arthroplasty: a randomized RSA and bone mineral densitometry study of 50 hips. Acta Orthop 2011;82(2):155–60.

85. Young AM, Sychterz CJ, Hopper RH Jr, et al. Effect of acetabular modularity on polyethylene wear and osteolysis in total hip arthroplasty. J Bone Joint Surg Am 2002;84-A(1):58–63.

86. Gonzalez Della Valle A, Su E, Zoppi A, et al. Wear and periprosthetic osteolysis in a match-paired study of modular and nonmodular uncemented acetabular cups. J Arthroplasty 2004;19(8):972–7.

87. Halma JJ, Vogely HC, Dhert WJ, et al. Do monoblock cups improve survivorship, decrease wear, or reduce osteolysis in uncemented total hip arthroplasty? Clin Orthop Relat Res 2013;471(11):3572–80.

88. Burroughs BR, Hallstrom B, Golladay GJ, et al. Range of motion and stability in total hip arthroplasty with 28-, 32-, 38-, and 44-mm femoral head sizes. J Arthroplasty 2005;20(1):11–9.

89. Howie DW, Holubowycz OT, Callary SA. The wear rate of highly cross-linked polyethylene in total hip replacement is not increased by large articulations: a randomized controlled trial. J Bone Joint Surg Am 2016;98(21):1786–93.

90. Hammerberg EM, Wan Z, Dastane M, et al. Wear and range of motion of different femoral head sizes. J Arthroplasty 2010;25(6):839–43.

91. Lachiewicz PF, Soileau ES, Martell JM. Wear and osteolysis of highly crosslinked polyethylene at 10 to 14 years: the effect of femoral head size. Clin Orthop Relat Res 2016;474(2):365–71.

92. Lanting B, Naudie DD, McCalden RW. Clinical impact of trunnion wear after total hip arthroplasty. JBJS Rev 2016;4(8) [pii:01874474-201608000-00003].

93. Jacobs JJ, Cooper HJ, Urban RM, et al. What do we know about taper corrosion in total hip arthroplasty? J Arthroplasty 2014;29(4):668–9.

94. Whitehouse MR, Endo M, Zachara S, et al. Adverse local tissue reactions in metal-on-polyethylene total hip arthroplasty due to trunnion corrosion: the risk of misdiagnosis. Bone Joint J 2015;97-b(8):1024–30.

95. Nassif NA, Nawabi DH, Stoner K, et al. Taper design affects failure of large-head metal-on-metal total hip replacements. Clin Orthop Relat Res 2014;472(2):564–71.

96. Gilbert JL, Buckley CA, Jacobs JJ. In vivo corrosion of modular hip prosthesis components in mixed and similar metal combinations. The effect of crevice, stress, motion, and alloy coupling. J Biomed Mater Res 1993;27(12):1533–44.

97. Tan SC, Teeter MG, Del Balso C, et al. Effect of taper design on trunnionosis in metal on polyethylene total hip arthroplasty. J Arthroplasty 2015;30(7):1269–72.

98. Del Balso C, Teeter MG, Tan SC, et al. Trunnionosis: does head size affect fretting and corrosion in total hip arthroplasty? J Arthroplasty 2016;31(10):2332–6.

99. Del Balso C, Teeter MG, Tan SC, et al. Taperosis: does head length affect fretting and corrosion in total hip arthroplasty? Bone Joint J 2015;97-b(7):911–6.

100. Lavernia CJ. Cost-effectiveness of early surgical intervention in silent osteolysis. J Arthroplasty 1998;13(3):277–9.

101. Dattani R. Femoral osteolysis following total hip replacement. Postgrad Med J 2007;83(979):312–6.

102. Brown JM, Mistry JB, Cherian JJ, et al. Femoral component revision of total hip arthroplasty. Orthopedics 2016;39(6):e1129–39.

103. Chang CY, Huang AJ, Palmer WE. Radiographic evaluation of hip implants. Semin Musculoskelet Radiol 2015;19(1):12–20.

104. Fritz J, Lurie B, Miller TT. Imaging of hip arthroplasty. Semin Musculoskelet Radiol 2013;17(3):316–27.

105. D'Antonio JA. Periprosthetic bone loss of the acetabulum. Classification and management. Orthop Clin North Am 1992;23(2):279–90.

106. Engelbrecht DJ, Weber FA, Sweet MB, et al. Long-term results of revision total hip arthroplasty. J Bone Joint Surg Br 1990;72(1):41–5.

107. Garbuz D, Morsi E, Mohamed N, et al. Classification and reconstruction in revision acetabular arthroplasty with bone stock deficiency. Clin Orthop Relat Res 1996;(324):98–107.

108. Paprosky WG, Perona PG, Lawrence JM. Acetabular defect classification and surgical

reconstruction in revision arthroplasty. A 6-year follow-up evaluation. J Arthroplasty 1994;9(1): 33–44.

109. Rubash HE, Sinha RK, Paprosky W, et al. A new classification system for the management of acetabular osteolysis after total hip arthroplasty. Instr Course Lect 1999;48:37–42.

110. Paprosky W, Sporer S, O'Rourke MR. The treatment of pelvic discontinuity with acetabular cages. Clin Orthop Relat Res 2006;453:183–7.

111. Berry DJ. Management of osteolysis around total hip arthroplasty. Orthopedics 1999;22(9): 805–8.

112. Chiang PP, Burke DW, Freiberg AA, et al. Osteolysis of the pelvis: evaluation and treatment. Clin Orthop Relat Res 2003;(417):164–74.

113. Claus AM, Walde TA, Leung SB, et al. Management of patients with acetabular socket wear and pelvic osteolysis. J Arthroplasty 2003;18(3 Suppl 1):112–7.

114. Hozack WJ, Bicalho PS, Eng K. Treatment of femoral osteolysis with cementless total hip revision. J Arthroplasty 1996;11(6):668–72.

115. Selvik G. Roentgen stereophotogrammetry. A method for the study of the kinematics of the skeletal system. Acta Orthop Scand Suppl 1989;232: 1–51.

116. Naudie DD, Engh CA Sr. Surgical management of polyethylene wear and pelvic osteolysis with modular uncemented acetabular components. J Arthroplasty 2004;19(4 Suppl 1):124–9.

117. Southwell DG, Bechtold JE, Lew WD, et al. Improving the detection of acetabular osteolysis using oblique radiographs. J Bone Joint Surg Br 1999;81(2):289–95.

118. Zimlich RH, Fehring TK. Underestimation of pelvic osteolysis: the value of the iliac oblique radiograph. J Arthroplasty 2000;15(6):796–801.

119. Walde TA, Weiland DE, Leung SB, et al. Comparison of CT, MRI, and radiographs in assessing pelvic osteolysis: a cadaveric study. Clin Orthop Relat Res 2005;(437):138–44.

120. Claus AM, Engh CA Jr, Sychterz CJ, et al. Radiographic definition of pelvic osteolysis following total hip arthroplasty. J Bone Joint Surg Am 2003; 85-A(8):1519–26.

121. Walde TA, Mohan V, Leung S, et al. Sensitivity and specificity of plain radiographs for detection of medial-wall perforation secondary to osteolysis. J Arthroplasty 2005;20(1):20–4.

122. Howie DW, Neale SD, Martin W, et al. Progression of periacetabular osteolytic lesions. J Bone Joint Surg Am 2012;94(16):e1171–6.

123. Puri L, Wixson RL, Stern SH, et al. Use of helical computed tomography for the assessment of acetabular osteolysis after total hip arthroplasty. J Bone Joint Surg Am 2002;84-A(4):609–14.

124. Stauffer RN. Ten-year follow-up study of total hip replacement. J Bone Joint Surg Am 1982;64(7): 983–90.

125. Brown GC, Lockshin MD, Salvati EA, et al. Sensitivity to metal as a possible cause of sterile loosening after cobalt-chromium total hip-replacement arthroplasty. J Bone Joint Surg Am 1977;59(2):164–8.

126. Maloney WJ. The surgical management of femoral osteolysis. J Arthroplasty 2005;20(4 Suppl 2):75–8.

127. Paprosky WG, Aribindi R. Hip replacement: treatment of femoral bone loss using distal bypass fixation. Instr Course Lect 2000;49:119–30.

128. Weeden SH, Paprosky WG. Minimal 11-year follow-up of extensively porous-coated stems in femoral revision total hip arthroplasty. J Arthroplasty 2002;17(4 Suppl 1):134–7.

129. Sinha RK, Shanbhag AS, Maloney WJ, et al. Osteolysis: cause and effect. Instr Course Lect 1998;47:307–20.

130. Kavanagh BF, Callaghan JJ, Leggon R, et al. Pelvic osteolysis associated with an uncemented acetabular component in total hip arthroplasty. Orthopedics 1996;19(2):159–63.

131. Harris WH. Wear and periprosthetic osteolysis: the problem. Clin Orthop Relat Res 2001;(393): 66–70.

132. Zicat B, Engh CA, Gokcen E. Patterns of osteolysis around total hip components inserted with and without cement. J Bone Joint Surg Am 1995; 77(3):432–9.

133. Schmalzried TP, Fowble VA, Amstutz HC. The fate of pelvic osteolysis after reoperation. No recurrence with lesional treatment. Clin Orthop Relat Res 1998;(350):128–37.

134. Mallory TH, Lombardi AV Jr, Fada RA, et al. Noncemented acetabular component removal in the presence of osteolysis: the affirmative. Clin Orthop Relat Res 2000;(381):120–8.

135. Maloney WJ, Paprosky W, Engh CA, et al. Surgical treatment of pelvic osteolysis. Clin Orthop Relat Res 2001;(393):78–84.

136. Maloney WJ, Peters P, Engh CA, et al. Severe osteolysis of the pelvic in association with acetabular replacement without cement. J Bone Joint Surg Am 1993;75(11):1627–35.

137. Rubash HE, Sinha RK, Maloney WJ, et al. Osteolysis: surgical treatment. Instr Course Lect 1998; 47:321–9.

138. Blaha JD. Well-fixed acetabular component retention or replacement: the whys and the wherefores. J Arthroplasty 2002;17(4 Suppl 1): 157–61.

139. Schwarz EM, Ritchlin CT. Clinical development of anti-RANKL therapy. Arthritis Res Ther 2007; 9(Suppl 1):S7.

140. Abu-Amer Y, Darwech I, Clohisy JC. Aseptic loosening of total joint replacements: mechanisms underlying osteolysis and potential therapies. Arthritis Res Ther 2007;9(Suppl 1):S6.

141. Schwarz EM, Implant Wear Symposium Biologic Work Group. What potential biologic treatments are available for osteolysis? J Am Acad Orthop Surg 2008;16(Suppl 1):S72–5.

142. St Pierre CA, Chan M, Iwakura Y, et al. Periprosthetic osteolysis: characterizing the innate immune response to titanium wear-particles. J Orthop Res 2010;28(11):1418–24.

143. Geng DC, Xu YZ, Yang HL, et al. Inhibition of titanium particle-induced inflammatory osteolysis through inactivation of cannabinoid receptor 2 by AM630. J Biomed Mater Res A 2010;95(1): 321–6.

144. Nichols CI, Vose JG. Clinical outcomes and costs within 90 days of primary or revision total joint arthroplasty. J Arthroplasty 2016;31(7): 1400–6.e3.

145. Shon WY, Gupta S, Biswal S, et al. Pelvic osteolysis relationship to radiographs and polyethylene wear. J Arthroplasty 2009;24(5): 743–50.

146. Heindel W, Gubitz R, Vieth V, et al. The diagnostic imaging of bone metastases. Dtsch Arztebl Int 2014;111(44):741–7.

Trauma

The Role of Value-Based Implants in Orthopedic Trauma

Kyle E. Lybrand, MD, Peter L. Althausen, MD, MBA*

KEYWORDS

• Value-based implants • Generic implants • Health care finance • Health care economics

---

KEY POINTS

- In this era of rapidly rising health care costs, it is the physician's moral and ethical responsibility to pursue value-based care options in orthopedics.
- Value-based and generic pharmaceutical options are widely accepted alternatives that have saved the health care system massive amounts of money with similar outcomes.
- Trauma patients are an underinsured patient population, and value-based care models involving care plans and decreased implant costs are needed to allow for the provision of quality care.
- Current research and US Food and Drug Administration regulations demonstrate that value-based implants are clinically equivalent to conventional implants; the only difference is cost.
- Gain sharing, comanagement, and bundled payment initiatives provide surgeons with incentive toward value-based care.

INTRODUCTION

Health care costs in the United States continue to increase, now accounting for more than $3.3 trillion, consuming 17.9% of the gross domestic product.[1] National health care spending is projected to grow at an average rate of 5.6% per year for 2016 to 2025, growing 1.2% points faster than the gross domestic product, resulting in continued escalation toward an unsustainable dollar amount.[2] Means of cost containment are being increasingly introduced on multiple levels by all parties. These include diagnosis-related group-based reimbursement to hospitals, bundling of payments for certain episodes of care, hospital use of matrix implant pricing, and reduced reimbursement for physicians.

Physicians, including orthopedic surgeons, have historically been poor stewards of cost containment and resource management. Several studies demonstrate that orthopedic surgeons often inaccurately estimate the cost of their implants and tend to underestimate the cost rather than overestimate.[3–5] New technology is commonly adopted by surgeons without the need and without strong evidence supporting improved outcomes. Historically, physician participation in hospital implant selection, screening, and pricing was uncommon. This allowed implant costs to increase unnecessarily exponentially. Failure to adhere to accepted preoperative screening guidelines and the practice of defensive medicine in orthopedic trauma are further examples of poor cost control by the medical community.[6–8] As costs continue to increase, so has transparency of pricing and cost increases, resulting in mounting pressure for physicians to be better stewards of the health care dollar.[9]

DISCUSSION

The total US orthopedic trauma implant market is estimated to be valued over $5.3 billion.[10] Implant costs are still the highest expense in

---

Disclosure: None.

Reno Orthopaedic Clinic, 555. North Arlington Avenue, Reno, NV 89503, USA

* Corresponding author.

E-mail address: Peteralthausen@outlook.com

Orthop Clin N Am 49 (2018) 437–443
https://doi.org/10.1016/j.ocl.2018.05.005

the operating room budget. Curtailing implant costs remains one the most straightforward ways to decrease costs in orthopedic trauma surgery. Much as generic alternatives to prescription medications become available as patents on existing brand medications expire, several orthopedic implant companies have emerged to distribute value-based orthopedic implants.

Value-Based Implant Background

In response to the rising economic pressure on the delivery of orthopedic care, several companies have entered the orthopedic implant market deploying various models that lower the cost of implant usage. These include decreasing the cost of implants themselves, eliminating sales representatives who utilize 42% of conventional implant company revenue, and utilizing single-use kits. These kits include all instrumentation, disposables, and implants required for a single small fragment fracture case. In this model, these vendors claim savings by eliminating the need for decontamination and sterilization of instrument and implant trays. The combination of eliminating sales representatives and utilizing value-based implants has the greatest potential to decrease costs.

Because of the massive financial impact value-based implants could have on the market, significant efforts are being undertaken by conventional companies to create an illusion of inferiority. Such techniques were attempted in the pharmaceutical industry and failed due to the US Food And Drug Administration (FDA) approval system. Like pharmaceuticals, the approval process to make and sell implants in the United States, outlined in section 510(k) of the Federal Food, Drug and Cosmetic Act, is the same for all. Vendors are required to submit criteria proving the likeness of its market-ready implant to preceding implants offered in the market by any vendor. Biomechanical testing data and implant design files are submitted for review by the FDA, and all vendors are held to the same standards by which the submitted data are measured. The FDA then provides the vendor with a letter stating that its findings indicate the device is substantially equivalent to the preceding device. The nature of the 510(k)-approval process highlights the fact that all implants brought to market in this fashion are generic, regardless of vendor.

It is also important to note the use of contract manufacturing in orthopedic implants. The entire US implant industry relies heavily on this process, which is an outsourced means of production that lowers manufacturing costs and quickens production. In the United States, contract manufacturing companies produce both brand name and value-based implants on the same machines, from the same medical-grade materials, and put them through the same quality assurance checks. Thus, both value-based and conventional implants are manufactured and produced in the same factories in the same way by the same people. Value-based implant companies now produce a variety of orthopedic trauma implants including cannulated screw systems, intramedullary nails, and locking plate systems.

Scientific Support

Hundreds of articles demonstrating the clinical equivalence of generic medications can be found in the literature; however, there is a paucity of literature comparing value-based implants with conventional implants. Waddell and colleagues[11] published a clinical trial involving 150 patients looking at generic total hip implants in Canada. Patients were followed for at least 2 years. These authors found no increased complication rates and general improvement in Harris hip scores with the use of generic implants. Another paper by Althausen and colleagues[12] evaluated the clinical and economic benefits of generic 7.3 mm cannulated screw use for the treatment of femoral neck fractures and percutaneous sacroiliac fixation. These authors demonstrated a 70% reduction in implant costs with no difference in the clinical outcomes of infection, nonunion, need for revision surgery, or mortality.

A third study by McPhillamy and colleagues evaluated generic locking plate utilization in a similar study. Operatively treated fractures evaluated included clavicle, proximal humerus, distal radius, proximal tibia, distal tibia pilon, and ankle fractures. These authors found a 56% reduction in implant costs with no differences in clinical outcomes of malunion, nonunion, implant failure, infection, and symptomatic implants requiring removal. The use of generic implants in this study resulted in an average cost savings of $1197 per case and a total amount saved of $458,080 over the study period.[13] Newer generic implant designs, such as intramedullary nails and external fixation, continue to be released and have the potential for significant cost savings as well; however, these implants have not been used long enough to study effectively at the current time.

Barriers to Value-Based Implant Utilization

Despite the economic pressures placed on care of the orthopedic trauma patient, biomechanical equivalence of value-based implants and published literature demonstrating no change in clinical outcomes, the adoption of value-based implants is slow. Multiple barriers to value-based implant use exist. These include

- Lack of surgeon confidence and reluctance to adopt nonconventional implants
- Conflicts of interest with industry
- Altered level of service provided by implant representatives
- Patient perceptions

In 2016, Walker and Althausen evaluated surgeon attitudes regarding the use of generic implants. These authors surveyed 52 orthopedic surgeons with active membership in the Orthopedic Trauma Association (OTA) for surgeon demographics, practice demographics, relationship of surgeons to industry, participation in other financial incentive programs, surgeon use of generic implants, surgeon perception of current health care spending, and the role of surgeons in cost containment.[14] Most surgeons were 35 to 54 years of age, had a well-distributed time in practice, had a varied practice setting, with 50% of participants in some form of academic practice and 25% in private practice. Most were employed in private practice or had an incentive program in addition to base salary. Surgeons had varied financial relationships with industry, their hospital, and their practices' financial endeavors. There was a relatively low level of involvement in comanagement and gain-sharing agreements; however, approximately 35% of surgeons had some form of employment tie to industry in the form of consultant or design surgeon. About 20% of surgeons indicated they owned stock in an orthopedic implant company, with 60% of those owning stock in a generic implant company.[14]

Interestingly, most surgeons in this study (77%) responded that sales representatives were present for most of their cases despite the fact that only 21% of these surgeons responded that they needed the representatives present for most of their cases. Few surgeons worked in a setting with representative-less implants and implant pricing. Most commonly cited reasons for needing an implant representative present include the need to assist the scrub technician with instrumentation and help with inventory. If surgeon reimbursement changed on the presence or absence of a representative, about half indicated that their opinion would change if it affected their reimbursement.[14]

Another interesting finding from the study by Walker and Althausen[14] was the use of generic medications and generic implants among surgeons. Approximately 73% of respondents had an awareness of generic implant availability and FDA approval status; however, only 25% used them in their practice. This is in stark contrast to the 96% of participating surgeons indicating that they routinely prescribe generic medications for their patients, and 87% indicating they and their family routinely use generic medications and medical supplies. Most surgeons cite they prescribe or use generic medications because they are less expensive. Most commonly cited reasons for why respondents had not tried generic implants were as follows: satisfaction with current implants (47%), lack of financial incentive to change (34%), and concern regarding the track record of generic implants (32%).

The findings of this study reinforce the idea that orthopedic surgeons are open to the use of generic products. The discrepancy between awareness and utilization of generic implants is certainly attributed to several different factors, one of which may be the relatively short history of generic orthopedic implants and concerns regarding lack of track record of such implants. However, surgeons routinely adopt new brand name implants long before any clinical data exist demonstrating their effectiveness or superiority in treating fractures. Data do exist demonstrating the clinical equivalency of generic implants,[11–13] but only 49% of surgeons indicated awareness of these publications.[14] Several studies have indicated that knowing the price of a given implant may affect surgeon choice of implant used.

One recent study by Okike and colleagues[15] evaluated the effectiveness of an implant selection tool (red-yellow-green) that guided surgeons toward more cost-effective implants, while minimally restricting surgeon choice. This institution selected 7 implant constructs that were commonly used: femoral intramedullary nail, tibial intramedullary nail, short cephalomedullary nail, long cephalomedullary nail, distal femoral plate, proximal tibial plate, and lower-extremity external fixator. Costs were determined for each implant type from each of 4 vendors. Based on costs, the implant supplied by each vendor was categorized as green (preferred vendor), yellow (midrange), or red (used for patient-specific requirements). This resulted in a red-yellow-green guidance tool that was posted in operating rooms frequented by orthopedic trauma surgeons to guide physician utilization in situations where more than one available system was determined clinically appropriate.

This study assessed preferred implant usage rates, vendor attitudes toward pricing structure, and hospital implant expenditures in a retrospective preintervention and postintervention design over a 12-month period. Overall, implant usage patterns changed significantly between preintervention and postintervention periods from 30% red, 56% yellow, and 14% green prior to intervention to 9% red, 21% yellow, and 70% green following the intervention (P<.0001). Specific vendor utilization went from 25% for vendor 1, 45% for vendor 2, and 30% for vendor 3 prior to the intervention to 20% for vendor 1, 60% for vendor 2, and 20% for vendor 3 after the intervention. Because of the intervention, implant prices were able to be renegotiated, with average price decreases ranging from 1.1% to 22.4%. Average implant expenditures decreased by 20%, representing a savings of $216,495 per year.[15]

Another study assessed the effect of price on surgeons' choice of implants for upper extremity fractures in a randomized controlled survey. A survey was distributed to orthopedic surgeons that consisted of 8 clinical cases of upper extremity fractures with a history and radiographs followed by surgical implant options. Surgeons selected an implant and ranked up to 3 factors affecting implant choice for each case including

What my mentor taught me
Recommended by colleagues
Shorter operating time
Less invasive
Most reliable fracture healing
Fewer complications or need for second surgery
Cost-effective/financially resourceful
Familiarity with implant
Higher reimbursement

Two versions of the survey were created: one with implant prices (price-aware group) and one without implant prices (price-naïve group).[16]

A total of 223 orthopedic surgeons completed the survey, including residents, fellows, and attending physicians from 6 continents. For the 6 cases that offered different classes of implants, implants selected were not significantly different between groups. However, for the 2 cases comparing models within the same implant class, implant choice significantly differed between the price-aware and the price-naïve survey groups. When offered 3 different models of distal radius locking plates, 25% of the price-naïve surgeons selected the most expensive plate compared with 7% of price-aware surgeons (P<.05). Similarly, the most expensive distal humerus plate

was selected by 25% of the price-naïve surgeons compared with 13% of the price-aware surgeons (P<.05). Across all cases, price-aware respondents were 1.4 times more likely than price-naïve respondents to rank cost as a factor (29% vs 21%, P<.05). The most common factors cited that drove implant choice included familiarity with the implant, evidence-based guidelines or literature, and reliable fracture healing. When choosing among same-class implants, cost was cited as an important factor (11%) in implant selection.[16]

These studies identify 1 potential factor that affects implant choices among surgeons. Previous work has shown that surgeons generally underestimate the cost of orthopedic implants, have poor awareness of implant costs, and underestimate the difference between high- and low-cost implants.[3,4] However, when knowledgeable of implant pricing, irrespective of company brand, surgeons may be more likely to choose a lower-cost implant when more than 1 option is available and deemed clinically appropriate. Awareness of implant cost is certainly not the only barrier facing the utilization of value-based implants.

Many surgeons have significant conflicts of interest with industry, as many are paid consultants or have royalty agreements with implant companies. This can make it difficult to incite change in many health care environments. Industry conflicts of interest and implant representatives in the operating room are closely intertwined. Perhaps at institutions where surgeons do not have consulting or royalty agreements with any of the major branded implant companies there may be an easier adoption of value-based implants. Conflicts of interest certainly arise when such relationships exist. This has been a major factor in recent US Department of Justice investigations of total hip and knee arthroplasty implant use. Many institutions receive significant research funding from industry, and there is considerable fear of loss of research funding. Money saved from utilization of value-based implants could be reappropriated toward research and service line reinvestment. This could potentially free institutions of manufacturer bias or single vendor support.

Another concern regarding implementation of value-based implants is the worry that existing conventional vendors and sales representatives would alter the level of service they provide or increase the prices on unique implants and instrumentation. Most surgeons cite the presence of an implant representative in the room; however, many admit they are not required for most cases.[14] The presence of an orthopedic implant representative for the most cases certainly leads to an unnecessary increase in implant costs. At the authors' institution, the use of value-based implant alternatives has resulted in better service from conventional companies that wish to preserve their market share. This finding was also seen in the red-yellow-green initiative described by Okike and colleagues[15] Value-based implant usage has the potential for dramatic implant savings and can provide the hospital with the ability to negotiate prices more effectively on conventional items such as intramedullary nails and plate constructs. Matrix pricing is another means to incur significant implant savings. This is a situation by which a hospital or health care system allows all companies to sell their implants, but they must meet a fixed price for each construct type.

Patient perceptions are another theoretic barrier to value-based implant used. An article by Sewell and colleagues[17] described this barrier regarding generic medication usage. Using generic medications in the underinsured population with similar efficacy to brand name medications clearly has its advantages. However, 4 focus groups with 30 community members (one-fourth uninsured, more than half with a high school education or less) revealed many misconceptions about generic medications. Common themes included perceptions that generics are not real medicine, that generics are only for minor illnesses, and that the medical system cannot be trusted. These authors concluded that although education about generics could help overcome misinformation, "overcoming mistrust of the medical system and the sense of having to settle for generics because of poverty may be more challenging." Although these perceptions exist, the World Health Organization states that strategies to promote generic substitution should be included in national medicine policies.[18]

Value-Based Savings

Despite these significant barriers to implementation of value-based implants, the need to do so and create change is paramount in the current US health care climate. Health care expenditures continue to increase to an unsustainable level, and means of cost containment are seriously being introduced and initiated by all parties on multiple levels. The orthopedic trauma implant market was estimated to be valued over $5.3 billion in 2016,[10] making the potential economic impact of value-based implant use as a cost-containment strategy among the hospital,

surgeon, patients, and payers significant. Previous studies have found a 40% to 60% reduction in implant costs[12,13] when value-based implants are utilized. If these cost savings were applied to the $5.5 billion trauma implant market, savings of over $3 billion would be realized. With these savings, and especially if these savings can be applied to other implants, such as intramedullary nails and external fixation, orthopedic surgeons could have a massive effect on cost containment in the health care crisis. Especially given the fact that many trauma patients are uninsured or underinsured, the authors believe orthopedic surgeons have a moral obligation to be cost conscious.

Gain Sharing and Comanagement Agreements

The most significant barrier to the implementation of value-based implant utilization is the surgeon. One might think that trauma surgeons would feel morally obligated to transition toward value-based care models. However, the previously mentioned studies show that ethics is not enough to convince physicians to change their practice patterns. Surgeons must be incentivized to change through economics.

Gain sharing and comanagement programs are both successful means of achieving physician buy-in for all cost containment programs in orthopedic surgery. Under comanagement agreements, physicians are reimbursed for their time and intellectual efforts in program and algorithm creation. The cost is minimal for the hospital in return for the millions of dollars in savings they achieve. Gain sharing models can incentivize physicians to quickly adopt cost-effective implant choices, care plans, and program development. Hospital systems keep most of the profits; patients and insurance carriers benefit from the cost savings, and physicians receive remuneration for their efforts. Careful attention must be paid to the legal issues surrounding the federal antikickback statute, the civil monetary penalty law, and the physician self-referral law when setting up these agreements. The keys to success for these programs are the presence of a physician champion, economic transparency for physicians and hospitals, accurate data collection, and adequate economic incentive for physicians to drive change in practice patterns.[19]

The bundled payments for care improvement (BPCI) initiative is the latest cost-saving program developed by the US Center for Medicare and Medicaid Innovation. It is essentially a government-approved form of gains haring. This model is intended to create a system for higher quality and more coordinated care at a lower cost to Medicare. It is currently an optional program for physician groups, hospitals, and postacute care providers to benefit financially from improved care models and cost containment measures. Under the initiative, organizations enter into payment arrangements that include financial and performance accountability for episodes of care. There are certain fraud and abuse waivers in place that allow gain sharing among BPCI organizations and approved providers so long as certain requirements are met.[20]

The authors' practice entered this initiative for total joint arthroplasty and hip and femur fracture episodes of care. The first-year experience demonstrated that a significant learning curve is required. Keys for success include appropriate patient selection for elective surgery, implant pricing control, adherence to preoperative and postoperative protocols, diligent postacute care management, and appropriate choice of metrics to maximize gain sharing potential. Ultimately, the BPCI program has been a successful venture, saving hospitals over $1.6 million in 2015. In the process, this provided an additional revenue stream for physicians while decreasing the overall cost of care.[20]

Despite the clear success of existing gain sharing and comanagement agreements, they are not as prevalent as one might think. The 2016 survey of Walker and Althausen found a relatively basic level of financial involvement and low level of financial incentives among participating surgeons. Few surgeons were involved in gainsharing or comanagement agreements with their hospitals, and several indicated they were unfamiliar that such agreements existed. Few surgeons indicated knowledge of the BPCI initiative.[14] Hospitals wishing to alter surgeon behavior or surgeons wishing to be compensated for active efforts in cost containment may want to consider the introduction of these financial incentives. One barrier to universal adoption of such agreements is that they take time to create. Surgeons and hospital administrators must have a basic business relationship. Hospitals must understand that they need to incentivize physicians, and physicians must be open to change and enter active hospital negotiations.

The Future

The rise of physician-owned surgery centers will clearly drive the value-based implant market in orthopedic trauma. In the past, most fracture patients were treated in the hospital setting. Many health care consultants now estimate that 80% of fracture care will be performed in outpatient centers by 2020. With better anesthetic techniques and nerve blocks, outpatient fracture and arthroplasty cases are regularly performed at surgeon-owned facilities across the United States. Unlike hospital-employed physicians, surgeons who own their own centers are highly incentivized to provide high quality care while controlling costs. This is the definition of the term value-based. As more data emerge of the clinical equivalence of value-based implants, conventional implant prices will be forced to drop as well. This will lower the cost of orthopedic trauma care in the United States and save millions for the health care system.

Health Insurance companies are also realizing the extremely high costs of orthopedic implants. Over the past 10 years, most insurance panels have already agreed to cover only generic medication alternatives as they have become available. The same path is sure to follow with orthopedic implants. Many orthopedic surgeons already receive a scorecard of cost and outcomes from their insurers. Soon it is likely that physician reimbursement rates will be linked to the cost-effectiveness of their implant choices. This will have a profound impact on the surgeons' perception of conventional implants and his or her need for sales representation.

SUMMARY

Health care costs in the United States continue to rise, and the economic pressures influencing the care of the orthopedic trauma patient have never been greater. Value-based health care is vital to the survival of the current health care system, and the use of value-based implants is a central component to success. Value-based implant usage has similar clinical outcomes to conventional implant utilization; however, multiple barriers to adoption exist. Despite biomechanical equivalence and significant cost savings, surgeons have difficultly changing implant use without financial incentive, fearing loss of consulting fees, companionship, or research support. The rise of physician-owned surgery centers, gain sharing, and comanagement agreements will likely drive this much needed change.

REFERENCES

1. Center for Medicare & Medicaid Services. National health expenditures 2016 highlights. 2016. Available at: https://www.cms.gov/research-statistics-data- and-systems/statistics-trends-and-reports/

nationalhealthexpenddata/downloads/highlights. pdf. Accessed January 8, 2018.

2. Center for Medicare & Medicaid Services. National Health Expenditure Projections 2016-2025. Available at: https://www.cms.gov/research-statistics-data- and-systems/statistics-trends-and-reports/nationalhealthexpenddata/downloads/highlights. pdf. Accessed January 8, 2018.

3. Okike K, O'Toole RV, Pollak AN, et al. Survey finds few orthopedic surgeons know the costs of the devices they implant. Health Aff (Millwood) 2014;33: 103–9.

4. Streit JJ, Youssef A, Coale RM, et al. Orthopaedic surgeons frequently underestimate the cost of orthopaedic implants. Clin Orthop Relat Res 2013; 471:744–9.

5. Luttrell K, Nana A. Effect of preoperative transthoracic echocardiogram on mortality and surgical timing in elderly adults with hip fracture. J Am Geriatr Soc 2015;63:2505–9.

6. Marcantonio A, Steen B, Kain M, et al. The clinical and economic impact of preoperative transthoracic echocardiography in elderly patients with hip fractures. Bull Hosp Jt Dis 2015;73:239–42.

7. Smeets SJ, Poeze M, Verbruggen JP. Preoperative cardiac evaluation of geriatric patients with hip fracture. Injury 2012;43:2146–51.

8. Stitgen A, Poludnianyk K, Dulaney-Cripe E, et al. Adherence to preoperative cardiac clearance guidelines in hip fracture patients. J Orthop Trauma 2015;29:500–3.

9. Okike K, Bozic KJ. Orthopaedic healthcare worldwide: the transparent pricing revolution in healthcare. Clin Orthop Relat Res 2014;472:2325–8.

10. U.S. Market for orthopedic trauma devices. Vancouver, BC, Canada: Data Research Inc. 2010. Available at: www.idataresearch.net. Accessed January 14, 2018.

11. Waddell JP, Morton J. Generic total hip arthroplasty. Clin Orthop Relat Res 1995;311:109–16.

12. Althausen PL, Shields T, Anderson SR. Clinical and economic impact of using generic 7.3-mm cannulated screws at a level II trauma center. Am J Orthop 2014;43(9):405–10.

13. Mcphillamy A, Gurnea TP, Moody AE, et al. The clinical and economic impact of generic locking plate utilization at a level II trauma center. J Orthop Trauma 2016;30:S32–6.

14. Walker JA, Althause PL. Surgeon attitudes regarding the use of generic implants: an OTA survey study. J Orthop Trauma 2016;30:S27–31.

15. Okike K, Pollak R, O'Toole RV, et al. "Red-Yellow-Green": effect of an initiative to guide surgeon choice of orthopaedic implants. J Bone Joint Surg Am 2017;99:e33 (1-6).

16. Wasterlain AS, Melamed E, Bello R, et al. The effect of price on surgeons' choice of implants: a randomized controlled survey. J Hand Surg Am 2017;42: 593–601.

17. Sewell K, Andreae S, Luke E, et al. Perceptions of and barriers to use of generic medications in a rural African American population, Alabama, 2011. Prev Chronic Dis 2012;9:E142.

18. Cameron A, Mantel-Teeuwisse AK, Leufkens HG, et al. Switching from originator brand medicines to generic equivalents in selected developing countries: how much could be saved? Value Health 2012;15(5):664–73.

19. McBride C, Althausen PL. Co-management and gainsharing opportunities for independent physicians. J Orthop Trauma 2016;30(Suppl 5): S45–9, 20.

20. Althausen PL, Mead L. Bundled payments for care improvement(BPCI): lessons learned in the first year. J Orthop Trauma 2016;30(Suppl 5):S50–3.

The Role of Business Education in the Orthopedic Curriculum

Peter L. Althausen, MD, MBA*, Kyle E. Lybrand, MD

KEYWORDS

- Business education • Health care finance • Health care economics • Orthopedic curriculum

---

KEY POINTS

- Business knowledge and education are important for success in orthopedics today.
- Practice management skills are vital for the creation of successful governance, contracting, financial management, and ancillary service development.
- Surgeons must be familiar with basic health care economic principles and the laws that surround them.
- Given the current status of the US health care system, value-based health care is the physician's moral and ethical responsibility.
- Understanding comanagement and gain sharing agreements is critical for hospital and physician negotiations.

INTRODUCTION

The field of orthopedics is becoming increasingly complex as the demands for success are not merely clinical competence and good interpersonal skills. Strategic planning, contract negotiation, health care law, practice management, health care economics, and personal finance are all needed skills to achieve stability. Unfortunately, most of these areas of professional growth require some basic background in business principles, 1 area that most recent residency graduates feel is neglected as a core educational competency. In these changing times, it is imperative that orthopedic residents and fellows obtain some formal business education.

Over the past decade, many graduates have taken hospital employed positions in part due to lack of business acumen and fear of running and maintaining a practice. The economic pressures on the health care system demonstrate that all orthopedic surgeons now find the need for business training. New government programs for bundled payments, opportunities for gain sharing and comanagement, and the trend toward value-based health care all require understanding and attention from physicians. If orthopedic training programs and current practicing surgeons do not accept the responsibility of teaching and learning the business aspects of medicine, physicians will gradually lose control of medicine and place the fate of surgeons and patients in the hands of government and hospital administrators.

With this goal in mind, The Reno Orthopedic Clinic Trauma Fellowship was conceived in 2007, accepting the first fellow for the 2010 to 2011 educational year. As a core dimension of this fellowship program, the authors designed a basic business curriculum in conjunction with business administrators employed within their hospital systems and the Reno Orthopedic Clinic (ROC) administrative team. Twenty basic orthopedic trauma business topics were identified, faculty and objectives assigned, syllabus and

---

Disclosure: None.
Reno Orthopaedic Clinic, 555 North Arlington Avenue, Reno, NV 89503, USA
* Corresponding author.
E-mail address: Peteralthausen@outlook.com

Orthop Clin N Am 49 (2018) 445–453
https://doi.org/10.1016/j.ocl.2018.05.006
0030-5898/18/© 2018 Elsevier Inc. All rights reserved.

reading materials suggested, and a faculty time-table created. The business curriculum is considered a critical element of the Reno Trauma Fellowship experience, occupying approximately 20% of the fellow's time. This syllabus has been published so that it can be used as a model for any orthopedic residency or training program.[1]

The underlying principle throughout the curriculum is to provide an orthopedic surgeon with the practical knowledge to participate in cost-efficient improvements in health care delivery. Through the ROC Trauma Fellowship Business curriculum, trainees learn that delivering health care in a manner that provides better outcomes for equal or lower costs is not only possible but a professional and ethical responsibility. However, instilling these values without providing actionable knowledge and programs would be insufficient and ineffective. For this reason, the core of the curriculum is based on individual teaching sessions with a wide array of hospital and private practice administrators. In addition, each section is equipped with a suggested reading list to maximize the learning experience.

There is no question that business training has a role in orthopedic education, and its objective is to empower orthopedic surgeons to

- Participate in strategic planning at both the hospital and practice level based on analysis of financial and clinical data
- Understand the function of health care systems at both a macro and micro level
- Possess the knowledge and skills to be strong leaders and effective communicators in the business lexicon of health care
- Be a partner and innovator in the improvement of the delivery of orthopedic services
- Combine scientific and strategic viewpoints to provide an evidence-based strategy for improving quality of care in a cost-efficient manner
- Understand the political, economic, and strategic basics of employed and private practice orthopedics

DISCUSSION
Business Basics
Although the primary goal of the orthopedic surgeon is to provide health care, there is no question that health care is a business. Any individual involved in business must learn the basic vocabulary and principles to function effectively.

Surgeons make clinical decisions based on data and numbers. businesspeople must make economic decisions based on data and numbers also. As members of the health care delivery system, physicians need to merge both clinical and economic decisions to be successful. Understanding generally accepted accounting principles and the interpretation of financial statements are necessary skills. It is imperative for all surgeons to read and interpret income statements, balance sheets, and cash flow statements in order to make credible business decisions regarding all aspects of their personal business. These 3 standard formats must be taught to evaluate the financial health of any entity or business decision.

The practicing orthopedic surgeon must have a sound knowledge of business fundamentals to be successful in the changing health care environment. Practice management encompasses multiple topics including governance, the financial aspects of billing and coding, physician extender management, ancillary service development, information technology (IT), transcription utilization, and marketing. Some of these are universal; however, several of these areas may be most applicable to the private practice of medicine. Attention to each component is vital to develop an understanding of the intricacies of practice management.

Governance
Understanding governance is key for any private or hospital-employed physician, because surgeons must know with whom to talk to obtain the correct information or outcome. Finding the decision makers is important to improve efficiency. All employees must understand the chain of command so that they know to whom they report and how to resolve problems as they arise. In a small private practice, this may be a simple decision tree; however, in a large private practice or hospital, the organizational chart can be complex. Depending on practice size, the practice may have several key employees serving the standard roles on major businesses such as the chief executive officer (CEO), chief financial officer (CFO), and chief operating officer (COO). It is important to understand the roles of each of these employees and their expectations.

Revenue Cycle Management
To understand practice financial performance, set measurable performance expectations, and monitor them, physicians should first understand revenue cycle management. They should

provide support for the implementation of practice-specific revenue cycle management strategies that will allow their practices to meet expectations. Reducing a physician practice's cost to collect requires the right technology, functionality, and staff. Three advanced collection techniques (denials management, contract compliance, and fee schedule management and maintenance) should be examined for their potential value in ensuring that a practice is paid correctly for every service. Although clearly important in private practice, attention to these details is also critical in an academic or employed setting to demonstrate productivity and justify resource allocation.

Billing and Coding

A sound understanding of billing and coding is vital to the financial viability of any orthopedic practice whether in a hospital or private practice. Most surgeons think this is just entering the correct current procedural terminology (CPT) code or international classification of disease, tenth (ICD-10) code. This is only the tip of the iceberg. Business education teaches the monetary loss associated with late or incomplete dictations, delayed charge submissions, and how improved attention to notes can massively affect hospital coding and revenue capture. The cost of collections is tremendous, and the right technology can help practices minimize the cost to collect and optimize reimbursement. To raise the level of IT sophistication in practices, certain functionality exists within practice management software to automate the 3 critical physician revenue cycle management processes: contract management, front-end claims editing, and denials management. If implemented and used correctly, newer capabilities such as workflow automation can also produce quantifiable operating efficiencies and cost reductions in specific revenue cycle activities. Workflow automation tools allow staff members to set parameters under which specific activities, such as accounts receivable(A/R) follow-up, will occur automatically. These tools also reduce the cost to collect by eliminating manual processes.

Salaries and benefits generally constitute the largest practice expense. Therefore, effectively hiring and, more important, retaining qualified billing staff are among the most effective ways to reduce a practice's cost to collect. As the rules and regulations surrounding provider reimbursement have increased dramatically over the past few years, so has the need for technology to automate processes that handle these complexities. As a result, the knowledge and expertise required of practice-based billing staff has increased exponentially. Practices now require virtually the same level of staff billing expertise as hospitals. Hospitals should avoid the temptation, however, to simply shift their own coders, billers, and collectors to their physician practices. Effective practice-based billing staff should have detailed knowledge of the billing rules for the medical specialties the practice provides. They should be able to understand and monitor specialty- and procedure-specific claims requirements for the payers that matter most to the practice.

Ancillary Services

Under current health care law, ancillary service income is available to orthopedic surgeons. In the era of decreasing physician reimbursement, these ancillaries are becoming more sought after revenue streams. In order to participate, it is essential to adhere to Medicare rules and physician self-referral laws. The ability to maintain these additional profit centers is regulated by both state and federal law. The laws are designed to keep the unethical surgeon from ordering unnecessary tests or therapy purely due to their own economic interest. If managed well, these additional services can generate a source of passive income for the orthopedic surgeons involved. Ancillary services now make up about one-third of physician income in a successful orthopedic practice. With sound business acumen, orthopedic surgeons can take full advantage of these options. Development of physician-owned surgery centers, imaging centers, physical therapy, durable medical equipment (DME) shops, and orthopedic urgent care clinics has been shown to be advantageous for patients and physicians alike. Improved patient outcomes, lower health care costs, improved efficiency, and increased physician reimbursement are found in each of these scenarios.[2]

Understanding of ancillary value also helps the hospital-employed physician leverage his or her contribution to the hospital's revenue in terms of radiographs, laboratory tests, physical therapy, and surgical income. This helps maintenance of service line reinvestment and salary targets and can greatly affect the outcomes of gain sharing and comanagement negotiations.[3]

Physician Extender Management

Because of the time constraints placed on surgeons and the increasing pressures of paperwork, good physician extender management is vital to the success of any practice and service line. If utilized appropriately, these individuals can help surgeons be more efficient in the clinic, spend more time with patients, and complete paperwork more accurately. In addition, they should function as another profit center for the orthopedic surgeon or the practice. Every year the American Academy of Orthopedic Surgeons (AAOS) annual meeting offers many symposia on the effective use of physician extenders for orthopedic practices. Certainly these individuals can assist in caring for large numbers of patients given appropriate physician oversight. In situations where surgeons cover several hospital emergency rooms in a single day, midlevel providers can be a key factor in improving response times and patient satisfaction and decreasing emergency room (ER) wait times, length of stay, and operating room (OR) transport times.[4] The scope of practice can be limited by state law, and each physician must be aware of limitations to maintain compliance with individual hospital by-laws also. Although some extenders can generate income from OR assist fees, most are more productive in the office setting. Using well-trained extenders in an orthopedic urgent care clinic has also been a successful model.[2]

Marketing
Competition is inherent in every business, and orthopedic surgery is no exception. The best marketing is word of mouth, clinical competence, and ethical behavior. However, times are changing rapidly as electronics and connectivity have blossomed. Business education has an important role to teach surgeons the different media of marketing, individual targets, legal constraints, and the costs associated with each choice. Knowing the difference between true marketing and goodwill is an important distinction. General business principles can guide surgeon practices on standard norms for what proportion of revenue should be directed toward marketing efforts. Knowing how to track the success of marketing efforts is important to avoid wasting money on useless campaigns. The use on Internet and social media is a growing marketing medium that has unlimited potential and competitive opportunities.

Understand the Value of Physician
Another objective of business education is to help the practicing surgeon understand his or her value to the health care system. Hospital administrators often attempt to convince surgeons that their contributions to the bottom line are smaller than reality. This allows them to decrease pay for hospital-employed physicians, decrease call pay, or fail to reimburse surgeons

for administrative duties. A sound business education shows physicians where to research their value. Many management companies have outlined the value of elective orthopedic practices to hospitals (Becker's, Medical Group Management Association [MGMA]). Several publications have outlined the value of orthopedic trauma surgeons and call takers to hospital systems.[3,5,6] In most hospitals, physicians are asked to serve on multiple committees without reimbursement. Decisions made on implant committees, operating room committees, and arthroplasty panels can save hospitals hundreds of thousands of dollars a year. Understanding the value of directorships and committee positions lets surgeons negotiate for appropriate reimbursement for their time and knowledge. Stipends to oversee specific programs, services, and departments to achieve certain metrics, help incentivize improvements, and improve clinical quality are justified. When appropriately structured, they allow physicians to be paid for their time and expertise. In turn, the hospital gains leadership, buy-in, and improved efficiency.

Understand Value-Based Health Care
The US health care system is at a tipping point. Health care costs in the United States continue to increase, now accounting for more than $2.9 trillion and consuming 17.4% of US gross domestic product. Although the rate of increase in health care spending has dropped in recent years, health care spending continues to escalate toward an unsustainable dollar amount. Cost-cutting measures are regularly being introduced on multiple levels by all parties and include measures such as diagnosis-related group-based reimbursement to hospitals, bundling of payments for certain episodes of care (BPCI), the comprehensive care for joint replacement model (CJR), hospital use of matrix implant pricing, and reduced reimbursement for physicians. Both practicing and graduating orthopedic surgeons need to be aware of these programs.

Orthopedic surgeons have historically been poor stewards of cost containment and resource management. Recent studies have demonstrated that orthopedic surgeons inaccurately estimate the cost of their implants and tend to underestimate the cost rather than overestimate. New technology is often adopted by surgeons without the need and without strong evidence supporting improved outcomes compared with older products. Until recently, physician participation in hospital implant selection, screening, and pricing was uncommon, allowing implant costs to balloon unnecessarily. Additionally, the practice of defensive medicine in orthopedic trauma and the failure of physicians to adhere to accepted preoperative screening guidelines are further examples of poor cost control by the medical community in general. As costs continue to escalate and the transparency of pricing and cost increases, pressure is mounting for physicians to be better stewards of the health care dollar. New programs have emerged to encourage such behavior and provide financial incentive to orthopedic surgeons for cost control. Implant costs remain the highest expense in the OR budget, and curtailing implant costs remains one of the most straightforward ways to decrease costs in orthopedic trauma surgery.

Generic alternatives to prescription medications have become available as patents on existing brand medications expire. These have massively reduced health care costs. Recently, several orthopedic implant companies have emerged, distributing generic or value-based orthopedic implants (Orthopedic Implant Company, Reno, Nevada; Impact Medical, Portland, Oregon). These implants are often hospital owned, and lack representative assistance, but provide US Food and Drug Administration–approved implants similar to the conventional implants at a discounted price to the hospital or health care system. As long as high-quality implants are used, a portion of that savings can be passed on to the surgeon by the way of gain sharing agreements. Despite the widespread availability and usage of lower-cost generic pharmaceuticals, the use of generic orthopedic surgical implants remains limited. Given the increasing concern over escalating health care costs and continuously decreasing physician and hospital reimbursement, lower-cost generic implants would seem to offer an attractive cost-containment option. The reasons for this limited acceptance include factors such as hospital reluctance to purchase implant systems because of the upfront cost of such systems, the limited number of products available, and surgeon factors.[7] Surgeons trained in business would better understand the need for cost savings and quickly adopt value-based measures to save money.

Gain Sharing and Comanagement

Recent experience and analysis indicates that physicians, patients, and hospital systems can all benefit from value-based care. However, it is clear that orthopedic surgeons need a basic understanding of health care finance and a financial incentive to change behavior. Gain sharing and comanagement programs are 2 successful means of achieving physician buy-in for cost containment programs in orthopedic surgery. In comanagement agreements, physicians are reimbursed for their time and intellectual efforts in program and algorithm creation. The cost is minimal for the hospital and often results in millions of dollars of savings. Gain sharing models incentivize physicians to quickly adopt cost-effective implant choices, care plans, and program development. Hospital systems retain the majority of the profits, while patients and insurance carriers benefit from the cost savings, and physicians receive remuneration for their efforts. Attention must be given to the legal issues surrounding the federal antikickback statute, the civil monetary penalty law, and the physician self-referral law when setting up these agreements. Keys to success for these programs include the presence of a physician champion, economic transparency for physicians and hospitals, accurate data collection, and adequate financial incentive for physicians to drive change in practice patterns.[8]

The Bundled Payments for Care Improvement (BPCI) initiative is a cost-saving program developed by the Centers for Medicare and Medicaid Innovation. It is a government-approved form of gain sharing that is now entering its second phase. This model was designed to create a system for higher quality and more coordinated care at a lower cost. It is currently an optional program for physician groups, hospitals, and postacute care providers to benefit financially from improved care models and cost containment measures. Under this initiative, organizations enter into payment arrangements that include financial and performance accountability for episodes of care for Medicare patients. Under this initiative, there are fraud and abuse waivers in place that allow gain sharing among BPCI organizations and approved providers so long as established requirements are adhered to. At its inception, the authors' orthopedic practice entered this initiative for total joint arthroplasty and hip and femur fracture episodes of care. The first year experience demonstrated a significant learning curve. Keys to success included strict adherence to appropriate patient selection for elective surgery, implant pricing control, preoperative and postoperative protocols, diligent postacute care management, and appropriate choice of metrics to maximize gain sharing potential. Ultimately, the BPCI program was a successful venture, saving the authors' hospital over $1.6 million in 2015. In the process, this provided an additional $1.3 million dollar revenue stream for physicians while decreasing the overall cost of care.[9] The following years 2016 and 2017 have resulted in similar economic success.

Understand Legal Issues Surrounding Orthopedic Care

There are several legal principles and laws that all orthopedic surgeons should understand in depth. These can have significant impact on the practice of medicine and the financial aspects of both hospital-employed and private practice orthopedics. There is a significant role for business education to teach the following legal statutes to all surgeons.

In a health care setting, the False Claims Act (FCA) states that it is "illegal to submit claims for payment to Medicare or Medicaid that you know or should know are false or fraudulent." The act does not distinguish between intentional and accidental violations. It is also important for physicians to know that the civil FCA created a "whistleblower provision that allows a private individual to file a lawsuit on behalf of the United States and entitles that whistleblower to a percentage of any recoveries." Whistleblowers can be anyone including "current or ex-business partners, hospital or office staff, or competitors." This is extremely important to understand for private practice and employed physicians. As value-based decisions increase, larger numbers of spurned sales representatives may incite frivolous claims to deter progress.

The Anti-kickback Statute is a law that makes it a criminal offense for physicians to "knowingly and willingly give or receive inducements or rewards for patient referrals or the generation of business involving any item or service payable by the Federal health care programs (eg, pharmaceuticals, supplies, services)." Inducements do not solely consist of money, but represent "anything of value (eg, free rent, vacations, meals, excessive compensation for medical directorships or consultancies)" This has significant importance in the development of ancillary services and negotiations and relationships with hospitals, physicians, and other health care providers. Along the same idea, The Beneficiary Inducement Statute is a law that imposes civil monetary penalties on physicians who offer remuneration to Medicare and Medicaid beneficiaries to influence them to use their services.

The Physician Self-referral (Stark) Law prohibits physicians from referring patients to receive "designated health services" payable by Medicare or Medicaid from entities with which the physician or an immediate family member has a financial relationship (with some exceptions). It is a strict liability statute. Intent to violate the law is not required. Financial relationships include both ownership and investment interests, as well as compensation arrangements. The list of possible designated health services is large and encompasses items such as clinical laboratory services, physical therapy, occupational therapy, outpatient speech therapy, radiology, DME and supplies, prosthetics, orthotics, prosthetic devices, home health services, and outpatient prescription drugs. Any practice with ancillary services or seeking to build them must know these statutes well.

Antitrust laws are designed to protect consumers by preventing boycotts, price fixing, and monopolies. In health care, the consumers are the patients. However, when patients are insured, it is the insurance company that pays the bill that is considered the consumer. These laws do protect doctors, but only as consumers and not as service providers. Physicians must be familiar with antitrust regulation not only to avoid scrutiny, but also to help protect their patients, practice, and communities from dominant insurance companies or hospital organizations. Compliance with antitrust laws is not enough. Improper behavior alone can be interpreted as a violation of antitrust law. Familiarity with anticompetitive behavior regulations is also required. These are often involved in hospital mergers, physician ownership issues, noncompete agreements, insurance contracting, and reimbursement rates.

The Emergency Medical Treatment and Labor Act (EMTALA) is an important law for any call taker or physician accepting transfers. It is jointly enforced by the Centers for Medicare & Medicaid Services (CMS) and the Office of Inspector General (OIG). It is often referred to as the "anti-dumping" law. It is not exclusive to just Medicare or Medicaid patients and ensures that patients can receive emergency care regardless of their ability to pay. Penalties for violation can be substantial with huge physician or hospital fines and civil lawsuits.

The Health Insurance Portability and Accountability Act (HIPAA) is designed to protect personal health information. A clear understanding of this law is important to anyone in the practice of orthopedics. It encompasses multiple areas of clinic management, medical records, disclosure, documentation, and research. IT, patient flow, and practice management all can be affected by this overreaching statute, and violations can be disastrous.

Creating a Strong on Call Contract or Trauma Service

Most orthopedic practices and departments have call responsibilities. The development of a strong on call contract or trauma program is clearly one of the most important facets of successful business development. Several recent publications have demonstrated that well-run trauma services can generate significant profits for both the hospital and the surgeons involved.[4–6] There are many aspects to this task that require constant attention and insight. Top notch patient care, efficiency, and cost-effective resource utilization are all important components that must be addressed while providing adequate physician compensation within the bounds of hospital financial constraints and the encompassing legal issues.

Independent of the trauma practice model, the AAOS and OTA have identified several requirements for the success of any orthopedic trauma service in their AAOS/OTA position statement (AAOS.com). These include:

- Emergency OR access 24/7/365
- OR availability for orthopedic trauma cases Monday through Saturday 7 a.m. to 5 p.m.
- Orthopedic OR nursing staff lead for organizing implants, instruments, and other materials
- 1 physician assistant/orthopedic trauma surgeon full time equivalent (FTE)
- Adequate numbers of reliable, functioning image intensifiers, and trained radiology technicians for OR support
- Funded call support coverage (ie, stipend)
- Available equipment and implant systems for intramedullary nailing, external fixation, plating, and arthroscopy
- Support for orthopedic trauma surgeon continuing medical education (CME)
- Clinic facilities to follow patients after discharge with adequate radiographic capacity, nurse staffing, and wheelchair/stretcher access
- Commitment from emergency department physician leadership to increase orthopedic injury triage capabilities
- Support for a research coordinator assigned to orthopedic trauma research in Level I and Level II centers corresponding to patient volumes
- Reimbursement for indigent care

In exchange for these resources provided by the hospital, orthopedic surgeons agree to provide several services, including quality assurance direction and leadership, responsibility for call schedule coverage, commitment to limit variation in implant usage, CME leadership and involvement for OR staff, staff physicians, floor nurses and clinic staff, and regular review of fiscal impact of the service with hospital administration. A formal business education would clearly assist in many of these tasks.

On call contract negotiations and patient care involve several of the legal issues addressed previously such as EMTALA, HIPPA, restraint of trade, noncompete agreements, collective bargaining, antitrust laws, and physician indemnity. Each of these issues can differ depending on state laws, precedent, and hospital by-laws. Understanding these laws and one's rights as a physician can result in better success when negotiating stipends and provision of care. Contract negotiation is always difficult. It is often said that at the end of a successful negotiation, both sides are never completely satisfied. In many cases, utilizing a mediator can be helpful to avoid adversarial interactions between physicians and hospital administration.

The key to any successful negotiation is knowing what each side wants and what each is willing to give up. Most hospitals are seeking consistent call coverage, efficient patient flow out of the emergency department, decreased length of stay, control of costly implants and materials, and development of physician-led quality measures. Most orthopedic surgeons seek acceptable compensation for providing services that are disruptive to an elective practice, compensation for services performed for indigent patients, and appropriate resources and personnel support to provide high quality care and compensation for participation in hospital committees and cost savings programs. Each of these requests will cost money, and to have successful negotiations physicians must know the numbers before entering into discussions with hospital administration. Familiarity with balance sheets, income statements, and other financial tools is vital.

Understand Government Programs

In order for a trauma surgeon to have an intelligent discussion with hospital administrators, health care plans, policy makers, or any other physicians, a basic understanding of the fundamentals of health care is paramount. It is truly shocking how many surgeons are unable to describe the difference between Medicare and Medicaid or describe how hospitals and physicians get paid. These topics may seem burdensome, but they are vital to all business decision making in the health care field.

Medicare and Medicaid are 2 federally financed health insurance programs. It is important to understand which patients qualify for these plans and the implications of caring for patients supported by each. Patients covered under these plans are all protected by strict regulations, and failure to be in compliance can have financial and criminal implications. Further, physician reimbursement is linked closely to Medicare rates. Understanding the difference between Medicare and Medicaid, who oversees these programs, and the role of government-sponsored health plans in hospital and physician bottom lines is an important topic. As CMS increases opportunities for physicians and hospitals to succeed and incentivize employees with gain sharing through BPCI and CJR, orthopedic surgeons need to be well versed in their options.

Teach Personal Financial Responsibility

Responsible personal finance management is a key component to the success of any physician. All surgeons understand that their clinical practice does not exist in a vacuum unaffected by circumstances and decisions in their personal life. Although some events that can negatively affect one's practice are random and unavoidable, consistently making sound decisions regarding one's personal life and finances will allow a physician to continue practicing at a high level. Most core principles of personal finance are common sense and do not involve high-level math. Although the concepts are straightforward, people including physicians, routinely fail to make good decisions at the most elementary level. The core common sense principles for financial success are simple. The role of any comprehensive business education should involve education on these principles. As physician salaries trend downward, it is imperative for surgeons to carefully protect what they have earned through sound investment principles, appropriate life and disability policies, incorporation, and trust documentation.

Motivate to Political Involvement

Surgeons have traditionally been passive with regard to politics. This is a luxury they can no longer afford. Political decisions have tremendous impact on a physician's ability to care for patients and can significantly impact one's business models. One significant role of business education is to empower surgeons to become involved in lobbying for the causes they know to be right. Understanding the importance of donation to the right causes, political action committees, and lobbies is vital to continued success. Involvement in state orthopedic societies and the AAOS should be mandatory for all practicing orthopedic surgeons. These entities need physicians with business understanding and motivation to protect careers and patients from the governmental, legal, and economic forces that oppose physicians' efforts.

SUMMARY

The examples provided should make it clear that business education does have a role in the training of orthopedic surgeons. In addition to clinical competence, physicians now must make a myriad of decisions regarding patient care, contract negotiation, practice management, and personal finances. Decision making in each of these areas is improved by some understanding of the business of health care. If orthopedic training programs and current practicing surgeons do not accept the responsibility of teaching and learning the business aspects of medicine, physicians will gradually lose control of medicine. The fate of surgeons and patients will be placed in the hands of government and hospital administrators and US health care will suffer.

REFERENCES

1. Althausen PL, Bray TJ, Hill AD. Reno orthopaedic trauma fellowship business curriculum. J Orthop Trauma 2014;28(7 Suppl):S3–11.
2. Anderson TJ, Althausen PL. The role of dedicated musculoskeletal urgent care centers in reducing cost and improving access to orthopaedic care. J Orthop Trauma 2016;30(Suppl 5):S3–6.
3. Hill A, Althausen PL, O'Mara TJ, et al. Why veteran orthopaedic trauma surgeons are being fired and what we can do about it? J Orthop Trauma 2013; 27(6):355–62.
4. Althausen PL, Shannon S, Coll D, et al. Impact of hospital employed physician assistants on a level II, community-based orthopaedic Trauma system. J Orthop Trauma 2013;27(4):e87–91.
5. Althausen PL, Coll D, Cvitash M, et al. Economic viability of a community-based level-II orthopaedic trauma system. J Bone Joint Surg Am 2009;91: 227–35.
6. Vallier HA, Patterson BM, Meehan CJ, et al. Orthopaedic traumatology: the hospital side of the ledger, defining the financial relationship between

physicians and hospitals. J Orthop Trauma 2008; 22(4):221–6.

7. Walker JA, Althausen PL. Surgeon attitudes regarding the use of generic implants: an OTA survey study. J Orthop Trauma 2016;30(Suppl 5): S27–31.

8. McBride C, Althausen PL. Co-management and gainsharing opportunities for independent physicians. J Orthop Trauma 2016;30(Suppl 5):S45–9.

9. Althausen PL, Mead L. Bundled payments for care improvement (BPCI):lessons learned in the first year. J Orthop Trauma 2016;30(Suppl 5):S50–3.

Pediatrics

MRI Safety with Orthopedic Implants

Zachary A. Mosher, MD, Jeffrey R. Sawyer, MD, Derek M. Kelly, MD*

KEYWORDS

- Magnetic resonance imaging • Radiofrequency-induced heating • Implant migration • Torque
- Safety

KEY POINTS

- This study reviews the current literature on MRI safety with orthopedic implants.
- MRI is safe in patients with orthopedic implants regarding migration and torque.
- Radiofrequency-induced heating of implants during MRI showed small differences among studies, although not clinically significant.
- Pediatric patients may be at an increased risk for thermal injury if anesthetized and/or unable to report temperature change during MRI.
- A risk-to-benefit ratio should be applied when using MRIs with orthopedic implants in pediatric patients requiring sedation.

INTRODUCTION

MRI is a valuable diagnostic tool, with utility in pediatric and musculoskeletal imaging due to its lack of ionizing radiation and excellent soft tissue contrast. A continual increase in MRI usage has been demonstrated in the United States, with a 5% rise annually, peaking at 118 examinations per 1000 population (64 in an ambulatory setting and 54 in an inpatient hospital setting).[1] Additionally, the United States has the second-most MRI units per capita, with a 188% increase since 1995, reaching 39 per 1 million population in 2015.[2,3] What makes MRI unique is the method by which the images are obtained. MRI uses a magnet to alter proton rotation, producing signals as the protons return to their baseline rotation at differing rates in various tissues of the body. The magnetic fields used to manipulate the protons during the imaging sequence come in varying strengths for different uses; however, nearly all clinically used scanners in the United States are under 3.0 T,[4] and only one 7.0-T scanner has received approval from the United States Food and Drug Administration for clinical use.[5] Scanners with strengths over 3.0 T are routinely used in research; however, this article's focus in on recommendations on clinically relevant field strengths.

MRI is considered safer and is generally preferred in the pediatric population compared with CT scans for advanced imaging because it does not use ionizing radiation. MRI is not without risk, however, and the Food and Drug Administration[6] receives reports of approximately 300 adverse events associated with these examinations annually. Second-degree burns are the most commonly reported problems and are often due to the formation of internal currents (via skin-to-skin contact)[7,8] or from external metallic objects contacting the body (electrocardiogram leads,[9] pulse oximeters,[10] microfiber tech clothing,[11] medical patches,[12] and so forth). Projectile events (objects drawn into the magnetic field), crush injury of the digits by the patient table, patient falls, and hearing loss or tinnitus are the next most commonly reported problems with MRI, all unrelated to the presence of an orthopedic

---

Disclosure Statement: The authors report no conflicts of interest in regard to this work.

Department of Orthopaedic Surgery and Biomedical Engineering, University of Tennessee, Campbell Clinic, 1211 Union Avenue, Suite 510, Memphis, TN 38104, USA

* Corresponding author.

E-mail address: dkelly@campbellclinic.com

implant. Additionally, pediatric patients requiring anesthesia to inhibit movement during the long MRI acquisition time are at higher risk of adverse events during the MRI sequence.[13–15] Over the past several decades, the safety, compatibility, and imaging artifact caused by surgical implants have been tested in numerous in vivo and ex vivo studies. Because MRI units use strong magnets, metal implants pose a particular hazard with their potential for dislodgment, heating of the implant, and possible damage to surrounding tissues. Although newer orthopedic implants seem safe for MRI, concerns remain with the increasing field strength of MRI scanners. Additionally, confusion remains regarding MRI use immediately postoperatively in patients with surgical implants. This study reviews the current literature concerning the safety of MRI in patients with orthopedic implants. Information was sought about displacement, torque, and radiofrequency-induced (RF) heating of orthopedic implants, paying special attention to any articles pertaining to pediatric orthopedics.

LITERATURE SEARCH

This study did not require institutional review board approval. PubMed was searched using the terms, "MRI and Safety and Orthopedic Implant"; "MRI and Safety and Surgical Implants"; "MRI and Safety and Medical Implants"; "MRI and Orthopedic Hardware and Soft Tissue"; "Magnetic Resonance Imaging and Radiofrequency Heating and Metal Implants"; "MRI and Safety and Pediatric and Orthopedics"; and "MRI and Safety and Spinal Implants." Google Scholar was also searched using these terms to capture relevant articles not listed on PubMed. Only articles published within the past decade were reviewed and only those that discussed MRI safety pertaining to orthopedics were included. In addition, the Web site mrisafety.com was reviewed.

LITERATURE SEARCH RESULTS

The PubMed search produced 402 articles. After narrowing the results to the past 10 years, 219 articles remained. After excluding duplicate articles, articles not pertaining to orthopedic implants, and articles discussing topics other than safety, 15 remained for review.[16–30] Implant displacement was discussed in 11 articles,[16–22,26–28,30] RF heating in 13,[16–21,23–25,27,28,30] and torque in 4.[21,22,26,27] Table 1 summarizes the results of the 15 studies.

Implant Displacement

Implant displacement in 1.5-T, 3.0-T, and 7.0-T scanners has been the focus of numerous studies.[16–22,26–28,30] The experimental studies examined the change in the hanging angle of implants in scanners during an imaging sequence compared with prior to imaging (Fig. 1). A displacement angle of 45° indicated that the translational force of the magnet was equivalent to the force of gravity, and an angle over 45° indicated a potential for implant displacement with MRI.[21,29] Overall, significant displacement in orthopedic implants was infrequent. Two studies reported deflection angles over 45° using a 7.0-T MRI.[21,22] In Feng and colleagues'[21] study, 2 stainless-steel implants showed deflection of more than 45° at 7.0 T. Dula and colleagues[22] reported a deflection angle of 55° for the Synergy Hip System (Smith and Nephew, Memphis, TN) (metal not reported). The deflection angle for all other implants reported was well below 45°, with most below 10° (see Table 1). Except for a known ferromagnetic posterior spinal implant with a deflection angle of 65°,[26] all other implants had no significant displacement in 1.5-T and 3.0-T scanners. All studies but 2[19,28] were performed in ex vivo conditions, and the 2 in vivo studies failed to demonstrate any clinically or radiographically significant implant migration. Two studies also found no detrimental effects of MRI on magnetic-controlled growing rods.[27,28]

Torque

Torque describes the rotational displacement and speed at which the implant aligns with the magnetic field. Only 4 studies reported torque values.[21,22,26,27] Feng and colleagues[21] reported 1+ (minimal) torque in 2 titanium implants and 1 titanium alloy implant. Dula and colleagues[22] reported 2+ (moderate) torque in a pyrocarbon knee implant, a Synergy Hip System, and a titanium alloy hip stem with a cobalt-chrome head stem. They also reported 1+ (minimal) torque in a cobalt-chrome staple and an oxidized zirconium knee implant. McComb and colleagues[26] reported 2+ (moderate) torque in 1 highly ferromagnetic posterior spinal implant but deemed the risk to patient safety minimal, given the rigid fixation of the implant.

Radiofrequency-induced Heating

RF heating of implants during MRI sequencing was discussed in 13 of the 15 articles,[16–21,23–25,27–30] with 8 showing a change

Table 1
Results of reviewed articles

Author	Implant	MRI Field Strength	Deflection Angle	Torque (1–4)	Temperature Change (°C)
Yang et al,[16] 2009	1 Charite (Depuy Spine, Raynham, MA)	<1.5 T	7.5°	NR	0.4
	1 ProDisc-L (Depuy Synthes, Raynham, MA)	<1.5 T	6.0°	NR	0.6
Zou et al,[17] 2015	7 Titanium plates and screws	1.5 T	4.28°	NR	0.48
	7 Stainless-steel plates and screws	1.5 T	7.74°a	NR	0.74b
Kumar et al,[18] 2006	6 Stainless-steel	0.25 T and 1.0 T	0°	NR	NR
	3 Femoral prostheses		0°		—
	1 Condylar blade plate		0°		—
	1 Femoral nail		Significant (at 1.0 T)		—
	1 Ex fix clamp		0°		NR
	5 Titanium		—		—
	1 Femoral prosthesis		—		—
	1 Shoulder hemiprosthesis		—		—
	1 Tibial buttress plate		—		—
	1 Femoral recon nail		—		—
	1 Tibial nail		0°		NR
	1 Cobalt-chrome femoral prosthesis		0°		—
	1 Carbon fiber ex fix rod		0°		NR
	2 Stainless-steel hip prostheses		NR		0.1–0.2
	1 Titanium plate		NR		0.1
Makhdom et al,[19] 2015	19 Stainless-steel Fassier-Duval rod (Pega Medical, Laval, Canada)	1.5 T	0°	NR	0

(continued on next page)

Author	Implant	MRI Field Strength	Deflection Angle	Torque (1–4)	Temperature Change (°C)
Tsukimura et al,[20] 2017	4 Pure titanium rods	3.0 T 7.0 T	1.0°–2.0° at 3.0 T 5.0°–6.2° at 7.0 T	NR	0.2–0.5 at 3T −0.2–0.4 at 7 T
	4 Titanium alloy rods		1.0°–2.3° at 3.0 T 5.7°–7.7° at 7.0 T		−0.3–0.3 at 3 T −0.2–0.2 at 7 T
	4 Cobalt-chrome rods		5.0°–6.0° at 3.0 T 17.8°–21° at 7.0 T		0.1–0.4 at 3 T 0–0.6 at 7T
	1 Titanium alloy/cobalt-chrome screw		3.2° at 3.0 T 10.0° at 7.0 T		0.2 at 3 T −0.3 at 7 T
	1 Titanium alloy cross-link bridge		2.2° at 3.0 T 6.7° at 7.0 T		0 at 3 T −0.2 at 7 T
Feng et al,[21] 2015	10 Stainless-steel	7.0 T	16°–47° (5 implants >44)	0	−0.54–0.41 (2 implants)
	6 Titanium		1°–44° (1 implant 44)	1 (2 implants)	0.21 (1 implant)
	4 Titanium alloy		0°–7°	—	—
	2 Cobalt-chrome		1°–2°	1 (1 implant)	—
	2 Aluminum oxide		0°–17°	—	—
	1 Vitallium		18°	—	—
Dula et al,[22] 2014	PEEK HTO plate	7.0 T	0°	0	NR
	PEEK distal radius plate		0°	0	
	Pyrocarbon knee implant		0°	2	
	Cobalt-chrome staple		23°	1	
	Oxidized zirconium knee implant		5°	1	
	Synergy Hip System		55°	2	
	Titanium alloy hip stem and cobalt-chrome-molybdenum hip stem		45°	2	
	Titanium and silver-plated cannulated screw		8°	0	

Study	Implant	Field strength	Deflection angle	Migration/torque	Heating (°C)
Muranaka et al,[23] 2011; Muranaka et al,[24] 2007; Muranaka et al,[25] 2010	Stainless-steel humeral implant 1 Cobalt-chrome hip implant 1 Titanium alloy hip implant	1.5 T	NR	NR	6.4–14.7 (depending on absorption rate, angle, and location) 9.0 5.3
McComb et al,[26] 2009	Posterior spinal fixator (Anatomica, Gothenburg, Sweden) with fixation blocks, expansion screws, and spindle bolt Highly ferromagnetic components	1.5 T and 3.0 T	65°	4	NR
Budd et al,[27] 2016	2 Magnetic-controlled growing rods	1.5 T	0°	0	No detectable heating
Schroeder et al,[28] 2018	28 Stainless-steel plates and screws in pediatric patients with DDH	1.5 T	No implant migration or loosening	NR	No thermal effects to soft-tissues noted
Poon et al,[29] 2017	3 Magnetic-controlled growing rods	1.5 T	NR	NR	0.39–1.51
Mansour et al,[30] 2009	4 Steinmann pins (varying sizes)	1.5 T	<10°	NR	<3
	Tractor bow (external for traction)		<45°	NR	1.9
	Kirschner wire bow (external for traction)		Highly ferromagnetic removed from study	—	—

Abbreviations: DDH, developmental hip dislocation; ex fix, external fixation; HTO, high tibial osteotomy; PEEK, polyetheretherketone; 1 torque, mild or low; 2 torque, moderate; greater than 3 torque, high; NR, not reported.

[a] The difference in value between the titanium implants and stainless-steel implants was significant (P<.001).

[b] There was an absence of blood circulation in the cadaver swine leg tested. In humans, this value would be lower.

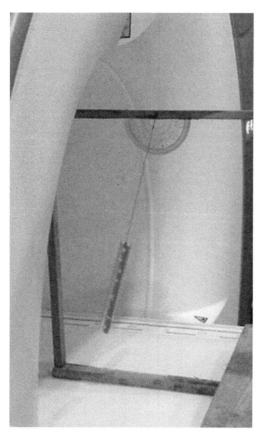

Fig. 1. Demonstration of the experimental setup used to assess hanging angle displacement of implants during an imaging sequence. (*From* Zou YF, Chu B, Wang CB, et al. Evaluation of MR issues for the latest standard brands of orthopedic metal implants: plates and screws. Eur J Radiol 2015;84(3):451; with permission.)

of less than 1°C.[16–21,27,28] Only 5 studies showed more than 1°C change.[23–25,29,30] Muranaka and colleagues[23–25] found increases from 5.3°C to 14.7°C in a stainless-steel humeral implant and cobalt-chrome and titanium hip implants. These experiments were performed in a laboratory setting using a tissue-equivalent, gel-filled polypropylene model. The humeral implant showed a 12.3°C increase at 2-cm depth after a 15-minute 1.5-T MRI sequence.[23] In these studies, implants deeper (6 cm) in the model had less temperature rise (<5.0°C), and the edges of the implants demonstrated the most volatile temperature increases (14.7°C). The maximum temperature rise was noted when the implant tip was parallel with the static magnetic field, and when the implant was moved away from the center of the irradiation coil (static magnetic field), less temperature rise was noted.

DISCUSSION

The concerns of MRI in patients with metal implants are centered on theoretic migration and RF heating of implants, causing damage to surrounding tissues. Numerous studies examining the safety of surgical implants have been published over the past 3 decades, concluding that most passive (no power associated with their operation) nonferromagnetic or weakly ferromagnetic implants are safe for patients in any setting requiring an MRI at 1.5 T or less.[31–34] The results of this review are similar. In general, MRI with field strengths up to 7.0 T can safely be used in patients with orthopedic implants, because the risk of implant-based complications is extremely low.

In this review, 3 of the studies cited areas of concern regarding displacement of orthopedic implants during MRI.[21,22,26] In total, 4 implants violated the previously stated goals for deflection angles being below 45°. The clinical relevance of orthopedic implant migration during MRI remains in doubt, however, and the results of this review support the assessment that in vivo orthopedic implants are likely unaffected by translational forces (even if they exceed 45° under experimental protocols) because they are firmly fixed to bone or are sutured in place, providing sufficient counter-force during imaging.[30] Additionally, in the 2 in vivo studies of this cohort, no clinical or radiographic evidence of implant migration was found after 1.5-T MRI sequencing in osteogenesis imperfecta patients with Fassier-Duval rods[19] or in 28 pediatric patients with developmental hip dysplasia treated with osteotomy and stainless-steel fixation,[28] thus supporting the hypothesis of rigid implant fixation being sufficient to secure the implants in place.

Concerns also exist in the literature regarding RF heating of orthopedic implants. RF heating theoretically occurs due to eddy currents in implants paralleling the static magnetic field of the scanner and causes heating and tissue damage.[17,18,25] Of this cohort, 5 studies reported temperature increases beyond the accepted range of 1°C, and 3 studies reported temperature increases of 5.3°C to 14.7°C.[23–25,29,30] These 3 outliers were ex vivo studies using a tissue-equivalent model with "the same electrical properties of muscle" and failed to document the baseline temperature change of the model during imaging without hardware implanted.[23–25] This lack of a control group calls into question if the temperature increases were due to baseline heating of the model or to RF heating of the implant. Although the results of these 3 studies are alarming, the insufficiencies in their methods breed skepticism regarding their clinical utility. All other studies of the cohort found the temperature change to be negligible, and both in vivo studies had zero patients reporting issues relating to RF heating or subjective burning.[19,28] In short, fears of temperature increases and subsequent tissue damage from RF heating may be unfounded, as suggested by the other studies.[19,28,30]

The effect of magnetic field strength has been studied. Although nearly all clinically used scanners in the United States are 3.0 T or below, 3 studies included in this cohort were performed at 7.0 T,[20–22] a strength often reserved for research purposes. Displacement forces generally increased with increasing magnetic field strength, but most implants remained in their accepted ranges at 7.0 T. RF heating was not associated with field strength, and did not demonstrate increases in temperature with increasing field strength.[20] With recent approval of the first clinical 7.0-T scanner in the United States,[5] little evidence supports limiting clinical use of MRI due to magnetic field strength.

Confusion remains regarding the use of MRI immediately postoperatively, and there is a paucity of recent literature discussing this issue in correlation with orthopedic implants. Shellock[31] stated that patients with passive nonferromagnetic implants can safely undergo MRI at 1.5 T or less immediately postoperatively, but if an implant Is weakly magnetic, practitioners should wait 6 weeks to 8 weeks after the procedure. This statement was referring to coils, filters, and stents, however, that could migrate due to their lack of rigid fixation, not orthopedic implants affixed to bone or when displacement is not a problem.[30] Furthermore, other articles have not reported adverse events related to early postoperative MRI (2 hours–1 day) in the presence of implants,[28,32] and early postoperative MRI remains the standard of care after spinal surgery in patients with postoperative neurologic changes.[35–37]

Image artifact in patients with metal implants does not pose a direct hazard to the patient but can lead to misinterpretation of the results. All metals generate image artifact regardless of their ferromagnetic properties and become an issue if the area of interest is near the implant. Although artifact was outside the scope of this study, 7 articles directly discussed artifact distortion with orthopedic implants.[16–19,23,27,28] In 2 in vivo studies,[19,28] image distortion was not present, although it was problematic in other studies.[16–18,23,27] Modifications of MR pulse sequences and optimization of scanning parameters, however, such as field of view, fast spin-echo, and short-tau inversion recovery, can minimize image distortion.[17,18] The ordering practitioner should weigh the benefits of each imaging sequence in relation to the possible image distortion of the implant. Also, the presence of bullets, shrapnel, and other foreign bodies was not examined in this study, but these articles may pose a threat of migration during imaging.[38–40] Clinical judgment and appropriate caution are warranted when foreign bodies are located near vital organs or the spine. As with all metallic implants, the composition of the foreign bodies affects the possible MRI interactions, with steel objects posing the greatest risk.

In the United States, the use of MRI continues to increase, with minimal associated adverse events. MRIs have a positive risk-to-benefit ratio, with 118 annual examinations per 1000 population in the United States[1] and only 300 adverse events.[6] Appropriate caution remains necessary, however, when ordering MRI in children. Pediatric patients are more likely to require sedation to inhibit movement, thus leaving them unable to express any possible issues that might arise during scanning or during recovery.[13–15]

The limitations of this study include that most of articles examined were laboratory-based studies, with only 2 retrospective clinical studies.[19,28] Additionally, only 2 studies[19,28] focused on pediatric patients. Lastly, zero reports of thermal burns via orthopedic implants or instances of implant migration have been published in the past 10 years, so the true risk of MRI is difficult to determine.

In summary, MRI is safe after orthopedic device implantation and can be performed postoperatively with little concern regarding implant migration. There is conflicting information regarding RF heating of implants, and various implant and patient-specific factors are involved with this phenomenon. Although implants pose minimal risk to patients, individual assessment of implant properties and MRI-related interactions is warranted and can be easily investigated. A risk-to-benefit ratio should be applied when deciding to use MRI in pediatric patients. If the information gained from the MRI is more valuable than the potential risk of anesthesia, migration, or heating, which is extremely low, then the study is likely warranted.

REFERENCES

1. Organization for Economic Cooperation and Development. Magnetic resonance imaging (MRI)

exams. [Web.]. 2017. Available at: https://data. oecd.org/healthcare/magnetic-resonance-imaging-mri-exams.htm. Accessed December 12, 2017.

2. Organization for Economic Cooperation and Development. Magnetic resonance imaging (MRI) units. [Web.]. 2016. Available at: https://data. oecd.org/healtheqt/magnetic-resonance-imaging-mri-units.htm. Accessed December 12, 2017.

3. Centers for Disease Control and Prevention. Table 123. Number of magnetic resonance imaging (MRI) units and computed tomography (CT) scanners: Selected countries, selected years 1990–2009. Health, United States, 2011 [Web.]. 2011. Available at: https://www.cdc.gov/nchs/hus/contents2011.htm#123. Accessed December 12, 2017.

4. Rinck P, editor. Facts and figures. magnetic resonance in medicine. A critical introduction. The basic textbook of the European magnetic resonance forum. 11th edition. 2017. Available at: http://magnetic-resonance.org/ch/21-01.html?q=facts. Accessed January 2, 2018.

5. Caccomo S. FDA clears first 7T magnetic resonance imaging device. [Web.]. 2017. Available at: https://www.fda.gov/NewsEvents/Newsroom/PressAnnouncements/ucm580154.htm. Accessed December 12, 2017.

6. United States Food and Drug Administration. MRI (Magnetic Resonance Imaging) Benefits and Risks. [Web.]. 2017. Available at: https://www.fda.gov/Radiation-EmittingProducts/RadiationEmittingProductsandProcedures/MedicalImaging/MRI/ucm482765. htm. Accessed December 12, 2017, 2017.

7. Eising EG, Hughes J, Nolte F, et al. Burn injury by nuclear magnetic resonance imaging. Clin Imaging 2010;34(4):293–7.

8. Friedstat JS, Moore ME, Goverman J, et al. An unusual burn during routine magnetic resonance imaging. J Burn Care Res 2013;34(2): e110–1.

9. Abdel-Rehim S, Bagirathan S, Al-Benna S, et al. Burns from ECG leads in an MRI scanner: case series and discussion of mechanisms. Ann Burns Fire Disasters 2014;27(4):215–8.

10. Haik J, Daniel S, Tessone A, et al. MRI induced fourth-degree burn in an extremity, leading to amputation. Burns 2009;35(2):294–6.

11. Pietryga JA, Fonder MA, Rogg JM, et al. Invisible metallic microfiber in clothing presents unrecognized MRI risk for cutaneous burn. AJNR Am J Neuroradiol 2013;34(5):E47–50.

12. Kuehn BM. FDA warning: remove drug patches before MRI to prevent burns to skin. JAMA 2009; 301(13):1328.

13. Kaila R, Chen X, Kannikeswaran N. Postdischarge adverse events related to sedation for diagnostic imaging in children. Pediatr Emerg Care 2012; 28(8):796–801.

14. Tith S, Lalwani K, Fu R. Complications of three deep sedation methods for magnetic resonance imaging. J Anaesthesiol Clin Pharmacol 2012;28(2):178–84.

15. Srinivasan M, Turmelle M, Depalma LM, et al. Procedural sedation for diagnostic imaging in children by pediatric hospitalists using propofol: analysis of the nature, frequency, and predictors of adverse events and interventions. J Pediatr 2012;160(5): 801–6.e1.

16. Yang CW, Liu L, Wang J, et al. Magnetic resonance imaging of artificial lumbar disks: safety and metal artifacts. Chin Med J (Engl) 2009;122(8):911–6.

17. Zou YF, Chu B, Wang CB, et al. Evaluation of MR issues for the latest standard brands of orthopedic metal implants: plates and screws. Eur J Radiol 2015;84(3):450–7.

18. Kumar R, Lerski RA, Gandy S, et al. Safety of orthopedic implants in magnetic resonance imaging: an experimental verification. J Orthop Res 2006;24(9): 1799–802.

19. Makhdom AM, Kishta W, Saran N, et al. Are Fassier-Duval rods at risk of migration in patients undergoing spine magnetic resonance imaging? J Pediatr Orthop 2015;35(3):323–7.

20. Tsukimura I, Murakami H, Sasaki M, et al. Assessment of magnetic field interactions and radiofrequency-radiation-induced heating of metallic spinal implants in 7 T field. J Orthop Res 2017;35(8):1831–7.

21. Feng DX, McCauley JP, Morgan-Curtis FK, et al. Evaluation of 39 medical implants at 7.0 T. Br J Radiol 2015;88(1056):20150633.

22. Dula AN, Virostko J, Shellock FG. Assessment of MRI issues at 7 T for 28 implants and other objects. AJR Am J Roentgenol 2014;202(2):401–5.

23. Muranaka H, Horiguchi T, Ueda Y, et al. Evaluation of RF heating due to various implants during MR procedures. Magn Reson Med Sci 2011;10(1):11–9.

24. Muranaka H, Horiguchi T, Usui S, et al. Dependence of RF heating on SAR and implant position in a 1.5T MR system. Magn Reson Med Sci 2007; 6(4):199–209.

25. Muranaka H, Horiguchi T, Ueda Y, et al. Evaluation of RF heating on hip joint implant in phantom during MRI examinations. Nihon Hoshasen Gijutsu Gakkai Zasshi 2010;66(7):725–33.

26. McComb C, Allan D, Condon B. Evaluation of the translational and rotational forces acting on a highly ferromagnetic orthopedic spinal implant in magnetic resonance imaging. J Magn Reson Imaging 2009;29(2):449–53.

27. Budd HR, Stokes OM, Meakin J, et al. Safety and compatibility of magnetic-controlled growing rods and magnetic resonance imaging. Eur Spine J 2016;25(2):578–82.

28. Schroeder KM, Haurno LS, Browne TS, et al. Evaluation of postoperative MRI in pediatric patients

after orthopaedic hardware implantation. Curr Orthop Pract 2018;29(2):140–3.

29. Poon S, Nixon R, Wendolowski S, et al. A pilot cadaveric study of temperature and adjacent tissue changes after exposure of magnetic-controlled growing rods to MRI. Eur Spine J 2017;26(6): 1618–23.

30. Mansour A, Block J, Obremskey W. A cadaveric simulation of distal femoral traction shows safety in magnetic resonance imaging. J Orthop Trauma 2009;23(9):658–62.

31. Shellock FG. Magnetic resonance safety update 2002: implants and devices. J Magn Reson Imaging 2002;16(5):485–96.

32. Shellock FG. MRISafety.com. [Web.]. 2017. Available at: http://www.mrisafety.com/. Accessed September 31, 2017.

33. Shellock FG. Biomedical implants and devices: assessment of magnetic field interactions with a 3.0-Tesla MR system. J Magn Reson Imag JMRI 2002;16(6):721–32.

34. Tsai LL, Grant AK, Mortele KJ, et al. A practical guide to MR imaging safety: what radiologists need to know. Radiographics 2015;35(6):1722–37.

35. Bommireddy R, Kamat A, Smith ET, et al. Magnetic resonance image findings in the early post-operative period after anterior cervical discectomy. Eur Spine J 2007;16(1):27–31.

36. Crocker M, Jones TL, Rich P, et al. The clinical value of early postoperative MRI after lumbar spine surgery. Br J Neurosurg 2010;24(1):46–50.

37. Leonardi MA, Zanetti M, Saupe N, et al. Early postoperative MRI in detecting hematoma and dural compression after lumbar spinal decompression: prospective study of asymptomatic patients in comparison to patients requiring surgical revision. Eur Spine J 2010;19(12):2216–22.

38. Martinez-del-Campo E, Rangel-Castilla L, Soriano-Baron H, et al. Magnetic resonance imaging in lumbar gunshot wounds: an absolute contraindication? Neursurg Focus 2014;37(1):E13.

39. Eshed I, Kushnir T, Shabshin N, et al. Is magnetic resonance imaging safe for patients with retained metal fragments from combat and terrorist attacks? Acta Radiol 2010;51(2):170–4.

40. Dedini RD, Karacozoff AM, Shellock FG, et al. MRI issues for ballistic objects: information obtained at 1.5-, 3- and 7-Tesla. Spine J 2013;13(7):815–22.

Perioperative Safety

Keeping Our Children Safe in the Operating Room

Kerwyn C. Jones, MD*, Todd Ritzman, MD

KEYWORDS

• Perioperative safety • Checklists • Huddles • Proficiency • Just Culture

---

KEY POINTS

- The surgeon functions as a team leader in the operating room. In this role, it is incumbent on the surgeon to act as a role model for ensuring patient safety. Several tools are necessary to achieve this safe environment. These include use of perioperative huddles, surgical checklists, operating room standardization, ensuring surgeon proficiency, and creating an environment that practices Just Culture.
- Perioperative huddles and checklists are modified to accommodate the needs of a patient population served by an institution. These are properly performed in a brief period of time, yet they create improved communication of team members.
- Standardized operating room teams familiar with the procedures performed and teams using standardized protocols provide increased quality of care and safety. This is especially evident when the team is functioning in an environment that is openly committed to Just Culture.

Surgery is one of the few times that parents relinquish all responsibility for their children's well-being to someone else. Thus, surgeons have a tremendous responsibility to their patients. To relinquish their child parents must assume that surgeons will provide their children as safe an environment as possible. Surgeons understand that the operating room (OR) is a highly complex environment with the constant potential for great risk. Therefore, it is incumbent on surgeons to understand the factors contributing to risk and to develop the necessary mechanisms to ensure as safe an environment as possible. There are many complex factors contributing to this risk. These include the following:

- Communication errors between team members[1]
- Inconsistency of team members
- Indifferent team members

- Surgeon proficiency
- Team members' lack of understanding of the procedure and its risks[2]
- Wide variation in procedures, techniques, equipment, and protocols
- Team hierarchy[3,4]

Although it is generally recognized that these risk factors cannot be completely eliminated it is also understood that they are mitigated by several necessary actions. Many surgeons believe that they have little control over many of these factors, attributing obstacles imposed by hospital leadership as impediments to change these behaviors. However, it is the belief of the authors that the surgeon, as a front-line leader, should be the key proponent to ensure safety for the patient in and around the OR. It is the responsibility of the surgeon to continuously challenge his/her staff and the administrative leadership to continually work together to

---

Disclosure Statement: Neither author has anything to disclose related to this article.

Department of Orthopedic Surgery, Akron Children's Hospital, 1 Perkins Square, Akron, OH 44308, USA

* Corresponding author.

E-mail address: kjones@akronchildrens.org

Orthop Clin N Am 49 (2018) 465–476

https://doi.org/10.1016/j.ocl.2018.05.008

optimize patient safety in and around the OR. Only through relentless pursuit is success achieved.

To optimize (ensure) this safety one must develop a consistent team that communicates well; is not afraid to speak openly about potential risks; is engaged in the process; has a baseline understanding of the procedures and events anticipated for the day; can follow standardized procedures, guidelines, and policies when applicable; and is led by a surgeon that promotes open discussion and is proficient in the surgical technique. Surgeon leaders in the OR can provide or at the least help team members work toward all of these necessary components of safe care. Evidence exists that team performance is most improved through a combined approach of using teamwork training with systems improvement.[5] All of these factors are established by instituting the following protocols in the OR:

- Preoperative huddles or briefings
- Surgical checklists
- OR team standardization
- Ensuring surgeon proficiency
- Just Culture

PERIOPERATIVE HUDDLES OR BRIEFINGS

Most successful sports teams huddle before every game or match and frequently at various times throughout. In the high stress situation of competition, huddles enable each member or the team to gain a better understanding of the game plan, help them to understand their roles for that given plan, give an opportunity to ask questions when the plan is not understood, potentially improve communication of team members, provide a feeling of team camaraderie for the members, and provide a mental model and common goal for the entire team.

Formal team briefings are also a mandatory part of high reliability teams functioning in high-risk processes, such as the airline industry.[6] Team huddles are currently being used in the health care setting in numerous venues. These include the use of huddles on inpatient floors, in labor and delivery, at the managerial or administrative level, and in the OR. Although it is difficult to demonstrate a direct relationship between perioperative or preoperative huddles and improved safety, there is evidence that the huddle improves the surgical teams' attitude toward safety.[7] It is also readily apparent that preoperative huddles decrease communication

errors[8] and improve team function,[9,10] which would certainly improve safety for patients. Furthermore, preoperative huddles are believed to be associated with reduced risk for wrong-site surgery and improved collaboration because of increased awareness of the surgical site and the side being operated on.[11]

In addition, there is a discrepancy in the perception of teamwork and communication among teams in the OR. Physicians tend to rate teamwork as high, whereas nurses at the same institution often rate the teamwork as mediocre.[12] This suggests that there may be a surgeon-centric opinion that he/she has a well-functioning team when in fact in Just Culture the team cannot function at its optimum unless all members of the team are empowered to speak up and possibly even "stop the system" if they believe there is inordinate risk to the patient or another team member.

The mechanics of the team huddle may differ slightly among institutions and is often dependent on the best time available, the availability of the team members, geographic space available in the perioperative space, and the previously determined poignant issues to discuss during the huddle. It is important that surgeons understand that they should be free to develop that huddle, along with input from their team, to accommodate these different parameters. However, there are some general key recommendations for huddles that all institutions should strive to perform.

The first consideration is the team members involved in the huddle. At a minimum there should be one representative of each service that will be present in the OR throughout the day. This typically involves one member each of anesthesia, OR nursing, surgical technicians, radiology technicians, and any other ancillary service to be used during the day. If feasible, it is also helpful to include preoperative and postoperative personnel because many issues carry over to and from each of these areas. In our experience, having the preoperative and postoperative team involved has led to markedly improved processing of the patients before and after surgery.

Second, it is necessary to follow a simple, scripted outline of the key considerations to be covered for the huddle. This varies from institution to institution dependent on many factors unique to each institution and the population that it cares for (Box 1).

Third, the script should include all cases of the day as they are reviewed in sequence one at

<table>
<tr><td>

Box 1
An example of the list of items discussed at a preoperative huddle

- Case: name, age
- Planned procedure and side
- Position
- Tourniquet (sterile or not)
- Essential equipment needed and size if applicable
- Radiograph needs (large or mini C arm)
- Antibiotics for the case
- Nerve block
- Estimated blood loss
- Estimated length of procedure
- Need for postoperative immobilization (splint, brace, cast)
- Special considerations
- Any questions?

Time required for huddle____

This can vary from institution to institution dependent on the surgeons' perception of the needs for their patient population.
From Jain AL, Jones KC, Simon J, et al. The impact of a daily pre-operative surgical huddle on interruptions, delays and surgeon satisfaction in an orthopedic operating room: a prospective study. Patient Saf Surg 2015;9:8; with permission.

</td></tr>
</table>

regarding "special considerations" and "equipment needs."[13] Some examples of such questions and concerns that we have experienced that have conceivably had a positive impact on the team were questions related to

- Staff confusion regarding equipment needed resulting in the wrong equipment being "pulled" for the procedure
- Recognition that the equipment or an implant was not readily available
- Notification that a patient had a miscalculated comorbidity
- The need for postoperative durable medical goods, such as a wheelchair, that have not been ordered preoperatively

In some scenarios recognition of these issues allowed the team to change the lineup order before first case in the morning to avoid a delay and to ensure that all safety considerations were addressed and limited. In the absence of a preoperative huddle these would not be recognized until the timeout with the patient already anesthetized or even in the middle of a case with an open surgical wound.

Using this system daily our surgeons reported improved satisfaction, improved flow for the day, and increased surgeon satisfaction because of numerous factors including fewer interruptions for questions during and between cases.[13] Surgical huddles also significantly decreased unexpected delays and the number of questions asked during the day. Perhaps most importantly, nursing staff experience was markedly improved. This was especially evident in such situations as after-hours emergent and urgent work where the operating team was not as familiar with orthopedic procedures and the instrumentation and implants.

Perhaps the biggest challenge for the use of preoperative huddles is the logistics of gathering one member of each team before the start of the day. Again, this is another example where surgeon buy-in and insistence can make this a routine part of the increased safety for patients.

In June 2008, the second part of the World Health Organization (WHO) Global Safety Challenges was launched in Washington, DC. This initiative introduced the surgery checklist requiring the checklist to be performed at sign in, time out, and sign out. The sign in is to be done some time between patient arrival in the OR and before induction of anesthesia, the timeout to be performed before incision or procedure start, and the sign out to be done before the patient leaves the OR.[14]

time using the script. If there are four cases then the script is used four times during the huddle. All of the cases in the entire lineup should be discussed in the preoperative huddle. Another essential consideration is that the huddle must be performed early enough to accommodate any issues identified during the huddle that require a change in the case. The best time to do this is before the start of the first case of the surgeon's lineup, before bringing the patient in the room because on a rare occasion we have even altered the order of the lineup for the day to improve the flow or increase patient safety. Although this seemingly is a lengthy process in reality our data show that the average time spent was 54 seconds per case. Therefore, an operative day with four cases would require an average of 3 minutes 36 seconds.[13]

Most importantly, team members should be asked at the end of each huddle if there are any questions or concerns that they would like to discuss. In our experience this is often the most valuable part of the huddle because it is unusual for nobody to have any comments at this time. The most common questions are

The WHO surgical checklist has been implemented worldwide and there is evidence that its use results in decreased morbidity and mortality for surgical patients.[15] Gawande[16] eloquently described for the lay public and medical personnel the impact of this tool. However, institution of the checklist alone is not adequate for success because checklist compliance is critically important for achieving these improved outcomes.[17,18] There is also a wide variation in checklist compliance and it is highly variable and dependent on the ways the checklist is introduced, its perceived relevance, and surgical team member engagement.[19,20] Multicenter studies reveal a wide variation in the quality and compliance with checklist guidelines. Forty percent of the cases had absent team members, an average of only two-thirds of the items were checked, and sign out only occurred in 39% of the cases. Most notably, the checklist performance was best when the surgeon led the discussion. This is just one more piece of clear evidence of the impact that surgeons can have on improved function of their teams that will ultimately lead to improved safety for patients.[21]

This raises the question as to whether the checklist actually can, if performed properly, improve safety for patients. There is some evidence specific to orthopedics that suggests that the WHO surgical checklist may not have any effect on improved patient safety. More than 900 percutaneous pinnings of supracondylar humerus fractures in children were assessed before and after institution of the checklist. The teams achieved 85% compliance with the checklist. There was a significant increase in returns to the OR in the prechecklist group but they were not believed to be caused by anything related to the checklist parameters, which may reflect the low complexity in terms of equipment/instrumentation in the surgical treatment of these injuries.[22] In Canada the administrative health care database was used to assess surgical complications in children before and after universal implementation of the checklist. More than 14,000 surgical procedures performed in pediatric patients were retrospectively reviewed before implementation and another 14,000 surgical procedures after implementation. There was no statistical difference in the adjusted odds for complications before and after the checklist was instituted.[23,24] Contrary to this, meta-analysis indicates an improved safety rate for patients with widespread use of the checklist.[25] Perhaps most importantly, a collaborative study at five academic institutions assessed efficacy of the WHO checklist in their patients. In this study particular attention was paid to completion of all three parts of the checklist (sign in, timeout, and sign out). When all three portions were performed there was a significant decrease in the percentage of complications. Furthermore, another 14% of the complications would have been prevented if all three parts of the checklist had been performed. This supports the point that the quality of the checklist is paramount for improved patient safety in the OR.[26]

The true incidence of wrong-site surgery is not known because it is not always reported. Recent studies have shown that 21% of hand surgeons, 50% of spinal surgeons, and 8.3% of knee surgeons surveyed have reported performing at least one wrong-site surgery during their career.[27]

The Joint Commission on the Accreditation of Health Care Organizations mandates that hospitals report wrong-site surgery and it therefore may be the best representation of the true incidence. Based on their data there has been a decrease in the numbers between 2011 and 2013. Further analysis of these data revealed that the most common primary causes were failure of team communication and lack of leadership, factors that are strongly influenced by the surgeon's leadership in the OR. The most common error was failure to perform a proper briefing before surgery.[1]

SURGEON PROFICIENCY

The link between repetitive performance of a task and achievement of skill is intuitive. Everyone has recollection of the repeating childhood mantra "practice makes perfect." Gladwell[28] famously reinforced this concept by quantitating the work requirement to achieve expertise: "researchers have settled on what they believe is the magic number for true expertise: ten thousand hours." Given the reality that parents trust their children in a surgeon's care during procedures with significant risk, one may argue that ethically this principle should be upheld even more stringently in the surgical profession. Without question, every surgeon has proven commitment to this principle through the decade plus of effort required to complete education and training. That being said, in the era of voluminous growth in surgical techniques, literature, and specialization, surgeons owe it to patients and parents to commit more deeply to achieving, ensuring, and maintaining expertise in the OR. This era of growth mandates that pediatric orthopedists, who traditionally pride themselves in being a specialized generalist competent to treat diverse anatomic locations and disorders, honestly assess individual and institutional expertise for the sake of patients' outcomes.

Skill Attainment: Surgical Learning Curve

A learning curve is simply defined as the number of times a task must be repeated before a steady state is achieved.[29] Gofton and colleagues[30,31] expand on this definition by describing three phases of a surgical learning curve: phase 1, in which skill development is slow and technical understanding is poor; phase 2, in which rapid skill acquisition occurs and understanding increases; and phase 3, in which the procedure is well learned and expert performance plateaus (Fig. 1). Ideally, patient safety is optimized by ensuring that all procedures are completed by surgeons who have completed the learning curve for a given procedure and acquired expertise. Additionally, ideal surgical training culminates in completion of the learning curve before independent practice. In a field as diverse as pediatric orthopedics, these ideals may not always be feasible or achievable, but it behooves one to focus on and strive toward these principles.

Extensive literature exists focusing on establishment of learning curves for various orthopedic subspecialities including sports medicine/arthroscopy,[31–34] arthroplasty,[35–41] hip preservation,[42–44] foot and ankle,[45] trauma,[40,46] and adult and pediatric spine.[47–62] Many of these publications attempt to quantify the minimum number of cases required for a specific procedure to ensure surgeon-obtained essential competence: optimized outcomes and operative efficiency

with minimized complications. For example, minimum threshold of cases to achieve a steady state of efficient operative time and minimize complications has been suggested as between 20 and 100 cases for knee ligament reconstruction,[31–33] 30 cases for hip arthroscopy,[34] 10 to 20 cases for Developmental Dysplasia of the Hip reduction,[63] 40 cases for Bernese periacetabular osteotomy,[42–44] 20 to 30 cases for hip fracture surgery,[63] 20 to 30 cases for minimally invasive spine decompression,[52] 20 to 30 cases for cervical fusions,[53] 40 cases for microdiscectomy, 45 cases for lumbar interbody fusion,[54] 30 to 80 cases for thoracic pedicle screw instrumentation,[56–58] and 50 to 80 cases for arthroplasty.[35,36,41] In an excellent review of this topic, Gofton and colleagues[64] generalized that 40 cases seems to be an important minimum threshold number, at least with respect to measures of surgical time and complications.'

Given the differing backgrounds, training, and inherent skill set of individual surgeons, these minimum threshold numbers are inexact. Nonetheless, the principle is sound, and consideration of these thresholds is prudent when onboarding new surgeons or when established surgeons incorporate new procedures at institutions. Strategies to be used to facilitate learning curve completion include cadaveric procedures, visiting professorships in which the visiting surgeon assists in procedures, site visits to expert surgeons, minifellowships, proctoring call cases during the first months of practice, and dual-surgeon cases with senior partner assistance. Each of these strategies has been used at the authors' institution to ensure the delivery of optimal patient safety and efficiency. It is the norm at our institution to have dual-attending participation for complex cases, such as multiligament knee reconstructions, hip preservation osteotomies, complex spine deformity, and single event multilevel cerebral palsy procedures. Additionally, weekly surgical indications conferences ensure that young surgeons benefit from the experience of their more experienced colleagues in preoperative planning and decision making.

Volume and Outcome

Numerous reports emphasize the relationship of individual surgeon and institutional volume and patient outcomes inclusive of all orthopedic subspecialties.[29,65–67] High-volume surgeons and institutions have been shown to outperform low-volume surgeons and institutions in efficiency, resource utilization/health care costs, and complication avoidance. This is evident for several orthopedic procedures including

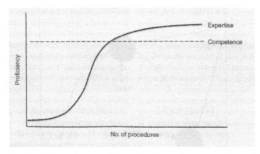

Fig. 1. Three phases of a surgical learning curve. Phase 1 (initial plateau): limited understanding, poor technical skill. Phase 2 (steeper section): improving understanding and rapid skill acquisition. Phase 3 (expertise plateau): expert understanding and skill mastery. (Reproduced with permission from Gofton WT, Papp SR, Gofton T, et al. Understanding and taking control of surgical learning curves. In: Throckmorton T, Gerlinger TL, editors. Instructional Course Lectures, volume 65. Rosemont (IL): American Academy of Orthopaedic Surgeons; 2016.)

arthroscopy,[31,34] arthroplasty,[35,37–40] cervical and lumbar decompression and fusion,[53,54] pediatric spine deformity,[55–57,60,68] and adult spine deformity.[62,69]

Skill Maintenance: Minimum Annual Rate of Performance

Not only is surgeon proficiency dependent on surpassing the learning curve for a procedure but also the ongoing case volume of the surgeon. It is necessary to ascend the learning curve and to practice the procedure regularly to maintain expertise.[63] In a database review of more than 6000 adolescent idiopathic scoliosis procedures, Paul and colleagues[60] demonstrated a definitive decrease in major complications among higher volume surgeons with concomitant lower cost/resource utilization despite that the higher volume surgeons have more complex procedural mix. High-volume surgeons were defined as maintaining a minimum practice volume of 20 cases annually. The odds ratios for this highest quartile of surgeons were 0.74 for surgical complications, 0.6 for mechanical complications, 0.36 for neurologic complications, and 0.75 for major complications (**Table 1**).[60] Similarly, Schoenfeld and colleagues[54] completed a database review of more than 187,000 spine procedures to provide meaningful volume-based benchmarks for common lumbar spine surgical procedures. In doing so, a volume threshold of 40 lumbar microdiscectomies annually, or about 1 discectomy a week, was exhibited to correlate with a significantly lower rate of complications. Surgeons who failed to meet that volume metric had a 56% increase in complications following discectomy.

Thus, surgeons and institutions must not only have a sufficient volume of cases to gain expertise through completion of the learning curve, but also must have ongoing procedural volume to maintain expertise and avoid skill degradation. For example, a volume of more than 40 adolescent idiopathic scoliosis surgeries annually should provide for consistent maintenance of expertise, avoidance of skills degradation, and optimize patient outcomes. However, despite a busy pediatric spine practice, pediatric spine surgeons rarely evaluate a patient who is a candidate for lumbar microdiscectomy in this age group. Given Schoenfeld's data,[54] it could be concluded that it is not appropriate to perform two to three lumbar discectomies annually when there are numerous adult spine surgeons in a community who perform more than 100 procedures annually (well higher than the volume benchmark for safety). In a subspecialty that prides itself in being a specialized generalist, these decisions are difficult for pediatric orthopedic surgeons. Institutional questions to be considered include the following:

- How many surgeons performing a complex procedure does our institutional volume permit? One may argue that for an institution with an annual volume of 80 adolescent idiopathic scoliosis cases, two surgeons performing 40 spine fusions each may provide better patient safety and surgical outcomes than six surgeons performing 10 to 15 fusions each.
- Individual surgeons may be faced with introspective questions of their personal procedural volume as it relates to outcomes. Anecdotally, if a surgeon performs 11 anterior cruciate ligament reconstructions annually and a colleague performs 90, who is most optimized from

Table 1
Odds ratio of complications in adolescent scoliosis exhibiting significant decrease in fourth quartile/high-volume surgical practices

Quartile	Any AHRQ Surgical Complications		Mechanical Complications		Neurologic Complications		Major Medical Complications	
	OR	95% CI	OR	95% CI	OR	95% CI	OR	95% CI
First	1.00	—	1.00	—	1.00	—	1.00	—
Second	1.17	1.111–1.239	0.58	0.511–0.659	1.65	1.337–2.037	1.03	0.916–1.145
Third	1.09	1.032–1.155	0.95	0.849–1.062	0.85	0.664–1.086	1.02	0.909–1.14
Fourth	0.74	0.695–0.785	0.60	0.527–0.681	0.36	0.264–0.481	0.75	0.662–0.846

Model: (Intercept), surgeon quartile adjusting for age, race, sex, neuromuscular scoliosis, operative complexity index, and comorbidities.
Abbreviations: AHRQ, Agency for Healthcare Research and Quality; CI, confidence interval; OR, odds ratio.
From Paul JC, Lonner BS, Toombs CS. Greater operative volume is associated with lower complication rates in adolescent spinal deformity surgery. Spine 2015;40(3):167; with permission.

a volume-outcome perspective to give that patient a good result? Perhaps he/she should stop performing anterior cruciate ligament reconstructions and refer them all to the higher volume partner.

- Does an institutional volume justify performance of a rare, high-risk procedure? For example, should a department perform surgical hip dislocations at a rate of two per year (lower than the threshold for learning curve completion or skill maintenance) when a regional center performs 25 procedures annually?

Undoubtedly, these are difficult questions to consider individually and departmentally. However, as the breadth of evidence grows linking the relationship between surgical volume and outcomes, they are ethically responsible questions to be addressed for the sake of optimized patient outcomes. Obviously, rural versus urban geography, department size/resources, institutional growth projections, and other variables are critical and unique for every surgeon and department when considering these issues.

TEAM STANDARDIZATION

The volume-outcome relationship does not only apply to surgeons, but also the entire team of caregivers who participate in a patient's surgical outcome. "Safety is influenced not only by the experience of the surgeon, but also by coordination among surgical and postoperative care staff with well-established protocols, which may be more likely to be well-tested in high-volume centers."[60] Familiarity with each other, a procedure, and a global treatment protocol certainly leads to improvements in efficiency and outcome in orthopedic surgery.[70–76] Patrick and colleagues[70] demonstrated 30-minute reduction in operative time when using a defined surgical team with limited staff turnover at an outpatient surgery center as compared with a rotating staff with high turnover at the inpatient setting. Mijaynji[75] demonstrated a significant decline in surgical site infections (odds ratio, 10 times less), operative time, length of stay, unplanned procedures, and allogeneic blood transfusions (odds ratio, 2.4 times less) after implementation of a multidisciplinary pediatric spine team. Flynn[76] corroborated this finding presenting a 30% reduction in operative time and average cost savings of almost $9000 per case after implementation of a dedicated pediatric spine deformity team inclusive of anesthesia, nursing, technicians, and surgeons.

As is true of the entire topic of volume-outcome relationships, these findings are intuitive. However, practicality of implementation can prove challenging. Anecdotally, the author's institution invested more than 12 months into the development of a comprehensive preoperative, intraoperative, postoperative spine deformity pathway with a multidisciplinary team-based approach. After 1 year of implementation of this pathway, length of stay has decreased from 6.2 to 3.3 days with zero readmissions, pediatric intensive care unit transfers, or surgical site infections and only one allogeneic blood transfusion (unpublished data). The administrative effort to institute standardized team approach to care is worth the reward. The evidence presented in this article may be used with hospital administration as impetus toward the development of operative/institutional team standardization for care.

JUST CULTURE: IT'S ALL ABOUT "WHAT" NOT "WHO"

Everyone wants to work on a team that has good communication, mutual respect among team members, and is universally successful. Lencioni[77] summarized the five parameters that he believed, based on his research, were most likely to result in a poorly cohesive team. The dysfunctions he described were

- Absence of trust
- Fear of conflict
- Lack of commitment and a failure to buy into decisions
- Failure to focus on achieving collective results
- Avoidance of accountability

Described in a reverse manner one can simply state that the keys to a functional team are a team that has developed trust in one another, is not afraid to speak up for fear of conflict, is committed to a common goal, is focused on achieving a collective result, and holds themselves and others accountable.

Just Culture was first described in 1997 by Reason[78] as a culture that creates an atmosphere of trust that encourages and rewards people for providing essential patient safety–related information. It was adopted first by the airline industry and in 2001 Marx[79] introduced it to the medical profession through the Agency for Health Related Quality. It is important to understand that Marx's Just Culture algorithm does not leave error mitigation to vague recommendations. Instead, he developed a clear algorithm to be used by team leaders when approaching the root cause of the error.

In many ways, what is described by Lencioni[77] is similar to the methodology for developing a team that practices Just Culture. It is the belief of these authors that most employees do not come to work planning to do a bad job. With rare exception, all employees have an inherent desire to perform well at their jobs. Therefore, when mistakes happen it is necessary to work toward a better understanding of why these employees make these mistakes when they had full intent to not do so. Just Culture helps focus on the question of "what" process or system can be modified to limit risk of error, rather than the "who" is to blame for the error.

he/she works.[81] The best way to support accountability is to involve the person making the mistake in the process of actively modifying or even developing a new system that mitigates the risk of future error.

A second tenet of Just Culture is that it differentiates between blame and accountability by asking four questions that summarize the employee's behavior:

- Was the individual impaired?
- Did the individual consciously decide to engage in an unsafe act?
- Did the caregiver make a mistake that other similar individuals would make in similar circumstances?
- Does the individual have a history of unsafe acts?

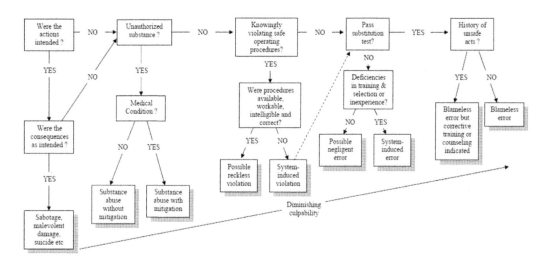

The primary advantage of Just Culture is that it provides a more effective method for an organization's ability to learn from its own mistakes and create an improved safety culture. One key tenet is that it provides a unique description of human error. It changes the concept of human error from a traditional view that the human component is the cause of the error to a newer concept that identifies human error as a symptom of a deeper problem within the system. Thus, in most cases the human error should not be treated in a punitive manner. This should not be used as an excuse to shirk one's responsibility in the source of the error.[80] After all, accountability is a key component of a true Just Culture. Rather, it strives to develop a better understanding of the direct relationship between the individual involved in the error and the systems within which

Asking these questions enables the team to understand the difference between an individual that committed human error and an individual that has at-risk behavior and/or reckless behavior. Human error is an inadvertent action that should be addressed by assessing/modifying and or redesigning processes, procedures, and environments, and providing additional education. At-risk behavior is one that is not recognized by the individual as being risky and can be corrected by removing the incentives for risky behavior and introducing institutional incentives for healthy behaviors. Reckless behavior involves a conscious disregard for unreasonable risk and generally requires punitive correction. This helps the institution understand the difference between "no blame" and blame, a total conscious disregard for doing the right thing.

Just Culture also mandates that every individual member of a team feel comfortable speaking up to bring attention to a potential risk without concern for personal repercussions. In an institution where Just Culture is truly embraced, any employee, from front line to executive, is enabled to "stop the line" when a patient is potentially going to experience undue harm. Achieving this type of embracement of Just Culture requires modeling by leadership. It also requires that the institution follow a specific process outlined by Dekker.[80] Additionally, it is imperative that the institution not directly punish the individual directly involved in the error provided that the behavior was not caused by an intentional disregard for protocol or conscious engagement in an unsafe act. Instead, the team recognizes that these errors are devastating to a well-intentioned team member's sense of self-worth. In fact, individuals often punish themselves for a negative outcome leading to significant self-imposed stress.[82]

One of the primary challenges in developing a Just Culture team is understanding the delicate balance between accountability and the concept of "no blame." If a team member acts out of accordance with standards of care and there are no repercussions then other team members may believe that it is permissible to do so. Contrarily, if the team member is publicly chastised and singled out for the outcome then the other team members will be reluctant to voluntarily speak up when concerning issues are recognized in the future.

Institutions with ingrained Just Culture have better morale, commitment to the organization, and job satisfaction.[83] A 2010 position statement from the American Nurses Association strongly supports the Just Culture concept and its application for health care to improve patient safety.[84] It is time that physicians not only accept it, but invest in the necessary leadership role that ultimately yields a functional team focused on the safest possible care for patients.

In summary, Just Culture embraces the following tenets:

- Emphasize quality and safety over blame and punishment
- Promote a process whereby mistakes/errors do not result in automatic punishment but a process to uncover the root cause of error
- Human errors that are not deliberate or malicious result in coaching, counseling, and education to decrease the likelihood of a repeated error
- Promote increased error reporting that leads to system improvements to create safer environments for patients and staff

SUMMARY

Surgeons are typically highly motivated human beings. They study medical journals, review patient outcomes, follow clinical practice guidelines, return to work in the middle of the night to care for the injured, and voluntarily educate other physicians and residents in training. All of this is done with the altruistic goal of providing the best possible outcomes for patients. Many, however, fail to understand that, perhaps the most important impact on outcomes is functioning as leaders for the surgical team in the OR. Surgeons have a tremendous influence over this team. It is critically important that they create an environment that enhances each person's feelings of team commitment and provides them with a safe environment where they feel comfortable looking out for the safety of patients. The tools to lead surgical teams include perioperative huddles, checklists, care standardization, development of specialized orthopedic team, Just Culture, and ensuring high-level surgeon proficiency for the procedures performed. Any of these in isolation may be inadequate for success, and one should constantly strive to achieve all of them. The onus is on surgeons to do this because patients come to surgeons, in large part, because they trust them to do so.

There is one final thought critical to success for a profession that desires the safest care possible for children in the OR. One must not forget that it is also incumbent on surgeons to train the next generation of surgeons to think about safety and to understand these methodologies.[85] The safety movement now has great inertia, and one can ensure that this momentum carries on in perpetuity by inspiring residents to think about these safety tools. Few residency programs involve residents in this type of training, yet there are numerous opportunities to do so. Residents have a tremendous amount of knowledge to acquire in a short and stress-filled period. Only by modeling these behaviors will they understand the importance of a thoughtful approach to patient surgeons. One can model the importance of these patient safety measures through incorporation of safety methodology into didactic lectures and conferences, discussions at morbidity and mortality conferences, involving residents in the peer review process, repetitive informal discussions at the scrub sink before surgery, and involvement of residents in orthopedic root cause analyses. When performed correctly, the root cause analyses can provide education for all individuals involved while also igniting them to become more thoughtful about processes that ensure safety for patients.

REFERENCES

1. A follow-up review of wrong site surgery. Sentinel Event Alert 2001;24:1–3.
2. Makary MA, Holzmueller CG, Thompson D, et al. Operating room briefings: working on the same page. Jt Comm J Qual Patient Saf 2006;32:351–5.
3. Christian CK, Gustafson ML, Roth EM, et al. A prospective study of patient safety in the operating room. Surgery 2006;139:159–73.
4. Lingard L, Espin S, Whyte S, et al. Communication failures in the operating room: an observational classification of recurrent types and effects. Qual Saf Health Care 2004;13:330–4.
5. McCulloch P, Morgan L, New S, et al. Combining systems and teamwork approaches to enhance the effectiveness of safety improvement interventions in surgery: the safer delivery of surgical services (S3) program. Ann Surg 2017;265:90–6.
6. Federal Aviation Administration Basic Pilot Briefings. Available at: https://www.faa.gov/about/office_org/headquarters_offices/ato/service_units/systemops/fs/alaskan/alaska/fai/pfpwb/. Accessed January 4, 2018.
7. Allard J, Bleakley A, Hobbs A, et al. Pre-surgery briefings and safety climate in the operating theatre. BMJ Qual Saf 2011;20:711–7.
8. Lingard L, Regehr G, Orser B, et al. Evaluation of a preoperative checklist and team briefing among surgeons, nurses, and anesthesiologists to reduce failures in communication. Arch Surg 2008;143:12–7.
9. Lingard L, Espin S, Rubin B, et al. Getting teams to talk: development and pilot implementation of a checklist to promote interprofessional communication in the OR. Qual Saf Health Care 2005;14:340–6.
10. Lingard L, Whyte S, Espin S, et al. Towards safer interprofessional communication: constructing a model of "utility" from preoperative team briefings. J Interprof Care 2006;20:471–83.
11. Makary MA, Mukherjee A, Sexton JB, et al. Operating room briefings and wrong-site surgery. J Am Coll Surg 2007;204:236–43.
12. Makary MA, Sexton JB, Freischlag JA, et al. Operating room teamwork among physicians and nurses: teamwork in the eye of the beholder. J Am Coll Surg 2006;202:746–52.
13. Jain AL, Jones KC, Simon J, et al. The impact of a daily pre-operative surgical huddle on interruptions, delays, and surgeon satisfaction in an orthopedic operating room: a prospective study. Patient Saf Surg 2015;9:8.
14. Wong DA, Lewis B, Herndon J, et al. Patient safety in North America: beyond "operate through your initials and" "sign your site". J Bone Joint Surg Am 2009;91:1534–41.
15. World Alliance for Patient Safety. Implementation manual–WHO surgical safety checklist. Safe surgery saves lives. Geneva (Switzerland): WHO Press; 2008.
16. Gawande A. The checklist manifesto: how to get things right. New York: Metropolitan Books;; 2010.
17. Haynes AB, Weiser TG, Berry WR, et al. A surgical safety checklist to reduce morbidity and mortality in a global population. N Engl J Med 2009;360:491–9.
18. van Klei WA, Hoff RG, van Aarnhem EE, et al. Effects of the introduction of the WHO "Surgical Safety Checklist" on in-hospital mortality: a cohort study. Ann Surg 2012;255:44–9.
19. Borchard A, Schwappach DL, Barbir A, et al. A systematic review of the effectiveness, compliance, and critical factors for implementation of safety checklists in surgery. Ann Surg 2012;256:925–33.
20. Conley DM, Singer SJ, Edmondson L, et al. Effective surgical safety checklist implementation. J Am Coll Surg 2011;212:873–9.
21. Russ S, Rout S, Caris J, et al. Measuring variation in use of the WHO surgical safety checklist in the operating room: a multicenter prospective cross-sectional study. J Am Coll Surg 2015;220:1–11.
22. Williams AK, Cotter RA, Bompadre V, et al. Patient safety checklists: do they improve patient safety for supracondylar humerus fractures? J Pediatr Orthop 2017;4(1):1–7.
23. O'Leary JD, Wijeysundera DN, Crawford MW. Effect of surgical safety checklists on pediatric surgical complications in Ontario. CMAJ 2016;188:E191–8.
24. Urbach DR, Govindarajan A, Saskin R, et al. Introduction of surgical safety checklists in Ontario, Canada. N Engl J Med 2014;370:1029–38.
25. Tang R, Ranmuthugala G, Cunningham F. Surgical safety checklists: a review. ANZ J Surg 2014;84:148–54.
26. Mayer EK, Sevdalis N, Rout S, et al. Surgical checklist implementation project: the impact of variable WHO checklist compliance on risk-adjusted clinical outcomes after national implementation: a longitudinal study. Ann Surg 2016;263:58–63.
27. Santiesteban L, Hutzler L, Bosco JA 3rd, et al. Wrong-site surgery in orthopaedics: prevalence, risk factors, and strategies for prevention. JBJS Rev 2016;4.
28. Gladwell M. Outliers: the story of success. New York: Little, Brown and Company; Hatchett Book Group; 2008.
29. Bookman J, Duffey R, Hutzler L, et al. The etiology of improved outcomes at high volume centers learning theory and the case of implant flashing. Bull Hosp Jt Dis (2013) 2016;74:155–9.

30. Gofton WT, Papp SR, Gofton T, et al. Understanding and taking control of surgical learning curves. Instr Course Lect 2016;65:623–31.

31. Hiemstra LA, Kerslake S, O'Brien CL, et al. Accuracy and learning curve of femoral tunnel placement in medial patellofemoral ligament reconstruction. J Knee Surg 2017;30:879–86.

32. Jackson WF, Khan T, Alvand A, et al. Learning and retaining simulated arthroscopic meniscal repair skills. J Bone Joint Surg Am 2012;94:e132.

33. Hohmann E, Bryant A, Tetsworth K. Tunnel positioning in anterior cruciate ligament reconstruction: how long is the learning curve? Knee Surg Sports Traumatol Arthrosc 2010;18:1576–82.

34. Hoppe DJ, de Sa D, Simunovic N, et al. The learning curve for hip arthroscopy: a systematic review. Arthroscopy 2014;30:389–97.

35. de Steiger RN, Lorimer M, Solomon M. What is the learning curve for the anterior approach for total hip arthroplasty? Clin Orthop Relat Res 2015;473:3860–6.

36. York PJ, Logterman SL, Hak DJ, et al. Orthopaedic trauma surgeons and direct anterior total hip arthroplasty: evaluation of learning curve at a level I academic institution. Eur J Orthop Surg Traumatol 2017;27:421–4.

37. Manley M, Ong K, Lau E, et al. Effect of volume on total hip arthroplasty revision rates in the United States Medicare population. J Bone Joint Surg Am 2008;90:2446–51.

38. Bozic KJ, Maselli J, Pekow PS, et al. The influence of procedure volumes and standardization of care on quality and efficiency in total joint replacement surgery. J Bone Joint Surg Am 2010;92:2643–52.

39. Sibley RA, Charubhumi V, Hutzler LH, et al. Joint replacement volume positively correlates with improved hospital performance on centers for Medicare and Medicaid services quality metrics. J Arthroplasty 2017;32:1409–13.

40. Maceroli M, Nikkel LE, Mahmood B, et al. Total hip arthroplasty for femoral neck fractures: improved outcomes with higher hospital volumes. J Orthop Trauma 2016;30:597–604.

41. Kempton LB, Ankerson E, Wiater JM. A complication-based learning curve from 200 reverse shoulder arthroplasties. Clin Orthop Relat Res 2011;469:2496–504.

42. Novais EN, Carry PM, Kestel LA, et al. Does surgeon experience impact the risk of complications after Bernese periacetabular osteotomy? Clin Orthop Relat Res 2017;475:1110–7.

43. Clohisy JC, Schutz AL, St John L, et al. Periacetabular osteotomy: a systematic literature review. Clin Orthop Relat Res 2009;467:2041–52.

44. Hussell JG, Rodriguez JA, Ganz R. Technical complications of the Bernese periacetabular osteotomy. Clin Orthop Relat Res 1999;363:81–92.

45. Usuelli FG, Maccario C, Pantalone A, et al. Identifying the learning curve for total ankle replacement using a mobile bearing prosthesis. Foot Ankle Surg 2017;23:76–83.

46. Pesenti S, Ecalle A, Peltier E, et al. Experience and volume are determinative factors for operative management of supracondylar humeral fractures in children. J Shoulder Elbow Surg 2018;27(3):404–10.

47. Mayo BC, Massel DH, Bohl DD, et al. Anterior cervical discectomy and fusion: the surgical learning curve. Spine (Phila Pa 1976) 2016;41:1580–5.

48. Lee JC, Jang HD, Shin BJ. Learning curve and clinical outcomes of minimally invasive transforaminal lumbar interbody fusion: our experience in 86 consecutive cases. Spine (Phila Pa 1976) 2012;37:1548–57.

49. Nandyala SV, Fineberg SJ, Pelton M, et al. Minimally invasive transforaminal lumbar interbody fusion: one surgeon's learning curve. Spine J 2014;14:1460–5.

50. Ahn J, Iqbal A, Manning BT, et al. Minimally invasive lumbar decompression-the surgical learning curve. Spine J 2016;16:909–16.

51. Sclafani JA, Kim CW. Complications associated with the initial learning curve of minimally invasive spine surgery: a systematic review. Clin Orthop Relat Res 2014;472:1711–7.

52. Nomura K, Yoshida M. Assessment of the learning curve for microendoscopic decompression surgery for lumbar spinal canal stenosis through an analysis of 480 cases involving a single surgeon. Global Spine J 2017;7:54–8.

53. Blais MB, Rider SM, Sturgeon DJ, et al. Establishing objective volume-outcome measures for anterior and posterior cervical spine fusion. Clin Neurol Neurosurg 2017;161:65–9.

54. Schoenfeld AJ, Sturgeon DJ, Burns CB, et al. Establishing benchmarks for the volume-outcome relationship for common lumbar spine surgical procedures. Spine J 2018;18:22–8.

55. Menger RP, Kalakoti P, Pugely AJ, et al. Adolescent idiopathic scoliosis: risk factors for complications and the effect of hospital volume on outcomes. Neurosurg Focus 2017;43:E3.

56. Lonner BS, Scharf C, Antonacci D, et al. The learning curve associated with thoracoscopic spinal instrumentation. Spine (Phila Pa 1976) 2005;30:2835–40.

57. Samdani AF, Ranade A, Sciubba DM, et al. Accuracy of free-hand placement of thoracic pedicle screws in adolescent idiopathic scoliosis: how much of a difference does surgeon experience make? Eur Spine J 2010;19:91–5.

58. Gonzalvo A, Fitt G, Liew S, et al. The learning curve of pedicle screw placement: how many screws are enough? Spine (Phila Pa 1976) 2009;34:E761–5.

59. Newton PO, Shea KG, Granlund KF. Defining the pediatric spinal thoracoscopy learning curve: sixty-five consecutive cases. Spine (Phila Pa 1976) 2000;25:1028–35.

60. Paul JC, Lonner BS, Toombs CS. Greater operative volume is associated with lower complication rates in adolescent spinal deformity surgery. Spine (Phila Pa 1976) 2015;40:162–70.

61. Rumalla K, Yarbrough CK, Pugely AJ, et al. Spinal fusion for pediatric neuromuscular scoliosis: national trends, complications, and in-hospital outcomes. J Neurosurg Spine 2016;25:500–8.

62. Paul JC, Lonner BS, Goz V, et al. An operative complexity index shows higher volume hospitals and surgeons perform more complex adult spine deformity operations. Bull Hosp Jt Dis (2013) 2016;74. 292–269.

63. Simpson AH, Howie CR, Norrie J. Surgical trial design: learning curve and surgeon volume: determining whether inferior results are due to the procedure itself, or delivery of the procedure by the surgeon. Bone Joint Res 2017;6:194–5.

64. Gofton WT, Solomon M, Gofton T, et al. What do reported learning curves mean for orthopaedic surgeons? Instr Course Lect 2016;65:633–43.

65. Finks JF, Osborne NH, Birkmeyer JD. Trends in hospital volume and operative mortality for high-risk surgery. N Engl J Med 2011;364:2128–37.

66. Birkmeyer JD, Stukel TA, Siewers AE, et al. Surgeon volume and operative mortality in the United States. N Engl J Med 2003;349:2117–27.

67. Chowdhury MM, Dagash H, Pierro A. A systematic review of the impact of volume of surgery and specialization on patient outcome. Br J Surg 2007; 94:145–61.

68. Cahill PJ, Pahys JM, Asghar J, et al. The effect of surgeon experience on outcomes of surgery for adolescent idiopathic scoliosis. J Bone Joint Surg Am 2014;96:1333–9.

69. Paul JC, Lonner BS, Goz V, et al. Complication rates are reduced for revision adult spine deformity surgery among high-volume hospitals and surgeons. Spine J 2015;15:1963–72.

70. Patrick NC, Kowalski CA, Hennrikus WL. Surgical efficiency of anterior cruciate ligament reconstruction in outpatient surgical center versus hospital operating room. Orthopedics 2017;40: 297–302.

71. Small TJ, Gad BV, Klika AK, et al. Dedicated orthopedic operating room unit improves operating room efficiency. J Arthroplasty 2013;28:1066–71.

72. Xu R, Carty MJ, Orgill DP, et al. The teaming curve: a longitudinal study of the influence of surgical team familiarity on operative time. Ann Surg 2013; 258:953–7.

73. Stepaniak PS, Vrijland WW, de Quelerij M, et al. Working with a fixed operating room team on consecutive similar cases and the effect on case duration and turnover time. Arch Surg 2010;145: 1165–70.

74. Maruthappu M, Duclos A, Zhou CD, et al. The impact of team familiarity and surgical experience on operative efficiency: a retrospective analysis. J R Soc Med 2016;109:147–53.

75. Mijaynji F. Implementing a team-based approach to pediatric spinal surgery significantly improves surgical and perioperative outcomes. Podium presentation SRS 51st Annual Meeting. Prague, Czech Republic, September 21–24, 2016.

76. Flynn JM. A dedicated pediatric spine deformity team significantly reduces surgical time and cost. Podium presentation SRS 52nd Annual Meeting. Philadelphia, PA, September 8, 2017.

77. Lencioni P. The five dysfunctions of a team summarized for busy people. New York: Wiley, John & Sons; 2014. Available at: https://quickpdf.gq/quickpdf/B00LYD3ONC-the-five-dysfunctions-of-a-team-summarized-for-busy-people.

78. Reason J. Understanding adverse events: human factor. Qual Health Care 1995;4:80–9.

79. Marx D. Patient safety and the Just Culture: a primer for health care executives. New York: Trustees of Columbia University; 2001.

80. Dekker S. Just Culture. Balancing safety and accountability. 2nd edition. Boca Raton (FL): CRC Press; 2012. p. 75–7.

81. Pellegrino ED. Prevention of medical error: where professional and organizational ethics meet. In: Sharpe VA, editor. Accountability: patient safety and policy reform. Washington, DC: Georgetown University Press; 2004. p. 83–98.

82. Berlinger N. After harm: medical error and the ethics of forgiveness. Baltimore (MD): Johns Hopkins University Press; 2005.

83. Cohen-Charash Y, Spector PE. The role of justice in organizations: a meta-analysis. Organ Behav Hum Decis Process 2001;86:278–321.

84. American Nurses Association. Position statement on Just Culture. Washington, DC: American Nurses Association; 2010. Available at: http://nursingworld.org/psjustculture. Accessed February 27, 2017.

85. Black KP, Armstrong AD, Hutzler L, et al. Quality and safety in orthopaedics: learning and teaching at the same time: AOA critical issues. J Bone Joint Surg Am 2015;97:1809–15.

Standardization of Care of Common Pediatric Fractures

Jaime Rice Denning, MD, MS*, Kevin J. Little, MD

KEYWORDS

- Quality improvement methodology • Supracondylar humerus fracture • Buckle fracture
- Standardization • Common pediatric fractures

KEY POINTS

- Quality improvement methodology is different than traditional research; done correctly, it is a regimented process, but is meant to be shared and implemented quickly.
- Using quality improvement methodology to implement an evidence-based protocol for surgical treatment of supracondylar humerus fractures, compliance among the 13 surgeons at the authors' institution increased from 0% to 85% over 2 months and was maintained for over 14 months.
- As a result of supracondylar fracture standardization, the authors also decreased the number of surgeon preference cards for this procedure from 13 to 1 and reduced variability in supply and surgical charges and charge per patient.
- Quality improvement methodology was used to implement Level-I evidence into clinical practice for treating distal radius buckle fractures.
- At 2 tertiary care institutions, the percentage of patients with distal radius buckle fractures treated with braces was increased from 34.8% to 84% over a 6-month intervention period.

INTRODUCTION

Distal radius fractures are the most common site of fracture in the pediatric population.[1–4] Supracondylar humerus (SCH) fractures are the most common surgically treated fracture of the pediatric elbow.[1–3,5] Although there is abundant literature discussing treatment and outcomes of these 2 common fractures, there is only emerging literature specifically discussing the variation in care among surgeons.[6] There is now a known need for standardization of these types of injuries to optimize the quality, safety, and value for patients. Quality Improvement (QI) methodology differs from traditional research in many important ways and is meant to be shared and used to implement changes

quickly.[7] This article will discuss the basic QI methodology and share 2 examples of specific programs that standardized the surgical care of SCH fractures at 1 institution and wrist buckle fracture care at 2 tertiary care orthopedic clinics.

QUALITY IMPROVEMENT METHODOLOGY

Over the last several years, a major focus of the health care industry has been to track the quality, safety, and value of medical care given by the health care system.[8] QI methodology is a formalized approach to analyze the performance of a health care delivery system, and to assess the impact and results of changes made to the system. A QI program involves systematic activities that are organized and implemented by a

---

Disclosure Statement: The authors have nothing to disclose.
Orthopaedic Surgery, Cincinnati Children's Hospital Medical Center, 3333 Burnet Avenue, ML 2017, Cincinnati, OH 45229, USA
* Corresponding author.
E-mail address: jaime.denning@cchmc.org

health care provider or team to monitor, assess, and improve the quality of health care being delivered. The QI methodology commonly used in health care is a framework called the Model for Improvement, and it is based on the 3 questions:

1. What are we trying to accomplish?
2. How will we know that a change is an improvement?
3. What changes can we make that will result in improvement?

There are many models of QI utilized in health care delivery, and the authors' institution adopted the System of Profound Knowledge, popularized by W. Edwards Deming.[9] This model involves the interrelationship of 4 main domains of quality improvement: the theory of knowledge, psychology, understanding variation, and the appreciation for a system (Fig. 1). The main concept of this model of QI is understanding that the system being studied has natural variability over time. By recognizing the natural, expected variability of the system over time (common cause variability), one can appreciate when unexpected variability (special cause variability) occurs, as well as track changes over time. The QI model then uses plan, do, study, act (PDSA) cycles to trial incremental changes and evaluate their effectiveness before implementing large-scale changes to the health care delivery system.[10] By utilizing this model, the system of health care delivery can be incrementally improved to maximize patient outcomes.

Although the QI methodology is a science and is performed systematically, it does differ from traditional hypothesis-driven research.[7,11] One of the important differences is that QI improves or reduces variability of a process by implementing a standardized approach to health care delivery, whereas the purpose of

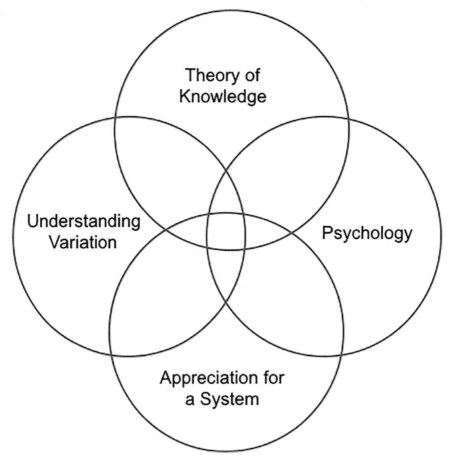

Fig. 1. The W. Edwards Deming model of quality improvement known as the system of profound knowledge. (*Data from* Lynn ML, Osborn DP. Deming's quality principles: a health care application. Hosp Health Serv Adm 1991;36(1):111–20; and Langley GJ, Moen RD, Nolan KM, et al. The improvement guide: a practical approach to enhancing organizational performance. 2nd edition. San Francisco (CA): Jossey-Bass; 2009.)

traditional research is to answer a question. QI methodology tests a process over time (usually months), and the hypothesis morphs throughout the testing, while traditional research often compares groups over a longer time course (usually years) and answers a fixed hypothesis. Additionally, the statistical methods differ between QI and traditional research. QI methodology incorporates a statistical understanding of the common cause variability of a given system with changes beyond the common cause more than 3 standard deviations away from the mean being significant (roughly equivalent to $P<.003$), whereas traditional research compares different groups with each other or similar groups before and after an intervention. QI projects do not require institutional review board (IRB) approval to begin (although it does need IRB to publish results) and is nonproprietary, with the intent of spreading improvement, whereas traditional research requires IRB approval, and the results are private until they are presented or published.

SMART Aim
As with most research projects, a QI study starts with a specific idea or problem that is noted within the health care delivery system. Within the model for improvement framework, any specific idea for improvement should begin with a SMART aim (Specific, Measureable, Actionable, Relevant, Time bound). At the authors' institution, the standard structure of a SMART aim is "we will increase/decrease (the key measure of the project) within a population from X (baseline %) to Y (goal %) by Z (target date)." This makes the aim specific. The process then has to have easily obtainable and measurable output data, such that real-time data collection can be used to help facilitate timely changes. The project team also should have a direct effect on the system such that their ideas are actionable and can lead to changes in the system output. The data collected also needs to be relevant to the aim and the global aim, such that changes in the data correlated with the expected shift in the health care delivery. Lastly, there should be a specified duration of the project, as a time-bound goal provides specificity and drive toward completion and avoids unnecessary delays. Usually if the SMART aim (and other related projects) is successfully implemented, a greater (global) aim can be achieved and sustained. All SMART aims should be developed in the context of a global aim, which incorporates how the SMART aim will fit within improving the health care system delivery.

Process Map
Once the SMART aim is fine-tuned, the next step in the QI framework is to assemble a team to create a process map. The team should consist of people involved in different areas of the process, such that different viewpoints and areas of expertise are included into the project design. There are several types of process maps, but regardless of the type, the team must critically observe the process to be studied and then list the chronologic steps in the process. In a high-level process map (the simplest kind), the beginning and ending steps are filled in first, and then the team brainstorms the 5 to 8 most important steps that occur in between the start and end points (including enough detail to identify improvement opportunities). Major decision points are marked out at each of these steps. The importance of doing this process mapping is to allow many steps to be viewed on a single page and help all the team members understand which steps may impact the outcome. It is a visual depiction that shows possible problem areas and where the possibilities for simplification or standardization may exist in the current system. It is important that the map gets shared with many different people involved in the process being studied, and the steps are edited as needed after seeking their input and further observation.

Simplified Failure Mode Effects Analysis
Failure mode effects analysis (FMEA) is a tool that can be used to identify problems or breakdowns in a process (an existing or new process) that may result in failure to achieve the desired outcome. The process map steps are filled into an FMEA, and then the team lists all of the ways that each step can fail along the bottom of the chart. Next, the members of the team address all of these failure modes by delineating all of the interventions that could be used to prevent them (**Fig. 2**).

Key Driver Diagram
Following the FMEA, the team then decides what are the key decision points that can affect changes to the system? These are included in the key driver diagram (KDD). Additional areas of intervention are identified and linked to each of the relevant key drivers along with their corresponding levels of reliability (LORs), where higher LORs are equated with more precision and standardization of the system. A KDD is a visual way of organizing the key elements that need to be in place for success of the SMART

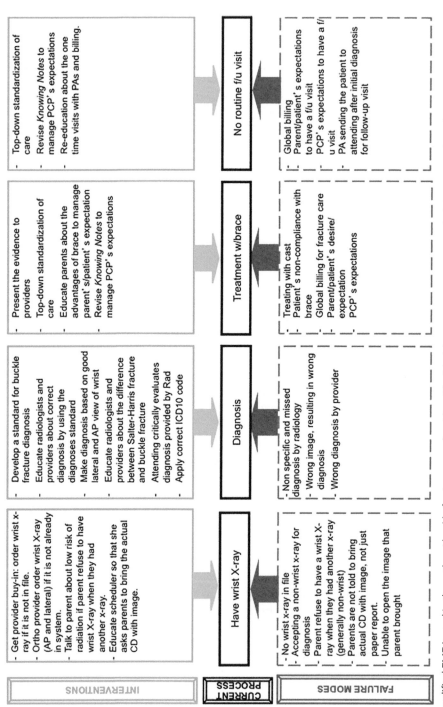

Fig. 2. The simplified FMEA used in the authors' buckle fracture care algorithm. The black boxes represent process decision points where failures may occur. The red boxes are modes of failure at each decision point, and the green boxes are ways to ameliorate these modes of failure.

aim and the actions or interventions that need to occur to assure that the key elements are in place (**Fig. 3**). Phrased another way, the key drivers are what needs to be in place for the SMART aim to succeed, and the interventions are how to achieve the necessary key drivers. The KDD is a dynamic chart that shows the organization and connections between key drivers and interventions and focuses the team on which interventions to test.

Plan-Do-Study-Act Cycles/Ramp

Once the KDD has been completed and sufficiently revised, the most important drivers of change should be tackled. The highest impact interventions are likely to be based on the highest frequency failure modes, be evidence-based, and be within the span of influence of members of the team. Oftentimes this can be accomplished by looking at the baseline data to identify areas of failure. These modes of failure can be categorized into different groups and a Pareto chart implemented. A Pareto chart will identify the most common causes of failures by organizing the modes of failures by decreasing frequency. In most cases, approximately 80% of the failures typically occur in about 20% of failure modes, and these are the failure modes that should be tackled first[12] (**Fig. 4**). PDSA cycles are then devised to address these areas of failure.

The first step is devising a plan of attack that should address the failure. The change is implemented on a small scale over a short time, and the results are studied. Based on the results of the implemented change, it can be acted upon, either by adopting it completely, adapting it into a new PDSA cycle, or abandoning or rejecting it completely. It should be noted that PDSA cycles that do not elicit change or promote negative change are often more useful and more insightful than those that elicit the expected change. There are no failed PDSA cycles, as learning opportunities are easily identified from all cycles. These cycles are organized into a ramp, where incremental changes are expanded upon to increase the scale, location, and time duration of the changes until measureable changes in the SMART aim are identified over time.

SUPRACONDYLAR HUMERUS FRACTURES

Because QI methodology can be a bit abstract, the best way to understand how to implement it is by showing examples. One of the global aims of the authors' hospital is to decrease the amount of variability (and cost) of common surgical procedures. The authors' division, therefore, chose to develop a care algorithm using QI methodology to standardize simple supracondylar fracture surgical care.

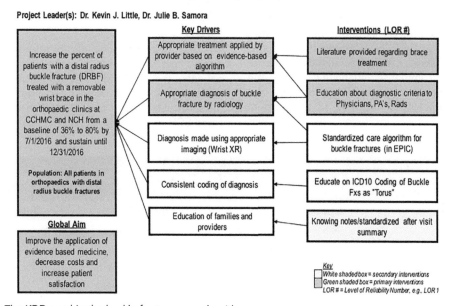

Fig. 3. The KDD used in the buckle fracture care algorithm.

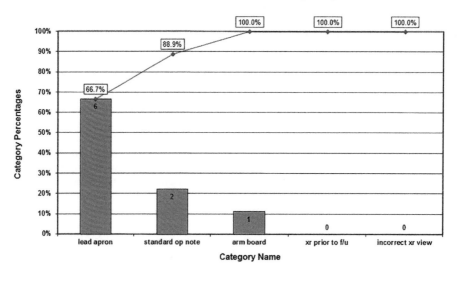

Fig. 4. Chart highlights the most common reasons for failure in compliance with the SCH fracture care algorithm.

Variation at Baseline

SCH fractures are the most common type of pediatric elbow fractures.[5] There is extreme variability among different hospitals and even among surgeons at the same hospital in the surgical treatment of this common injury. The American Board of Orthopedic Surgery (ABOS) has realized the need for improving quality, safety, and value of orthopedic care and has developed a performance improvement questionnaire (PIQ) for surgeons who treat SCH. Using this ABOS PIQ as part of a larger survey, Iobst and colleagues[6] found that uniform consensus among 35 surgeons at 6 hospitals was only 27%. Consensus among the surgeons within 1 hospital group was slightly better at 49%, but this immense variability illustrates the need for standardization. To understand the practice variability among the 13 surgeons at the authors' own institution, a survey was

conducted, which showed that there was no consensus regarding positioning (using an arm board vs using the portable c-arm as a table), draping (draping out the entire upper extremity vs draping out only the flexed elbow), timing of postoperative visits (1 week vs 4 weeks vs other), timing of postoperative radiographs (1 week vs 4 weeks vs other), and postoperative immobilization (cast vs splint vs other form of immobilization). The operating room (OR) staff had 13 different preference cards (one for each surgeon) for this 1 common procedure (Table 1).

SMART Aim

Working toward a global aim of improving efficiency, cost and quality of care for orthopedic patients, the study aim was to develop and implement a standardized care algorithm for the surgical treatment of patients with uncomplicated SCH to decrease the cost of care, number

Table 1
Prestandardization survey results showing the variability of 13 surgeons' preferences for the treatment of SCH fractures at the authors' institution

Component	Option 1	Option 2	Option 3
Positioning	44% - green arm board	27% - C-arm	
Draping	72% - whole arm	27% - Other	
Postoperative visits	27% −1 week	45% - 4 week	27% - Other
Radiographs	27% - @ 1 week	18% - @ 4 week	55% - Other
Cast versus splint	43% - cast	43% - splint	14% - Other

of visits, and radiation exposure (intra- and post-operatively). The authors defined uncomplicated SCH as a type II or III SCH requiring closed reduction and percutaneous pinning (CRPP). The authors excluded patients who needed open reduction, internal fixation (ORIF), or vascular/nerve exploration. The main process metric that they measured was "percentage of SCH fracture patients treated according to the standard care algorithm," but they also measured percentage of component compliance with each of the 4 components of the algorithm. Using the standard format, the SMART aim was "we will increase the percentage of uncomplicated SCH fracture patients treated according to the standard care algorithm from baseline of 0% to goal of 80% by 3 months from now."

Process Map

Working with a team made up of 3 attending orthopedic surgeons who care for supracondylar humerus fractures, 1 orthopedic business director, 2 ambulatory nurses, 1 OR circulating nurse, 2 research associates, and 2 quality improvement consultants, the authors outlined the process for an uncomplicated type II or type III supracondylar humerus fracture treated with CRPP (**Fig. 5**). The authors then decided on the key decision points, including whether the patient was positioned with the appropriate arm board, if the lead apron was placed under the patient's body, whether the standard operative note template was used, if the patient followed at the appropriate time point based on his or her postoperative immobilization (cast vs splint), and whether the appropriate radiographs (2-view elbow) were taken at the correct interval from surgery.

Consensus

At the start of algorithm development, a literature search was performed to identify areas for

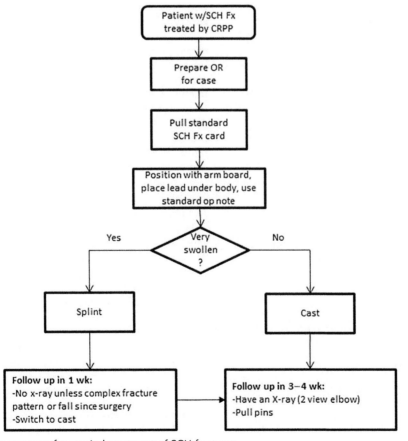

Care Algorithm for Surgical Treatment of Uncomplicated Supracondylar Humerus Fractures (SCH Fx)

Fig. 5. Process map for surgical treatment of SCH fractures.

potential practice standardization. This initial evidence-based algorithm was tested with 5 attending surgeons over a 2-month period. The algorithm recommendations were edited based on concerns about radiation exposure (related to positioning of the C-arm), leading to a recommendation that the lead be placed underneath the patient during the procedure.[13,14] Consensus discussions took place at academic faculty meetings, and once the final algorithm for treatment of uncomplicated supracondylar fractures was presented, this algorithm achieved 100% consensus among attending physicians in the division of orthopedics (13 surgeons).

Measures

The primary outcome was the overall adherence to the supracondylar care algorithm, defined as the percentage of patients diagnosed with an SCH fracture who were treated with CRPP according to all of the algorithm recommendations (appropriate positioning on the arm board, placement of lead shield under the patient, use of standardized operative note, no radiographs between operative fluoroscopy and 3- 4-week follow-up visit, and use of 2-view elbow radiograph). Adherence was measured for groups of 10 consecutive patients, to account for seasonal variability in volume. This was tracked on a P-chart using weekly and monthly data collection of the number of patients with SCH treated with CRPP. Secondary outcomes included the type of imaging performed at the follow-up visit, time to follow-up and whether it was completed, and surgical and overall charges per patient. All patients were followed until union to verify that there were no malunions or nonunions.

Key Driver Diagram

The team identified the key drivers as:

1. Effective care algorithm to treat uncomplicated SCH fractures
2. High provider buy-in to follow the algorithm
3. Availability of a standardized preference card for SCH fractures
4. Preoccupation with patient safety

Once these key drivers were outlined, appropriate interventions were identified to facilitate adoption of these drivers (Fig. 6).

Plan, Do, Study, Act Testing

Five (of the 13 total) surgeons trialed the care algorithm on an average of 2 patients each over a 2-month period. During trialing, concerns were expressed about possible increased radiation exposure as a result of C-arm placement and

deflection from the lead being placed over the patient. This is reflected in the Pareto chart (see Fig. 4) as lead apron being the most frequent mode of failure during early testing. Discussion with the hospital/radiology physicist revealed that deflection would not be an issue if the lead was placed on the table and under the patient. The protocol was modified to include these instructions. Monthly faculty meetings were used to discuss perceived difficulties with the protocol, so when there was trouble correctly placing patient's arm on the armboard, the team provided training material to the OR staff with pictures showing the correct placement.

After the initial trial period, the algorithm was trialed on a larger scale by the entire department. A 1-page document detailing the care algorithm was created to streamline education. The orthopedic attending physicians received ongoing reminders and compliance data regarding the care algorithm during monthly faculty meetings. The team leader educated fellows, advanced practice nurses (APRNs), and residents at the beginning of their rotations. For OR staff, in-person education was provided, and the 1-page document was posted in the ORs and the supply room to serve as a visual reminder.

The team worked with the OR and sterile processing department to decrease the number of doctor preference cards from 13 to 1, and a single surgical supply pack was created for SCH fracture CRPP. The team worked with the EPIC team to create a standardized template for the operative note for CRPP for SCH, which assisted providers in accurate documentation and facilitated accurate data collection for algorithm compliance.

Results

The percentage of patients with uncomplicated SCH who were treated according to the SCH care algorithm went from 0% at baseline to 85% at the end of the study period. This constituted a significant change defined by a change in the baseline data of 7 consecutive data points above the previous median (Fig. 7).

Sustainability

Once the project reached a steady state of greater than 80% compliance, a sustainability plan was enacted. The key steps to this plan were

- Continuous tracking of data for 12 months, followed by quarterly tracking of 10 to 20 patients in order to ensure maintained

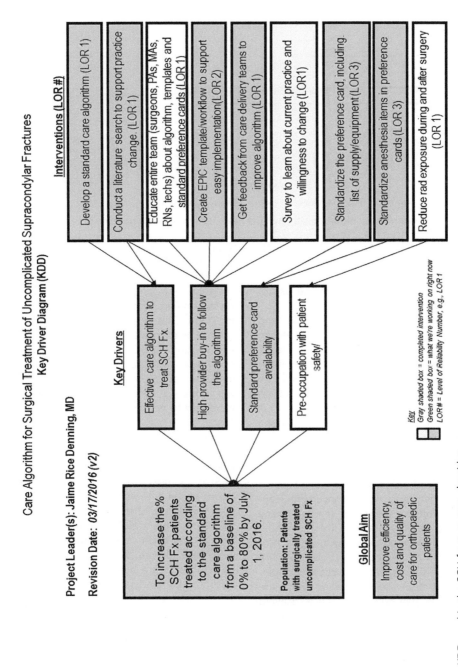

Fig. 6. The KDD used in the SCH fracture care algorithm.

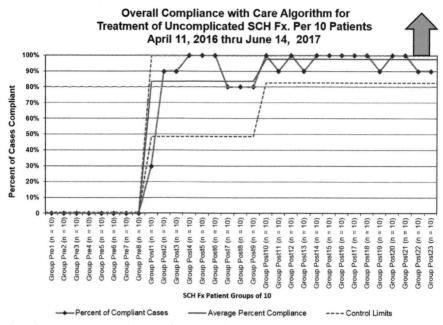

Fig. 7. P-chart demonstrating compliance with the SCH fracture surgical care algorithm.

compliance. The most recent quarterly data (21 months after implementation) showed 100% algorithm compliance.

- New hires will be trained on the use of care algorithm.
- Control charts for clinical, process, and financial outcomes will be reviewed at quarterly team meetings and at faculty meetings until the end of the calendar year. The cause of failures will be investigated by the team, and actions will be taken appropriately.
- Key measures will be maintained on a dashboard as part of the existing ongoing performance monitoring process.

Lessons Learned/Next Steps

From this project and other concurrent standardization projects, the team learned many techniques to help create positive change in the hospital. By starting slowly with a few providers and then ramping up as problems were addressed with the algorithm, successful implementation was step-wise but steady up to the goal of greater than 80% compliance. Staying focused on 1 common orthopedic condition (without the involvement of other divisions) helped the team with standardization. Compliance data were difficult to collect automatically, so the criteria included in the algorithm had to be limited to use resources efficiently; the standardized operative note helped make data collection easier, but implementing the

standardized operative note took a long time due to EPIC resource allocation. There was buy-in from OR staff, because they appreciate the value of having 1 algorithm for all surgeons for a common procedure. There were some unintended consequences of the standard algorithm. For example, an adequate neurovascular examination for SCH patients was documented only about 20% to 30% of the time prior to implementation of the algorithm, but with the standard operative note, documentation increased to nearly 100%.

Summary

Using QI methodology to implement an evidence-based protocol for surgical treatment of SCH fractures, compliance among the 13 surgeons at the authors' institution increased from 0% to 85% over 2 months and was maintained for over 14 months. This model of health care change has been used in multiple other ways within the authors' division and throughout the hospital to create positive change and increase quality, value, and safety for patients.

BUCKLE FRACTURES
Variation at Baseline

Distal radius fractures are the most common fracture in children. Buckle fractures, where the cortical bone crumples but remains intact with metaphyseal trabecular fracturing, are stable variants of pediatric buckle fractures. As such, there are many treatment methods that result in timely healing, including braces, splints, elastic bandages, and casts for a recommended period of 1 to 4 weeks. Numerous randomized, controlled trials have demonstrated that removable braces or splints provide similar outcomes to casting, and provide for improved patient satisfaction, decreased medical costs, and a faster return to function. However, a survey of pediatric orthopedists demonstrated that only 29% routinely prescribed braces for these fractures.[15] A survey of data from 2 tertiary care facilities demonstrated a similar baseline finding, with only 36% of pediatric buckle fractures treated in removable braces combined.

SMART Aim

Working toward a global aim of improving efficiency, cost, and quality of care for orthopedic patients, the study aim was to develop and implement a standardized care algorithm for the treatment of patients with distal radial buckle fractures in order to reduce the variability of the care received, as well as the cost of care and the number of visits necessary for healing beginning in December of 2015. The authors included all pediatric buckle fractures, and defined a buckle fracture as an incomplete fracture of the distal radius metaphysis or metadiaphysis without cortical discontinuity and with buckling on at least 1 view, with at least 2 points of inflection.[16] Excluded were patients with fracture lines heading toward the physis or any cortical discontinuity. The main process metric measured was the percentage of distal radius buckle fractures treated according to the standard care algorithm, including the use of a removable brace, no follow-up visit and no

further imaging needed to verify healing. Using the standard format, the authors' SMART aim was "we will increase the percentage of buckle fracture patients treated according to the standard care algorithm from baseline of 36% to goal of 80% by July 1, 2016."

Process Map

Working with a team from 2 tertiary care medical centers, made up of 4 attending orthopedic surgeons, a hand surgery fellow, a physician assistant, 3 research associates and 3 quality improvement consultants, the authors outlined the process for a clinical visit for a patient with a distal radius buckle fracture. The authors then decided on the key decision points, including if they had appropriate wrist radiographs from their initial diagnostic visit, met diagnostic criteria for a buckle fracture, and if they were treated in a brace with no follow-up. The authors included their strict definition of a buckle fracture (**Fig. 8**).

Consensus

Consensus discussions took place at academic faculty meetings for both institutions. The authors used a PowerPoint presentation to help define the diagnostic criteria and treatment choices available for the treatment of buckle fractures and highlighted the relevant literature demonstrating superior patient satisfaction and lower medical costs with removable brace treatment compared with castings. At 1 institution, 8 of 11 attending physicians agreed to implement the algorithm, with 2 additional attending physicians participating partially and 1 attending physician abstaining. At the second institution, all 7 of the faculty members agreed to

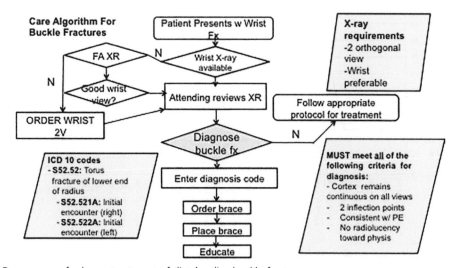

Fig. 8. Process map for brace treatment of distal radius buckle fractures.

participate. Overall, 15 of 18 providers routinely (>67% of the time) prescribed braces for distal radius buckle fractures, and only 1 provider continued to prescribe casts with 3- to 4-week follow-up for all buckle fracture patients.

Measures

The primary outcome was the overall adherence to the care algorithm, defined as the percentage of patients who were diagnosed with a buckle fracture and were treated with a brace and no follow-up appointment. This was tracked on a P-chart using weekly and monthly data collection of the number of patients with buckle fractures treated at both institutions (Fig. 9). Additionally, 1 attending physician at each institution tracked all distal radius fractures treated in the clinic and underwent a blinded review of the radiographs to confirm the correct diagnosis and to ensure that more severe fracture patterns (ie, complete fractures, or physeal fractures) were inappropriately treated in removable splints. Secondary outcomes measures included the costs of each treatment episode and the number of radiographs obtained for each treatment episode. Additionally, patients were tracked for 90 days to ensure that no unexpected return visits for were made for their buckle fracture care.

Key Driver Diagram

The 2 institutions developed a combined KDD to identify the key components to the care algorithm to drive the change identified in the SMART aim. The identified key drivers were

1. Appropriate treatment applied by providers based on evidence-based algorithm
2. Appropriate diagnosis of buckle fracture by radiology and provider
3. Diagnosis made with appropriate imaging (AP and lateral view wrist radiographs)
4. Consistent ICD-10 (International Classification of Diseases) coding of diagnosis at clinical visit
5. Education of families and providers

Once these drivers were identified, appropriate interventions were designed to facilitate adoption of the key drivers (see Fig. 3).

Plan, Do, Study, Act Testing

The first PDSA cycle included the orthopedic fellow attending fracture clinics with providers who were low on buckle fracture compliance during baseline data collection. The fellow assisted in identifying patients with buckle fractures and educating providers on the appropriate ICD-10 codes and treatment methods. This was then spread to multiple providers during fracture clinics, then to all providers in all clinics during PDSA cycles at both institutions. Monthly faculty meetings were used as a platform for eliciting feedback from providers in order to facilitate changes to the algorithm or clinic processes and aid in the appropriate diagnosis, coding, and treatment of buckle fractures. Regular compliance updates were provided to both individuals and in the form of P-charts and provider-specific bar charts. For those providers with lower compliance, a member of the care algorithm team would

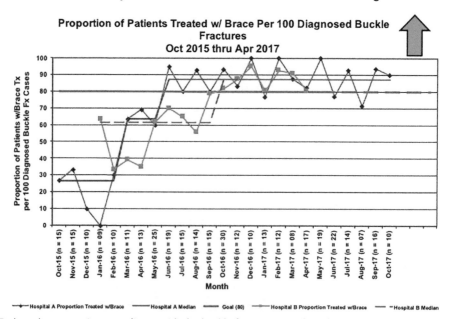

Fig. 9. P-chart demonstrating compliance with the buckle fracture care algorithm at 2 tertiary care institutions.

privately contact that individual provider to elicit feedback from them and to discuss concerns and understand impediments to brace treatment. Repeated education on the algorithm and correct identification of buckle fractures along with additional evidence-based literature were provided to low-compliance providers and their staff as indicated. The most commonly cited reason for providing cast treatment was patient or family choice. Patients and families who professed an interest in casting as compared to a removable brace were given an overview of the evidence behind brace treatment, the costs associated with both treatment regimens, and the need for follow-up if they chose a cast. The authors amended the care algorithm such that, for patients/families professing a desire for casting despite the educational resources given to them, these would not be counted as failures, since the appropriate treatment was offered.

Results

The percentage of patients with a distal radius buckle fracture treated in a brace went from a combined 34.8% to 84% at the end of the study period. This constituted a significant change as defined by a change in the baseline data corresponding to 7 consecutive data points above the previous median. The chance of 7 consecutive data points being above the median through normal data variability is approximately 0.3%, or about 3 standard deviations from the mean, roughly equivalent to a P value of about .003. Additionally, the authors only noted a 2% rate of unexpected follow-up visits associated with brace treatment, mostly due to patient noncompliance once they left the physician's office (see **Fig. 9**).

Sustainability

Once the project reached a steady state of greater than 80% compliance, a sustainability plan was enacted. The 4 key steps to this plan were

- Continuous tracking of data for 6 months, followed by quarterly tracking of 10 to 20 patients in order to ensure maintained compliance
- Quarterly presentation of P-charts and provider compliance at administrative meetings during dashboard reviews
- Elicit concerns with the algorithm at administrative meetings
- Physician-to-physician private discussions with providers demonstrating low compliance to elicit private feedback and influence change

Lessons Learned/Next Steps

Over the duration of the project, the authors learned many lessons that will help influence positive change in the future. By starting slowly with single clinics and single providers and then ramping up, the algorithm could be put into place in real time, while allowing time to adjust the algorithm and create time for provider buy-in. Additionally, meeting individually with the entire care provider's group (physician, physician assistant, nurse practitioner, medical assistant, registered nurse) allowed the authors to address team-specific concerns and needs during the implementation phase of the project. Working with families and providers to understand the risks, benefits, and costs associated with each treatment option helped present a stronger argument for brace treatment, which could help sway families and providers who were initially hesitant. One of the hardest lessons learned was that many providers are reluctant to accept changes to their practice, but also that physician buy-in to the change can be influenced by the change in practice patterns of their colleagues.

SUMMARY

This project demonstrated that QI methodology can be used to help implement Level 1 evidence into clinical practice by using a coordinated effort of monitoring, tracking, and presenting data to those practitioners who can create the desired change in practice. The process requires making small changes slowly over time and influencing those people who are initially hesitant to change their practice. This model of health care change can be used in almost any situation to improve patient outcomes, decrease costs, and improve the efficiency of health care delivery.

ACKNOWLEDGMENTS

The authors would like to thank their colleagues who were immeasurably helpful in keeping them on track and making these projects successful. This includes Roger Cornwall, Jenna Godfrey, Julie Samora, Matt Frazier, Setenay Kara-Tuncel, Nate Hanlon, Jennifer Anadio, Sandy Singleton, Jeanne Barth, Mary Hughett, Sandra Girten, and Jim McCarthy.

REFERENCES

1. Cooper C, Dennison EM, Leufkens HG, et al. Epidemiology of childhood fractures in britain: a study using the general practice research database. J Bone Miner Res 2004;19(12):1976–81.
2. Landin LA. Epidemiology of children's fractures. J Pediatr Orthop B 1997;6(2):79–83.

3. Hedström EM, Svensson O, Bergström U, et al. Epidemiology of fractures in children and adolescents. Acta Orthop 2010;81(1):148–53.

4. Bailey DA, Wedge JH, McCulloch RG, et al. Epidemiology of fractures of the distal end of the radius in children as associated with growth. J Bone Joint Surg Am 1989;71(8):1225–31.

5. Landin LA, Danielsson LG. Elbow fractures in children. An epidemiological analysis of 589 cases. Acta Orthop Scand 1986;57(4):309–12.

6. Iobst CA, Stillwagon M, Ryan D, et al. Assessing quality and safety in pediatric supracondylar humerus fracture care. J Pediatr Orthop 2017;37(5):e303–7.

7. McCarthy JJ, Alessandrini EA, Schoettker PJ. POSNA quality, safety, value initiative 3 years old and growing strong POSNA precourse 2014. J Pediatr Orthop 2015;35(5 Suppl 1):S5–8.

8. Brighton BK. National surgical quality improvement program-pediatric (NSQIP) and the quality of surgical care in pediatric orthopaedics. J Pediatr Orthop 2015;35(5):S48–50.

9. Lynn ML, Osborn DP. Deming's quality principles: a health care application. Hosp Health Serv Adm 1991;36(1):111–20.

10. Langley G, Moen RD, Nolan KM, et al. The improvement guide: a practical approach to enhancing organizational performance. San Francisco (CA): Jossey-Bass Publishers; 2009. https://doi.org/10.1002/ptr.3379.

11. Solberg LI, Mosser G, McDonald S. The three faces of performance measurement: improvement, accountability, and research. Jt Comm J Qual Improv 1997;23(3):135–47.

12. Best M, Neuhauser D. Joseph Juran: overcoming resistance to organisational change. Qual Saf Health Care 2006;15(5):380–2.

13. Hsu RY, Lareau CR, Kim JS, et al. The effect of C-arm position on radiation exposure during fixation of pediatric supracondylar fractures of the humerus. J Bone Joint Surg Am 2014;96(15):e129.

14. Kaplan DJ, Patel JN, Liporace FA, et al. Intraoperative radiation safety in orthopaedics: a review of the ALARA (As low as reasonably achievable) principle. Patient Saf Surg 2016;10(1). https://doi.org/10.1186/s13037-016-0115-8.

15. Boutis K, Howard A, Constantine E, et al. Evidence into practice: pediatric orthopaedic surgeon use of removable splints for common pediatric fractures. J Pediatr Orthop 2015;35(1):18–23.

16. TerreBlanche B, Eismann E, Laor T, et al. Distal radius buckle fracture misdiagnosis in children. 2016 Annual Meeting American Association for Hand Surgery. Scottsdale (AZ), January 13–16, 2016.

Quality, Safety, and Value in Pediatric Spine Surgery

Bayard C. Carlson, MD, Todd A. Milbrandt, MD, MS, A. Noelle Larson, MD*

KEYWORDS

- Infection • Implant density • Cost • Scoliosis

KEY POINTS

- Progress has been made toward the elimination of surgical site infections in pediatric spine surgery with the use of topical antibiotic powder and multidisciplinary pathways.
- Reducing the length of stay following pediatric spine surgery has been shown to provide modest cost savings and may provide positive clinical benefits for patients.
- Given the potential financial impact and clinical benefit for patients, the appropriate pedicle screw density should be used for patients undergoing pediatric spine surgery.
- A variety of intraoperative techniques from tactile sensation to computed-tomography (CT)–guided navigation can help surgeons minimize the risk of pedicle screw malposition and its associated consequences.
- Physicians should implement strategies designed to reduce radiation exposure with posteroanterior versus anteroposterior imaging, low-dose CT, and minimization of radiographs.

Quality, safety, and value initiatives (QSVIs) have increasingly been implemented in orthopedic centers. A review of the reported outcomes following pediatric spine surgery quickly shows the need for improvement (Table 1). For all pediatric spine surgeries, the Scoliosis Research Society's Morbidity and Mortality database reports overall complications rates at 8.5%, infection rates at 2.7%, and new neurologic deficits at 1.4%.[1] For scoliosis surgery in particular, there was a 10% complication rate, 0.7% new neurologic deficit for patients treated with pedicle screws, 0.3% mortality for congenital and neuromuscular scoliosis, and 0.02% mortality for idiopathic scoliosis.[2] Outcomes at 30 days postoperatively from patients entered in the National Surgical Quality Improvement Program's (NSQIP) database show a 10% complication rate, 0.15% mortality, and 3.7% reoperation rate.[3] Morbidity was highest in neuromuscular patients at 13.0% and lowest in the idiopathic cohort (5.7%).[3] For adolescent idiopathic scoliosis, the 2-year return to the operating room (OR) for all pedicle screw constructs is high at 3.5%[4] and the 5-year follow-up was reported at 7.5% return to the OR.[5] With the advent of quality initiatives, major progress has been made to decrease the length of stay, lower blood transfusion rates, and reduce infection rates; but further comprehensive work is needed.

Many of the quality premises now being used in medicine are taken from other industries, including aviation and manufacturing. A multidisciplinary approach is key, engaging teams in the

---

Funding: A.N. Larson was supported by an NIH grant from the National Institute of Arthritis and Musculoskeletal and Skin Diseases (R03 AR 66342).

Disclosures: A.N. Larson has received research support from the Scoliosis Research Society, Orthopedic Research and Education Foundation, and research support through consulting fees/honorarium from K2M and Orthopediatrics. T.A. Milbrandt and A.N. Larson have received research support from POSNA. T.A. Milbrandt has received research support through consulting fees from Orthopediatrics. B.C. Carlson has no disclosures.

Department of Orthopedic Surgery, Mayo Clinic Rochester, Mayo Clinic, 200 First Street Southwest, Rochester, MN 55905, USA

* Corresponding author.

E-mail address: larson.noelle@mayo.edu

Orthop Clin N Am 49 (2018) 491–501

https://doi.org/10.1016/j.ocl.2018.05.007

Table 1 Complications in pediatric spine surgery	
Major Complication Rate	
Fu[1]	
Rate for all pediatric spine surgery	8.5%
Reames[2]	
Rate for all diagnoses	10%
Rate for neuromuscular scoliosis	17.9%
Rate for congenital scoliosis	10.6%
Rate for idiopathic scoliosis	6.3%
Pugley[3]	
Rate for all diagnoses	10%
Infection Rate	
Fu[1]	
Rate for all pediatric spine surgery	2.7%
Pugley[3]	
Rate for neuromuscular scoliosis	1.5%
Rate for congenital scoliosis	0%
Rate for idiopathic scoliosis	1.4%
Marks[8]	
Rate for idiopathic scoliosis	1.6%
Mackenzie[9]	
Rate for neuromuscular scoliosis	9.2%
Rate for syndromic scoliosis	8.4%
Rate for congenital scoliosis	3.9%
Rate for idiopathic scoliosis	2.6%
Neurologic Deficit	
Fu[1]	
Rate for all pediatric spine surgery	1.4%
Reames[2]	
Rate for congenital scoliosis	2.0%
Rate for neuromuscular scoliosis	1.1%
Rate for idiopathic scoliosis	0.8%
Return to the Operating Room	
Pugley[3]	
Rate for all diagnoses	3.7%
Rate for congenital scoliosis	6.2%
Rate for neuromuscular scoliosis	5.5%
Rate for idiopathic scoliosis	2.8%
Samdani[4]	
2-y rate for idiopathic scoliosis	3.5%
Ramo[5]	
5-y rate for idiopathic scoliosis	7.5%

Plan-Do-Study-Act cycle. In addition, multiple interventions are undertaken at once, including bundles to address a specific topic, such as surgical site infection, from different angles concomitantly. Although this results in rapid implementation, the downside is that it is difficult to determine which dosing, timing, and screening strategies are most effective. The very nature of QSVI entails simultaneous implementation of multiple quality improvement measures, which allows little room for scientific method to determine which interventions are worthwhile. Thus, quality initiatives must work in tandem with high-quality research to determine which interventions should be implemented on a large scale and which patient populations may most benefit. Clear areas for quality improvement in the realm of pediatric spine surgery include lowering the infection risk, reducing the length of stay, maximizing value by achieving optimal screw numbers for fusion surgeries, eliminating the return to the OR for pedicle screw malposition, and improving patient safety by reducing radiation exposure and neurologic events. This article summarizes the recent developments in each of these areas.

INFECTION

Surgical site infections (SSIs) following surgery for pediatric spinal deformity are significant complications with rates ranging from 0.5% to 2.6% in idiopathic scoliosis and up to 40% in patients undergoing surgery for early onset scoliosis.[6–9] There is a paucity of level 1 evidence to help guide physicians in the prevention and management of SSIs following pediatric spinal surgery. Because infections are relatively rare, it is difficult to perform a randomized controlled trial with SSI as the outcome, as many patients would need to be prospectively enrolled. Most series are retrospective, case control studies, or based on registry or administrative data sets.[10] Thus, practices vary among surgeons and institutions. A recent survey illustrated the variability in clinical strategies for infection prevention among physicians managing patients with early onset scoliosis with growth-friendly spinal procedures.[11] To some extent, literature from the adult spinal deformity population can be applied to children; but comorbidities and patient considerations may differ.

Several meta-analyses have been performed to help summarize the existing literature and to provide evidence-based recommendations regarding the prevention of SSIs in pediatric spine patients. A recent literature review found that patients with underlying diseases, such as neuromuscular disease, as well as urinary or bowel incontinence have an increased risk of SSI.[12] Medical comorbidities, cardiac disease, congenital and neuromuscular scoliosis, and poor nutrition along with obesity are associated with SSI and wound complications.[12,13] Furthermore, these patients often require instrumentation constructs that extend to the pelvis, which has also been shown to increase the infection risk.[12,13,14]

There are several preventative steps shown in the literature that surgeons can take to reduce the infection risk. One modifiable risk factor for SSIs includes appropriate antibiotic dosing.[12] The current standard of care for perioperative infection prevention involves the provision of a first-generation cephalosporin within 1 hour of incision and continued for 24 hours postoperatively.[12] Noncompliance with the appropriate dosing and timing of perioperative antibiotics is a risk factor for SSI in pediatric spine surgery.[12,15] Further, topical vancomycin powder is now routinely being placed on spinal wounds before closure, despite warnings from the Centers for Disease Control and Prevention against prophylactic use of vancomycin due to concerns of inducing resistance.[16] Studies have shown that vancomycin power placed on the wound seems to be safe in the pediatric population, with no detectible serum levels or change in creatinine and only rare allergic side effects.[10,17,18] Preoperative chlorhexidine wipes are commonly recommended, although a recent cervical spine study showed no benefit, but only 16 patients were included in this study.[19–21] Other larger trials have shown decreased bacterial colonization rates and decreased infection risks for high-risk total knee arthroplasty after preoperative use.[19–21]

Similarly, there are high-quality studies in adult spine patients regarding the role of intraoperative irrigation, particularly a dilute betadine soak for nonallergic patients.[22,23] To date, there are limited studies in the pediatric literature that address intraoperative irrigation. There is also insufficient evidence that preoperative nasal swabs, preoperative education sheets, limited OR access, plastic surgery assistance with wound closure, or the use of ultraviolet lights have any influence on the rate of SSI specifically in pediatric spine patients.[12] Maintenance of an occlusive postoperative dressing type for several days postoperatively may also reduce postoperative wound infection.[24] A meta-analysis has found no clear evidence whether postoperative drains reduced infection risk, but drains do decrease the incidence of saturated postoperative dressings.[14,25] Recent data have shown that stainless steel implants may have a higher delayed infection rate and that, once established, it is more difficult to retain implants and eradicate the infection in patients with stainless steel instrumentation.[26] Patients with adolescent idiopathic scoliosis (AIS) with prominent implants may have a higher risk of SSI.[14]

Study groups have formulated best practice guidelines for the prevention of SSI based on level 4 evidence, or expert opinion.[6,7] Patients with early onset scoliosis are at particularly high risk of infection, given multiple operative procedures and associated comorbidities (**Fig. 1**). For patients with early onset scoliosis, preoperative assessment should include a nutrition and pulmonary evaluation if there is a history of respiratory problems. Based on expert opinion, patients should have a chlorhexidine skin wash the night before surgery, the OR access should be limited, perioperative antimicrobial guidelines should strictly be followed, including perioperative intravenous (IV) prophylaxis for gram-negative bacilli

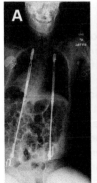
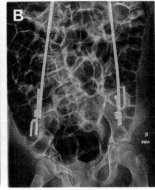
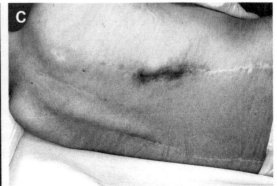

Fig. 1. (*A*) A 15-year-old patient who had a rib-based prosthesis implanted at 5 years of age for the management of neuromuscular scoliosis. After more than 15 surgeries, (*B*) he sustained a right-sided rod failure and (*C*) developed a deep fungal infection. Implant removal and final fusion is indicated.

in neuromuscular patients. Intraoperatively, the fascia/muscle incisions should not be made over the planned implant sites, intraoperative wound irrigation should be performed before closure, and topical vancomycin powder should be applied as well as an impervious bandage. Prevention and eradication of pediatric spine infection is an area that requires continued research, as SSIs remain a prevalent and expensive problem.

LENGTH OF STAY

Hospital length of stay following posterior spinal fusion (PSF) is an area for cost savings in the treatment of AIS.[27–30] Length of stay averages between 4 and 9 days for patients in North America.[28,31,32] Based in large part on the tenets imparted by projects to reduce the length of stay following other major orthopedic procedures, several centers have worked to implement systems designed to decrease hospital stays following pediatric spinal surgery.[27,28,30,33] In 2014, Fletcher and colleagues[28] published on their experience with an accelerated discharge pathway for patients following PSF for AIS. This pathway was designed to promote early mobilization and focused on early interventions, including drain and Foley catheter removal, diet initiation, aggressive pain control, and immediate mobilization.[28] When assessing the efficacy of this pathway, the investigators found that patients in the accelerated discharge pathway averaged 31.7% fewer days in the hospital (2.92 days vs 4.28 days, $P < .0001$). This decrease allowed for a 33% decrease in hospital room charges and an 11% decrease in physical therapy costs.[28] A follow-up study showed that this pathway allows for a significantly decreased hospital stay (2.17 days vs 4.21 days, $P < .0001$).[27] There was no difference between the discharge pathways in regard to readmissions or wound complications.[27,30] An accelerated discharge corresponded to a 22% decrease in postoperative hospital charges ($18,360 vs $23,640, $P < .0001$), although this does not take into account intraoperative charges, which comprise most of the cost for AIS surgery.[30,32] Implant charges alone frequently comprise greater than 50% of the total cost of AIS surgery.[34] Raudenbush and colleagues[29] argue that although accelerated discharge protocols can successfully decrease the length of hospital stays, intraoperative variables, such as spinal instrumentation and bone graft utilization, contribute far more to surgical costs. Although other variables may play a

more important role in cost containment strategies, it is important to recognize that decreasing hospital length of stay has other positive implications, including minimizing exposure to nosocomial infections, potentially an earlier return to work for parents, as well as a faster transition to the home setting for patients and their families.[27,35] Overall, decreasing the hospital length of stay following PSF seems to have positive clinical and economic benefits.

CHOOSING THE RIGHT NUMBER AND DISTRIBUTION OF PEDICLE SCREWS

Pedicle screws are the standard of care for pediatric spine instrumentation because of improved 3-dimensional (3D) correction of spinal deformity, long-term maintenance of correction, and lower revision rates due to reduced pseudarthroses.[4,36] Optimizing screw number and position is a promising target for quality improvement. Implants comprise from 30% to 50% of the total surgical cost.[32,34] A small reduction in the number of implants could easily yield as much cost savings as markedly decreasing the length of stay with potentially minimal impact on patient experience.[37] In addition to cost savings, fewer screws may result in decreased operative time, blood loss, and risk of screw malposition. If too few screws are used, however, there may be a risk of pseudoarthrosis and implant failure, potentially increasing the revision rates. Also, if fewer screws are to be used, ideal positioning in the construct and in the pedicle should be used to achieve optimal biomechanics and correction.

In decades past, hybrid fixation entailed a careful study of implant positioning, in that hooks were directional and functioned in groupings to bring about corrective forces. Screws provide better fixation; but, in contrast to hook fixation, there are less data available regarding where the screws should be positioned within the construct.[38] Early adopters of pedicle screw placement recommended high-density constructs with 2 screws per level fused.[39] Recently, based on expert consensus, a study group recommended an intermediate screw density (1.6 screws per levels fused).[40] Other reports have shown no significant difference in outcomes between high- and low-density constructs, although these studies were underpowered.[41,42] Variables contributing to curve correction include number and position of implants, rod diameter and contour, curve stiffness, and correction maneuvers. Increased implant density at the apical vertebra has shown to be correlated with curve correction in a large multicenter scoliosis database.[43] The ideal location for pedicle screw dropout is in the periapical regions. Computerized models of curve correction using both a Cotrel-Dubousset rod derotation and using cantilever bending correction technology have shown that correction does not depend on implant density. Using Cotrel-Dubousset derotation, implant density on the apical concavity is associated with rod correction.[38,44,45] Using cantilever bending, then left/right screw density does not make a difference. Further, in a counterintuitive fashion, bone-implant stresses are actually found to be higher when an increased number of implants are used because of the forces from engaging the rod in so many screw heads.[45] Thus, further work is needed to determine the optimum number and position of pedicle screws.

ELIMINATING PEDICLE SCREW MALPOSITION

Using fewer screws may reduce the risk of screw malposition. Up to 5% to 15% of pedicle screws placed with freehand or fluoroscopy are known to be malpositioned.[46–48] The consequence and recommended treatment of malpositioned is not well-agreed on in the literature.[49] Some surgeons think that asymptomatic malpositioned screws can safely be ignored. Asymptomatic medial breeches in neurologically intact patients may likely be safely observed, although delayed headache due to cerebrospinal fluid leak and acquired Chiari malposition has been described due to upper thoracic screw malposition.[49] Kim and colleagues[50] rated pedicle screw breeches as mild (<2 mm), moderate (2–4 mm), or severe (>4 mm), whereas Ughwanogho and colleagues[46] used a slightly different methodology. Based on volumetric analysis that a pedicle or laminar hook intruded into the canal several millimeters, medial breeches less than 4 mm are thought to be safe.[51] Cadaveric dissection shows a layer of thick periosteum on the anterior vertebral body, and similarly anterior breeches less than 4 mm are likely well tolerated.[51] Lateral or anterior breeches adjacent to the great vessels hold the concern for delayed erosion of the screws into the vessels and resultant pseudoaneurysm or hemorrhage. Delayed vascular and esophageal injury have also been reported due to pedicle screw malposition. The most frequent consequence of screw malposition is return to the OR for screw removal or revision, which is reported in up to 0.66% to 3.0% of operative cases.[52–55] Neurologic complications due to pedicle screw position have been reported in

0.15% of patients.[52] In this era of health care payment for quality not quantity, the concept of never events has been advanced for SSIs, urinary tract infections, and readmission, none of which seem completely preventable. However, returning to the OR for screw malposition could also be declared a never event.

Multiple advanced technologies are available to decrease the rate of screw malposition. First-generation techniques include the use of a ball-tip ped probe to feel the pedicle, which has an accuracy of 80% for an attending surgeon and 60% to 70% for a trainee.[56] Screw stimulation or a stimulated pedicle probe can be used in conjunction with neuromonitoring where low measured resistance points to a pedicle screw breech. Fluoroscopy can be used, and fluoroscopic times vary widely. The region at most risk for screw malposition is in the upper thoracic spine (T3–T8), where the pedicles are smallest,[57,58] so if adjunct safety measures are to be used, the upper thoracic levels deserve the most attention. Robotic assistance can be used with a robotic arm directing a drill guide based on preoperative computed tomography (CT) imaging.[59] A 3D model or preprinted drill guides can be custom-printed to help guide screw placement. A range of CT-guided navigation options exist as well.

CT-guided navigation has been shown to improve screw accuracy from 85% to 90% up to 95% to 99%.[60–62] Either an intraoperative CT can be performed to provide computer-assisted navigation or a CT check spin can be performed to verify correct screw position before or after rod placement. Thus, further work is underway to reduce the return to OR for screw malposition, which is a measurable phenomenon. It will be difficult to show a change in the rare catastrophic cases of neurologic compromise or vascular injuries, because the reported literature really only includes case reports; but metrics including return to the OR due to screw malposition likely can be reduced by advanced intraoperative techniques.

New technology has its drawbacks. Downsides of intraoperative CT include expense to obtain and maintain the machine as well as personnel to operate the device. Infection rates, blood loss, and operative times have not been shown to be affected by intraoperative navigation or robotics. Another concern includes radiation exposure to patients and the OR team.

REDUCING RADIATION EXPOSURE

Many of the aforementioned navigation techniques require either a preoperative or an intraoperative CT scan, resulting in increased radiation exposure to patients. In addition, patients with scoliosis are known to have significant cumulative exposure to radiation, which historically resulted in increased cancer risk in adulthood.[63–66]

A pediatric dose setting should be used for every intraoperative CT navigation setup. A variety of protocols have been described in the literature, most commonly reducing the setting to 80 kV, 20 mA, and 80 mAs for patients less than 80 kg without stainless steel implants in place.[67–70] For more than 80 kg and with stainless implants in place, higher settings are typically needed. One low-dose CT scan represents approximately 85 thoracic spine fluoroscopy images, an intraoperative posteroanterior (PA)/lateral 2-view spine series, or 0.65 mSv.[67] Annual background radiation is around 3 mSv, and a chest radiograph is 0.1 mSv. Millisieverts measure the effect of radiation on the entire body. This unit was initially developed to quantify occupational risk. Up to 20 mSv of annual occupational radiation exposure is allowable, and up to 1 mSv of annual environmental exposure to the general population is acceptable without notification (ie, nuclear plant operating next to a town).

In contrast to adolescent patients, patients with early onset scoliosis are exposed to very high amounts of radiation, with one-half of the exposure due to x-rays. Two investigators reported extreme levels of exposure, including 87 mSv cumulative radiation dose and 22.5 mSv in the year before growing rod surgery.[71,72] Interestingly, patients with early onset scoliosis may have more exposure due to x-rays than from axial imaging.

Cumulative radiation exposure for patients with nonoperative and operative AIS would typically experience during the course of scoliosis treatment has been evaluated.[73] In general, lateral radiographs result in more radiation exposure than PA or anteroposterior radiographs (Table 2). PA radiographs are preferable in that there is reduced radiation exposure to the breast, testes, and thyroid, which are considered radiosensitive organs. Use of biplanar slot scanning imaging may reduce cumulative radiation exposure from serial radiographs from 5.38 mSv to 2.66 mSv.[73,74] Further introduction of the microdose may result in another 70% to 80% reduction in cumulative radiation exposure, bringing the total dose down to 0.2 mSv for the entire course of treatment.[75] Whether these further reductions are clinically meaningful and ultimately result in decreased

cancer risk will be difficult to detect. Highlights of biplanar slot scanning imaging include the ability to build 3D reconstructions and improved radiology workflow, whereas the downsides include cost, increased space needs than a traditional x-ray machine (higher ceiling height), and potential for motion artifact, because children have to stand very still for approximately 6 seconds.[76]

NEUROLOGIC EVENTS

Paralysis or neurologic deficit is a catastrophic complication following pediatric spine surgery. Historical data included only the wake-up test or somatosensory evoked potentials. More recent data include motor evoked potentials, which are more sensitive, resulting in an increased frequency of alerts but essentially no false-negative events. In the last decades, the complexity of spine surgery has increased. Previously, procedures were primarily fusions, and the degree of correction with second-generation implants, including hooks and wires, limited the amount of forces that could be placed on the spine. Now in the era of pedicle screws, much more force can be applied to the spine. Osteotomies are commonly performed. Ponte osteotomies have been shown to increase the rate of neurologic alerts in adolescent idiopathic scoliosis surgery. They are routinely performed as part of the procedure at some centers with the goal of optimizing 3D deformity correction. However, many surgeons find adequate correction of routine AIS deformity without Ponte osteotomies.

Three column osteotomies provide powerful correction but have an even higher rate of neurologic events. As prospective data become available on this topic, it may be that some patients find the risks of surgery outweigh the benefits of the proposed deformity correction. Neurologic events are also frequent with growing spine surgery. Spine-based proximal fixation can result in migration of the proximal screws resulting in a neurologic deficit. Rib prosthetic devices have been associated with brachial plexus palsy, particularly when placed on the first rib. Surgical treatment of congenital kyphosis holds the highest risk of neurologic deficit. Large pediatric registries, such as NSQIP, have been used to validate these reported numbers.

Decreasing the rate of neurologic deficit following pediatric spine surgery must be part of global quality initiatives. Checklists have been created for intraoperative use in the event of

Table 2
Common scoliosis x-ray radiation dosing to organs and overall effective dose

	Microdose EOS Posteroanterior[75]	EOS Anteroposterior[73,a]	Estimated Dose Posteroanterior[73,a]			Estimated Dose Lateral[73,a]		
			EOS Posteroanterior	Scoliosis X-ray	Intraoperative Thoracic Spine	EOS Lateral	Scoliosis X-ray	Intraoperative Thoracic Spine
Thyroid (mGy)	0.0008	0.19	0.05	0.09	0.03	0.24	0.51	0.13
Lung (mGy)	0.0053	—	—	—	—	—	—	—
Reproductive organ (mGy)	0.0020	—	—	—	—	—	—	—
Breast (mGy)	—	0.19	0.02	0.08	0.05	0.16	0.21	1.70
Ovary (mGy)	—	0.08	0.08	0.27	0.00	0.09	0.25	0.00
Testicles (mGy)	—	0.25	0.04	0.02	0.00	0.05	0.02	0.00
Active bone marrow (mGy)	—	0.05	0.10	0.32	0.15	0.09	0.29	0.39
Effective dose ICRP 103, (mSv)[74]	0.0026	0.121	0.069	0.215	0.119	0.121	0.295	0.712

Abbreviations: EOS, bipolar slot scanning imaging; ICRP, International Commission on Radiological Protection.
[a] For assumed 56-kg patient, no copper filter used in standard EOS films.

neurologic monitoring change. Interventions include warming patients, increasing the blood pressure, checking for technical monitoring issues, checking for surgical issues, such as compression on neurologic structures, implant malposition, or reducing force on the implants or removing rods or implants. If available, intraoperative CT may provide a rapid assessment. Other alternatives include a wake-up test or aborting the case. Every neurologic monitoring event must be taken seriously with appropriate steps. Failure to rapidly act on neurologic monitoring events can lead to a permanent neurologic deficit.

In summary, this article addresses patient safety topics in spine surgery, including infection, length of stay, instrumentation strategies, pedicle screw malposition, radiation exposure, and neurologic events. Quality, safety, and value are concepts that are practical, easy to understand, and can be implemented on any scale and may be matched to individual practices. Further, with quality improvement, there is a culture shift to openly share information, protocols, and strategies so that more patients can rapidly benefit. The increasing costs of health care and unacceptable levels of complications demand the attention of every physician to control costs, improve safety, and increase value per dollar. If surgeons do not regulate the medical practice and take initiative, others who are not as closely connected to the needs of the patients will take over these leadership roles. The authors hope this article may serve to promote projects to reduce unplanned returns to the OR, SSIs, and neurologic events while improving long-term safety in patient care.

REFERENCES

1. Fu KM, Smith JS, Polly DW, et al, Scoliosis Research Society Morbidity and Mortality Committee. Morbidity and mortality associated with spinal surgery in children: a review of the Scoliosis Research Society morbidity and mortality database. J Neurosurg Pediatr 2011;7(1):37–41.

2. Reames DL, Smith JS, Fu KM, et al. Complications in the surgical treatment of 19,360 cases of pediatric scoliosis: a review of the Scoliosis Research Society Morbidity and Mortality database. Spine 2011;36(18):1484–91.

3. Pugely AJ, Martin CT, Gao Y, et al. The incidence and risk factors for short-term morbidity and mortality in pediatric deformity spinal surgery: an analysis of the NSQIP pediatric database. Spine (Phila Pa 1976) 2014;39(15):1225–34.

4. Samdani AF, Belin EJ, Bennett JT, et al. Unplanned return to the operating room in patients with adolescent idiopathic scoliosis: are we doing better with pedicle screws? Spine (Phila Pa 1976) 2013; 38(21):1842–7.

5. Ramo BA, Richards BS. Repeat surgical interventions following "definitive" instrumentation and fusion for idiopathic scoliosis: five-year update on a previously published cohort. Spine (Phila Pa 1976) 2012;37(14):1211–7.

6. Glotzbecker MP, St Hilaire TA, Pawelek JB, et al, Children's Spine Study Group, Growing Spine Study Group. Best practice guidelines for surgical site infection prevention with surgical treatment of early onset scoliosis. J Pediatr Orthop 2017. https://doi.org/10.1097/BPO.0000000000001079.

7. Vitale MG, Riedel MD, Glotzbecker MP, et al. Building consensus: development of a Best Practice Guideline (BPG) for surgical site infection (SSI) prevention in high-risk pediatric spine surgery. J Pediatr Orthop 2013;33(5):471–8.

8. Marks MC, Newton PO, Bastrom TP, et al, Harms Study Group. Surgical site infection in adolescent idiopathic scoliosis surgery. Spine Deform 2013; 1(5):352–8.

9. Mackenzie WG, Matsumoto H, Williams BA, et al. Surgical site infection following spinal instrumentation for scoliosis: a multicenter analysis of rates, risk factors, and pathogens. J Bone Joint Surg Am 2013;95(9):800–6. S1-2.

10. Gans I, Dormans JP, Spiegel DA, et al. Adjunctive vancomycin powder in pediatric spine surgery is safe. Spine (Phila Pa 1976) 2013;38(19):1703–7.

11. Glotzbecker MP, Garg S, Akbarnia BA, et al. Surgeon practices regarding infection prevention for growth friendly spinal procedures. J Child Orthop 2014;8(3):245–50.

12. Glotzbecker MP, Riedel MD, Vitale MG, et al. What's the evidence? Systematic literature review of risk factors and preventive strategies for surgical site infection following pediatric spine surgery. J Pediatr Orthop 2013;33(5):479–87.

13. Martin CT, Pugely AJ, Gao Y, et al. Incidence and risk factors for early wound complications after spinal arthrodesis in children: analysis of 30-day follow-up data from the ACS-NSQIP. Spine (Phila Pa 1976) 2014;39(18):1463–70.

14. Mistovich RJ, Jacobs LJ, Campbell RM, et al. Infection control in pediatric spinal deformity surgery: a systematic and critical analysis review. JBJS Rev 2017;5(5):e3.

15. Vandenberg C, Niswander C, Carry P, et al. Compliance with a comprehensive antibiotic protocol improves infection incidence in pediatric spine surgery. J Pediatr Orthop 2018;38(5): 287–92.

16. CDC, Committee HICPA. Recommendations for preventing the spread of vancomycin resistance. Morb Mortal Wkly Rep 1995;44(RR-12).

17. DeFrancesco CJ, Flynn JM, Smith JT, et al, Children's Spine Study Group. Clinically apparent adverse reactions to intra-wound vancomycin powder in early onset scoliosis are rare. J Child Orthop 2017;11(6):414–8.

18. Armaghani SJ, Menge TJ, Lovejoy SA, et al. Safety of topical vancomycin for pediatric spinal deformity: nontoxic serum levels with supratherapeutic drain levels. Spine (Phila Pa 1976) 2014;39(20): 1683–7.

19. Makhni MC, Jegede K, Lombardi J, et al. No clear benefit of chlorhexidine use at home before surgical preparation. J Am Acad Orthop Surg 2018; 26(2):e39–47.

20. Murray MR, Saltzman MD, Gryzlo SM, et al. Efficacy of preoperative home use of 2% chlorhexidine gluconate cloth before shoulder surgery. J Shoulder Elbow Surg 2011;20(6):928–33.

21. Kapadia BH, Zhou PL, Jauregui JJ, et al. Does pre-admission cutaneous chlorhexidine preparation reduce surgical site infections after total knee arthroplasty? Clin Orthop Relat Res 2016;474(7): 1592–8.

22. Tomov M, Mitsunaga L, Durbin-Johnson B, et al. Reducing surgical site infection in spinal surgery with betadine irrigation and intrawound vancomycin powder. Spine (Phila Pa 1976) 2015;40(7):491–9.

23. Cheng MT, Chang MC, Wang ST, et al. Efficacy of dilute betadine solution irrigation in the prevention of postoperative infection of spinal surgery. Spine (Phila Pa 1976) 2005;30(15):1689–93.

24. Bains RS, Kardile M, Mitsunaga LK, et al. Postoperative spine dressing changes are unnecessary. Spine Deform 2017;5(6):396–400.

25. Liu Y, Li Y, Miao J. Wound drains in posterior spinal surgery: a meta-analysis. J Orthop Surg Res 2016; 11:16.

26. Glotzbecker MP, Gomez JA, Miller PE, et al. Management of spinal implants in acute pediatric surgical site infections: a multicenter study. Spine Deform 2016;4(4):277–82.

27. Fletcher ND, Andras LM, Lazarus DE, et al. Use of a novel pathway for early discharge was associated with a 48% shorter length of stay after posterior spinal fusion for adolescent idiopathic scoliosis. J Pediatr Orthop 2017;37(2):92–7.

28. Fletcher ND, Shourbaji N, Mitchell PM, et al. Clinical and economic implications of early discharge following posterior spinal fusion for adolescent idiopathic scoliosis. J Child Orthop 2014;8(3): 257–63.

29. Raudenbush BL, Gurd DP, Goodwin RC, et al. Cost analysis of adolescent idiopathic scoliosis surgery: early discharge decreases hospital costs much less than intraoperative variables under the control of the surgeon. J Spine Surg 2017; 3(1):50–7.

30. Sanders AE, Andras LM, Sousa T, et al. Accelerated discharge protocol for posterior spinal fusion patients with adolescent idiopathic scoliosis decreases hospital postoperative charges 22. Spine (Phila Pa 1976) 2017;42(2):92–7.

31. Daffner SD, Beimesch CF, Wang JC. Geographic and demographic variability of cost and surgical treatment of idiopathic scoliosis. Spine (Phila Pa 1976) 2010;35(11):1165–9.

32. Kamerlink JR, Quirno M, Auerbach JD, et al. Hospital cost analysis of adolescent idiopathic scoliosis correction surgery in 125 consecutive cases. J Bone Joint Surg Am 2010;92(5):1097–104.

33. Husted H. Fast-track hip and knee arthroplasty: clinical and organizational aspects. Acta Orthop Suppl 2012;83(346):1–39.

34. Martin CT, Pugely AJ, Gao Y, et al. Increasing hospital charges for adolescent idiopathic scoliosis in the United States. Spine (Phila Pa 1976) 2014; 39(20):1676–82.

35. Rao RR, Hayes M, Lewis C, et al. Mapping the road to recovery: shorter stays and satisfied patients in posterior spinal fusion. J Pediatr Orthop 2017; 37(8):e536–42.

36. Kuklo TR, Potter BK, Lenke LG, et al. Surgical revision rates of hooks versus hybrid versus screws versus combined anteroposterior spinal fusion for adolescent idiopathic scoliosis. Spine (Phila Pa 1976) 2007;32(20):2258–64.

37. Larson AN, Polly DW Jr, Ackerman SJ, et al, Minimize Implants Maximize Outcomes Study Group. What would be the annual cost savings if fewer screws were used in adolescent idiopathic scoliosis treatment in the US? J Neurosurg Spine 2016;24(1): 116–23.

38. Wang X, Larson AN, Crandall DG, et al. Biomechanical effect of pedicle screw distribution in AIS instrumentation using a segmental translation technique: computer modeling and simulation. Scoliosis Spinal Disord 2017;12:13.

39. Suk SI, Lee CK, Kim WJ, et al. Segmental pedicle screw fixation in the treatment of thoracic idiopathic scoliosis. Spine (Phila Pa 1976) 1995;20(12): 1399–405.

40. de Kleuver M, Lewis SJ, Germscheid NM, et al. Optimal surgical care for adolescent idiopathic scoliosis: an international consensus. Eur Spine J 2014;23(12):2603–18.

41. Larson AN, Polly DW Jr, Diamond B, et al. Does higher anchor density result in increased curve correction and improved clinical outcomes in Adolescent Idiopathic Scoliosis (AIS)? Spine 2014. https://doi.org/10.1097/BRS.0000000000000204.

42. Larson AN, Aubin CE, Polly DW, et al. Are more screws better? A systematic review of anchor density and curve correction in adolescent idiopathic scoliosis. Spine Deform 2013;1(4):237–47.

43. Le Naveaux F, Aubin CE, Larson AN, et al. Implant distribution in surgically instrumented Lenke 1 adolescent idiopathic scoliosis: does it affect curve correction? Spine (Phila Pa 1976) 2015;40(7):462–8.

44. Delikaris A, Wang X, Boyer L, et al. Implant density at the apex is more important than overall implant density for 3D correction in thoracic adolescent idiopathic scoliosis using rod derotation and en bloc vertebral derotation technique. Spine (Phila Pa 1976) 2018;43(11):E639–47.

45. Le Naveaux F, Larson AN, Labelle H, et al. How does implant distribution affect 3D correction and bone-screw forces in thoracic adolescent idiopathic scoliosis spinal instrumentation? Clin Biomech (Bristol, Avon) 2016;39:25–31.

46. Ughwanogho E, Patel NM, Baldwin KD, et al. Computed tomography-guided navigation of thoracic pedicle screws for adolescent idiopathic scoliosis results in more accurate placement and less screw removal. Spine 2012;37(8):E473–8.

47. Ledonio CG, Polly DW Jr, Vitale MG, et al. Pediatric pedicle screws: comparative effectiveness and safety: a systematic literature review from the Scoliosis Research Society and the Pediatric Orthopaedic Society of North America task force. J Bone Joint Surg Am 2011;93(13):1227–34.

48. Baghdadi YM, Larson AN, McIntosh AL, et al. Complications of pedicle screws in children 10 years or younger: a case control study. Spine (Phila Pa 1976) 2013;38(7):E386–93.

49. Floccari LV, Larson AN, Crawford CH 3rd, et al, Minimize Implants Maximize Outcomes Study Group. Which malpositioned pedicle screws should be revised? J Pediatr Orthop 2018;38(2):110–5.

50. Kim YJ, Lenke LG, Kim J, et al. Comparative analysis of pedicle screw versus hybrid instrumentation in posterior spinal fusion of adolescent idiopathic scoliosis. Spine (Phila Pa 1976) 2006;31(3):291–8.

51. Polly DW Jr, Potter BK, Kuklo T, et al. Volumetric spinal canal intrusion: a comparison between thoracic pedicle screws and thoracic hooks. Spine (Phila Pa 1976) 2004;29(1):63–9.

52. Diab M, Smith AR, Kuklo TR. Neural complications in the surgical treatment of adolescent idiopathic scoliosis. Spine (Phila Pa 1976) 2007;32(24):2759–63.

53. Parker SL, McGirt MJ, Farber SH, et al. Accuracy of free-hand pedicle screws in the thoracic and lumbar spine: analysis of 6816 consecutive screws. Neurosurgery 2011;68(1):170–8 [discussion: 8].

54. Hicks JM, Singla A, Shen FH, et al. Complications of pedicle screw fixation in scoliosis surgery: a systematic review. Spine (Phila Pa 1976) 2010;35(11):E465–70.

55. Di Silvestre M, Parisini P, Lolli F, et al. Complications of thoracic pedicle screws in scoliosis treatment. Spine 2007;32(15):1655–61.

56. Lehman RA, Potter BK, Kuklo TR, et al. Probing for thoracic pedicle screw tract violation(s): is it valid? J Spinal Disord Tech 2004;17(4):277–83.

57. Heidenreich M, Baghdadi YM, McIntosh AL, et al. At what levels are freehand pedicle screws more frequently malpositioned in children? Spine Deformity 2015;3(4):332.

58. Zindrick MR, Knight GW, Sartori MJ, et al. Pedicle morphology of the immature thoracolumbar spine. Spine (Phila Pa 1976) 2000;25(21):2726–35.

59. Macke JJ, Woo R, Varich L. Accuracy of robot-assisted pedicle screw placement for adolescent idiopathic scoliosis in the pediatric population. J Robot Surg 2016;10(2):145–50.

60. Larson AN, Polly DW Jr, Guidera KJ, et al. The accuracy of navigation and 3D image-guided placement for the placement of pedicle screws in congenital spine deformity. J Pediatr Orthop 2012;32(6):e23–9.

61. Larson AN, Santos ER, Polly DW Jr, et al. Pediatric pedicle screw placement using intraoperative computed tomography and 3-dimensional image-guided navigation. Spine 2012;37(3):E188–94.

62. Luo TD, Polly DW Jr, Ledonio CG, et al. Accuracy of pedicle screw placement in children 10 years or younger using navigation and intraoperative CT. Clin Spine Surg 2016;29(3):E135–8.

63. Ronckers CM, Land CE, Miller JS, et al. Cancer mortality among women frequently exposed to radiographic examinations for spinal disorders. Radiat Res 2010;174(1):83–90.

64. Ronckers CM, Doody MM, Lonstein JE, et al. Multiple diagnostic X-rays for spine deformities and risk of breast cancer. Cancer Epidemiol Biomarkers Prev 2008;17(3):605–13.

65. Doody MM, Lonstein JE, Stovall M, et al. Breast cancer mortality after diagnostic radiography: findings from the U.S. Scoliosis Cohort Study. Spine (Phila Pa 1976) 2000;25(16):2052–63.

66. Simony A, Hansen EJ, Christensen SB, et al. Incidence of cancer in adolescent idiopathic scoliosis patients treated 25 years previously. Eur Spine J 2016;25(10):3366–70.

67. Su AW, McIntosh AL, Schueler BA, et al. How does patient radiation exposure compare with low-dose o-arm versus fluoroscopy for pedicle screw placement in idiopathic scoliosis? J Pediatr Orthop 2017;37(3):171–7.

68. Su AW, Luo TD, McIntosh AL, et al. Switching to a pediatric dose o-arm protocol in spine surgery significantly reduced patient radiation exposure. J Pediatr Orthop 2016;36(6):621–6.

69. Abul-Kasim K, Soderberg M, Selariu E, et al. Optimization of radiation exposure and image quality of the cone-beam O-arm intraoperative imaging system in spinal surgery. J Spinal Disord Tech 2012;25(1):52–8.

70. Sarwahi V, Payares M, Wendolowski S, et al. Low-dose radiation 3D intraoperative imaging: how low can we go? An O-arm, CT scan, cadaveric study. Spine (Phila Pa 1976) 2017;42(22):E1311–7.

71. Cannon TA, Neto NA, Kelly DM, et al. Characterization of radiation exposure in early-onset scoliosis patients treated with the vertical expandable prosthetic titanium rib (VEPTR). J Pediatr Orthopedics 2014;34(2):179–84.

72. Mundis GM Jr, Pawelek JB, Nomoto EK, et al. Longitudinal pilot analysis of radiation exposure during the course of growing rod treatment for early-onset scoliosis. Spine Deform 2016;4(1):55–8.

73. Luo TD, Stans AA, Schueler BA, et al. Cumulative radiation exposure with EOS imaging compared with standard spine radiographs. Spine Deformity 2015;3(2):144–50.

74. The 2007 recommendations of the International Commission on Radiological Protection. ICRP publication 103. Ann ICRP 2007;37(2–4):1–332.

75. Hui SC, Pialasse JP, Wong JY, et al. Radiation dose of digital radiography (DR) versus micro-dose x-ray (EOS) on patients with adolescent idiopathic scoliosis: 2016 SOSORT- IRSSD "John Sevastic Award" Winner in Imaging Research. Scoliosis Spinal Disord 2016;11:46.

76. Simon AL, Ferrero E, Noelle Larson A, et al. Stereo-radiography imaging motion artifact: does it affect radiographic measures after spinal instrumentation? Eur Spine J 2018;27(5):1105–11.

Hand and Wrist

Cost, Value, and Patient Satisfaction in Carpal Tunnel Surgery

Joseph Ingram, MD*, Benjamin M. Mauck, MD,
Norfleet B. Thompson, MD, James H. Calandruccio, MD

KEYWORDS

- Carpal tunnel release • Costs • Endoscopic • Open • Complications • Outcome
- Patient satisfaction

KEY POINTS

- The cost of carpal tunnel release (CTR) surgery can be significantly reduced by changes in location (freestanding ambulatory surgery center vs hospital) and technique (open vs endoscopic).
- The use of electrodiagnostics in the diagnosis of carpal tunnel syndrome remains a matter of controversy.
- Because of the infrequent occurrence of infection after CTR, perioperative antibiotics do not appear to be indicated.
- Patient satisfaction may relate more to shorter waiting times and the quality of the interaction with the surgeon than with the quantity of time spent.

INTRODUCTION

Carpal tunnel release (CTR) is one of the most frequently done hand/wrist procedures, with approximately 600,000 CTR procedures done each year. Approximately 2% of men and 4% of women will have CTR during their lifetimes.[1] The treatment costs associated with CTR represent a large cost to the health care system. Identifying quality, value, and safety issues associated with CTR may help identify factors that can be extrapolated to other hand and wrist procedures.

LOCATION

A number of methods for reducing costs of hand procedures have been proposed. Van Demark and colleagues[2] suggested using "minor field sterility" and wide-awake local anesthesia no tourniquet (WALNAT) to decrease costs while maintaining patient safety and satisfaction.

Others also have evaluated the use of a minor procedure room rather than a standard operating room (OR).[3–7] Leblanc and colleagues[6] reported a 0.4% rate of superficial infection and no deep infections after CTR with "field sterility." In their protocol, field sterility was obtained by preparing the hand with iodine or chlorhexidine and using the equivalent of a single drape and a sterile tray with modest instruments. Sterile gloves and masks are used, but surgeons are not gowned. No prophylactic antibiotics are given. The use of the procedure room was found to be more than twice as time-efficient and cost 73% less per case than procedures done in the OR. In a later detailed cost and efficiency analysis, they determined that open CTR done in the procedure room cost 32% less than in the OR, with similar postoperative pain control, satisfaction scores, and frequency of infection. Savings of 85% with the use of WALNAT in a

---

Campbell Clinic-University of Tennessee, Department of Orthopaedic Surgery and Biomedical Engineering, 1211 Union Avenue, Suite 510, Memphis, TN 38104, USA
* Corresponding author.
E-mail address: Jingram@campbellclinic.com

procedure room rather than the main OR for CTR were reported by Rhee and colleagues[8]

TECHNIQUE

In addition to the location of CTR, the technique used can make a marked difference in cost. Law and colleagues[9] compared 507,924 open CTRs to 68,758 endoscopic procedures in Medicare patients. Contrary to previous literature, they found that endoscopic CTR had lower charges and higher reimbursement rates than open CTR. Similar differences in reimbursement were reported by Zhang and colleagues[10]: reimbursement fees for endoscopic CTR ($2602) were significantly higher than for open CTR ($1751), primarily because of higher facility fees for endoscopic CTR. Because of the lack of clear evidence of the superiority of one procedure over the other, however, these investigators suggested that value-based health care models may favor open CTR for delivery of high-quality care while minimizing costs. Using a large database of 576,692 patients, Hubbard and colleagues[11] also found that annual charges were significantly higher for open CTR than endoscopic CTR, but reimbursements paid by Medicare were higher for endoscopic CTR. More recently, however, Kazmers and colleagues[5] compared open CTR with endoscopic CTR done in the OR procedure room and found that open CTR done with local anesthetic in the procedure room significantly minimized costs relative to other surgical methods (endoscopic CTR) and anesthetic methods (Bier block, monitored anesthesia care, general). The cost-savings of open CTR compared with endoscopic CTR have been confirmed in other studies.[3,7,12]

PREOPERATIVE AND POSTOPERATIVE PROTOCOLS

Costs of CTR may be affected not only by location and technique, but also by preoperative and postoperative protocols. The use of electrodiagnostic studies, such as nerve conduction studies, and imaging studies, such as MRI, remains a controversial topic, with proponents for and against these.[13–18] Although these additional tests undoubtedly contribute to the cost of treatment of carpal tunnel syndrome, some argue that confirming its existence before CTR actually is cost-effective in that it avoids unnecessary surgery.[16,19] However, Glowacki and colleagues[15] compared the outcomes of open carpal tunnel release in 2 patient cohorts: one with a clinical diagnosis of carpal tunnel syndrome confirmed using nerve conduction study (NCS) and one without NCS before surgery. Outcomes were similar between the groups, and the investigators concluded that routine NCS before surgery was not indicated. Fowler and colleagues[13,14] compared ultrasound, NCS, and the 6-item carpal tunnel symptoms scale (CTS-6) for the diagnosis of carpal tunnel syndrome and found similar sensitivity and specificity among the 3. NCS had the lowest sensitivity and specificity. The diagnostic accuracy of MRI compared with electrodiagnostic studies is only moderate in evaluating patients with carpal tunnel syndrome (CTS). MRI may be useful in helping to predict which patients will respond best to medical or surgical treatment.

Because surgical site infections often are used as a performance metric in assessing the quality of health care, prophylactic antibiotics are commonly used perioperatively. Johnson and colleagues[20] hypothesized that prophylactic antibiotics are overused in clean soft tissue hand procedures (open or endoscopic CTR, trigger finger release, de Quervain release, and wrist ganglion excision). In their study, approximately 20% of patients who had clean soft tissue hand procedures had preoperative or postoperative antibiotic administration. Younger age, male gender, lower income, and obesity were factors leading to more frequent antibiotic use. The investigators estimated that $1.6 million could have been saved without this use of prophylactic antibiotics. They also noted that this represents a fraction of total costs, which may include the treatment of allergic reactions, *Clostridium difficile* complications, widespread antimicrobial resistance, and the costs associated with purchasing, storing, and administering the antibiotic. Harness and colleagues,[21] likewise, found that antibiotic use did not decrease the risk of infection in patients with CTR, including patients with diabetes. They suggested that the routine use of antibiotic prophylaxis is not indicated.

Postoperative pain control is another area in which cost reductions are possible. Dwyer and colleagues,[22] in a study of 121 CTRs, reported that written guidelines for surgeons and educational handouts for patients significantly reduced the number of prescribed opioid pills by 25% to 55%, while achieving high patient satisfaction and a low refill rate. They recommended 5 to 10 opioid pills after surgery. Pain catastrophizing has been shown to be associated with greater opioid consumption[22]; recognition of this behavior may help target patients for additional support, such as counseling or behavioral therapy. Several other studies have found that many more opioids were prescribed than needed after CTR.[23–25] Rodgers and colleagues[25] found that overprescribing opioids (30 tablets per patient) for 250 patients resulted in 4639 unused tablets. They recommended 15 tablets with 1 refill of a Schedule III opioid analgesic for elective outpatient upper extremity procedures.

COMPLICATIONS

With the advent of bundled payment plans and other payment models, complications have an important financial impact. Although rare, complications, such as postoperative infection and pain or persistent or recurrent symptoms, can be devastating. The overall complication rate after CTR is low (<1%). Goyal and colleagues[4] reported a 0.2% rate of adverse events in 28,737 CTRs done in an ambulatory surgery center (ASC). Seven complications (0.1%) requiring reoperation and/or unplanned admission within 30 days of surgery in 7254 CTRs were reported by Goodman and colleagues.[26] Harness and colleagues,[21] in a multicenter, retrospective review of complications after CTR, found a 0.23% frequency of deep infections that required return to the OR. Endoscopic CTR has been reported to be associated with fewer postoperative complications than open CTR, although at a greater cost.[27]

Intraoperative complications may include injury to the medial or ulnar nerves, but this occurs in fewer than 1% of cases. Nerve injury can lead to persistent paresthesias or painful neuroma formation and is generally more frequent after endoscopic CTR than open CTR; most are temporary neurapraxias.

Failure of treatment (no improvement in symptoms over 12 months or clinical deterioration) requiring secondary surgery has been reported in 7% to 12% of patients. Revision surgery includes nerve exploration and repeat release, and augmentation with local or free-tissue grafting may be needed. Outcomes after revision CTR are generally reported to be worse than after primary CTR.

Although cost estimates vary in the literature, most investigators agree that open CTR costs less than endoscopic CTR, the clinic procedure room is cheaper than the ASC which is less than the hospital, and that costs should include cost to society for missed work and complications.

PATIENT SATISFACTION

Patient satisfaction is increasingly used as a metric of quality of care and is an important component of reimbursement programs. Kim and Kim[28] identified 4 attributes associated with patient satisfaction after hand surgery: board certification status, distance from patient's residence, medical cost, and waiting time for surgery. The most important attribute was the physician's board certification, followed by distance from the patient's residence to the hospital, waiting time, and costs. Time spent with the hand surgeon has been shown to not be associated with patient satisfaction measured directly after the visit, whereas longer time waiting to see the physician correlated with decreased patient satisfaction.[29] Patient satisfaction among patients undergoing hand surgery may relate more to shorter time in the waiting room and to the quality more than the quantity of time spent with the patient.[29] In their study, Parrish and colleagues[30] found that patient satisfaction was not associated with perceived visit duration but did correlate strongly with patient-rated surgeon empathy. Efforts to make hand surgery office visits more patient-centered should focus on improving dialogue quality, and not necessarily on making visits longer.

The resolution of their symptoms, especially pain and numbness, is a key component of patient satisfaction. CTR is an effective treatment with a high success rate: in patients younger than 50 years, 92% of men and 99% of women have resolution of daytime numbness by 6 months.[31] In a long-term follow-up study (mean follow-up of 9 years), complete resolution of symptoms was reported in 94% of patients.[32]

Patient psychological status (depression, anxiety) also has been associated with symptom severity and postoperative patient satisfaction.[33,34] Shin and colleagues[34] found that patients' depression levels and pain anxiety were significantly associated with CTS symptoms preoperatively and postoperatively. Vranceanu and colleagues[35] found that depression was the sole predictor of both disability and pain intensity after CTR in 39 patients. Parrish and colleagues[30] identified greater symptoms of depression and lower-rated surgeon empathy as independently associated with patient dissatisfaction. These findings suggest that some of the disproportionate pain and disability after otherwise uncomplicated and objectively successful surgery, such as CTR, may be a function of untreated depressive symptoms. Wilkens and colleagues[36] suggested that catastrophic thinking and kinesophobia, along with less effective coping strategies, can hinder recovery. They recommended that surgeons learn to recognize signs of these conditions and treat them with compassion, empathy, and patience and be prepared to add formal support (eg, cognitive-behavioral therapy) to help facilitate recovery. Park and colleagues,[37] however, questioned the association between psychological factors and patient satisfaction, noting that, although a systematic review found depression correlated with postoperative pain, the association was less clear between psychological factors and outcomes such as satisfaction, perceived levels of symptoms and function, and physical measures of recovery.[38,39] Because pain may not be a primary symptom or outcome of CTS, these authors did not consider the current literature as providing strong support for an association between psychological factors and outcomes of CTR.

Patients have always sought value in health care, but the definition of "value" has been nebulous. Currently, the most accepted definition is a health care outcome achieved per dollar spent to achieve that outcome. Patient-reported outcome measures (PROM) are frequently used to evaluate outcomes; with more routine use of PROMs, more attention will need to be paid to the factors that have the strongest influence on these scores: depression, anxiety, and ineffective coping strategies.

REFERENCES

1. Pourmemari MH, Heliövaara M, Viikari-Juntura E, et al. Carpal tunnel release: lifetime prevalence, annual incidence, and risk factors. Muscle Nerve 2018. [Epub ahead of print].

2. Van Demark RE Jr, Becker HA, Anderson MC, et al. Wide-awake anesthesia in the in-office procedure room: lessons learned. Hand (N Y) 2018;13(4): 481–5.

3. Chatterjee A, McCarthy JE, Montagne SA, et al. A cost, profit, and efficiency analysis of performing carpal tunnel surgery in the operating room versus the clinic setting in the United States. Ann Plast Surg 2011;66(3):245–8.

4. Goyal KS, Jain S, Buterbaugh GA, et al. The safety of hand and upper-extremity surgical procedures at a freestanding ambulatory surgery center. A review of 28,737 cases. J Bone Joint Surg Am 2016; 98:700–4.

5. Kazmers NH, Presson AP, Xu Y, et al. Cost implications of varying the surgical technique, surgical setting, and anesthesia type for carpal tunnel release surgery. J Hand Surg Am 2018. [Epub ahead of print].

6. Leblanc MR, Lalonde DH, Thoma A, et al. Is main operating room sterility really necessary in carpal tunnel surgery? A multicenter prospective study of minor procedure room field sterility surgery. Hand (N Y) 2011;6:60–3.

7. Nguyen C, Milstein A, Hernandez-Boussard T, et al. The effect of moving carpal tunnel releases out of hospitals on reducing United States health care charges. J Hand Surg Am 2015;40(8):1657–62.

8. Rhee PC, Fischer MM, Rhee LS, et al. Cost savings and patient experiences of a clinic-based, wide-awake hand surgery program at a military medical center: a critical analysis of the first 100 procedures. J Hand Surg Am 2017;42:e139–47.

9. Law TY, Rosas S, Hubbard ZS, et al. Trends in open and endoscopic carpal tunnel release utilization in the Medicare patient population. J Surg Res 2017;214:9–13.

10. Zhang S, Vora M, Harris AHS, et al. Cost-minimization analysis of open and endoscopic carpal tunnel release. J Bone Joint Surg Am 2016;92:1970–7.

11. Hubbard ZS, Law TY, Rosas S, et al. Economic benefit of carpal tunnel release in the Medicare patient population. Neurosurg Focus 2018;44:E16.

12. Gould D, Kulber D, Kuschner S, et al. Our surgical experience: open versus endoscopic carpal tunnel surgery. J Hand Surg Am 2018. [Epub ahead of print].

13. Fowler JR. Nerve conduction studies for carpal tunnel syndrome: gold standard or unnecessary evil? Orthopedics 2017;40:141–2.

14. Fowler JR, Cipolli W, Hanson T. A comparison of three diagnostic tests for carpal tunnel syndrome using latent class analysis. J Bone Joint Surg Am 2015;97:1958–61.

15. Glowacki KA, Breen CJ, Sachar K, et al. Electrodiagnostic testing and carpal tunnel release outcome. J Hand Surg Am 1996;21:117–21.

16. Keith MW, Masear V, Chung K, et al. Diagnosis of carpal tunnel syndrome. J Am Acad Orthop Surg 2009;17:389–96.

17. Kerasnoudis A. Ultrasound and MRI in carpal tunnel syndrome: the dilemma of simplifying the approach to a complex disease or making complex assessments of a simple problem. J Hand Surg Am 2012;37:2200–1.

18. Sears ED, Lu YT, Wood SM, et al. Diagnostic testing requested before surgical evaluation for carpal tunnel syndrome. J Hand Surg Am 2017;42: 623–9.

19. Hameso A, Bland JD. Prevalence of decompression surgery in patients with carpal tunnel syndrome 8 years after initial treatment with a local corticosteroid injection. J Hand Surg Eur Vol 2017;42:275–80.

20. Johnson SP, Zhong L, Chung KC, et al. Perioperative antibiotics for clean hand surgery: a national study. J Hand Surg Am 2018;43:407–16.

21. Harness NG, Inacio FF, Fleil FF, et al. Rate of infection after carpal tunnel release surgery and effect of

antibiotic prophylaxis. J Hand Surg Am 2010;35: 189–96.

22. Dwyer C, Soong M, Hunter A, et al. Prospective evaluation of an opioid reduction protocol in hand surgery. J Hand Surg Am 2018;43:516–22.e1.

23. Chapman T, Kim N, Maltenfort M, et al. Prospective evaluation of opioid consumption following carpal tunnel release surgery. Hand (N Y) 2017; 12:e39–42.

24. Miller A, Kim N, Zmistowski B, et al. Postoperative pain management following carpal tunnel release: a prospective cohort evaluation. Hand (N Y) 2017; 12:541–5.

25. Rodgers J, Cunningham K, Fitzgerald K, et al. Opioid consumption following outpatient upper extremity surgery. J Hand Surg Am 2012;37: 645–50.

26. Goodman AD, Gil JA, Starr AM, et al. Thirty-day reoperation and/or admission after elective hand surgery in adults: a 10-year review. J Hand Surg 43(4):383.e1–383.e7.

27. Devana SK, Jensen AR, Yamaguchi KT, et al. Trends and complications in open versus endoscopic carpal tunnel release in private payer and Medicare patient population. Hand (N Y) 2018. [Epub ahead of print].

28. Kim JK, Kim YK. Predictors of scar pain after open carpal tunnel release. J Hand Surg 2011; 36:1042–6.

29. Teunis T, Thornton ER, Jayakumar P, et al. Time seeing a hand surgeon is not associated with patient satisfaction. Clin Orthop Relat Res 2015;473: 2362–8.

30. Parrish RC II, Menendez ME, Mudgal CS, et al. Patient satisfaction and its relation to perceived visit duration with a hand surgeon. J Hand Surg Am 2016;41:257–62.

31. Watchmaker JD, Watchmaker GP. Independent variable affecting outcome of carpal tunnel surgery. Hand (N Y) 2017. [Epub ahead of print].

32. Tang CQY, Lai SWH, Tay SC. Long-term outcome of carpal tunnel release surgery in patients with severe carpal tunnel syndrome. Bone Joint J 2017;99-B:1348–53.

33. Crijns TJ, Bernstein DN, Ring D, et al. Depression and pain interference correlate with physical function in patients recovering from hand surgery. Hand (N Y) 2018. [Epub ahead of print].

34. Shin YH, Yoon JO, Kim YK, et al. Psychological status is associated with symptom severity in patients with carpal tunnel syndrome. J Hand Surg Am 2018; 43:484.e1-8.

35. Vranceanu AM, Jupiter JB, Mudgal CS, et al. Predictors of pain intensity and disability after minor hand surgery. J Hand Surg Am 2010;35:956–60.

36. Wilkens SC, Lans J, Bargon C, et al. Hand posturing is a nonverbal indicator of catastrophic thinking for finger, hand, or wrist injury. Clin Orthop Relat Res 2018;476:706–13.

37. Park JW, Gong HS, Rhee SH, et al. The effect of psychological factors on the outcomes of carpal tunnel release: a systematic review. J Hand Surg Asian Pac Vol 2017;22:131–7.

38. Hobby JL, Venkatesh R, Motkur P. The effect of psychological disturbance on symptoms, self-reported disability and surgical outcomes in carpal tunnel syndrome. J Bone Joint Surg Br 2005;87:198–200.

39. Katz JN, Losina E, Amick BC 3rd, et al. Predictors of outcomes of carpal tunnel release. Arthritis Rheum 2001;44:1184–93.

Shoulder and Elbow

Practicing Cost-Conscious Shoulder Surgery

Eric K. Bonness, MD[a],*, Laurence D. Higgins, MD, MBA[b]

KEYWORDS

• Shoulder • Value • Cost-effectiveness • Surgery

KEY POINTS

- Health care sector costs will continue to increase through 2025 because of advances in expensive technology and aging populations.
- Universal reporting of outcomes and costs, and an integration of systematic improvements, will be crucial to successfully revamping the US health care system.
- By practicing evidence-based methods for improved outcomes at lower costs, providers can increase both efficiency and profitability, while patients experience better care and higher satisfaction.

INTRODUCTION

Health care costs in the United States continue to increase with advances in expensive technologies and an aging patient population. These costs are unsustainable, leading to an increased focus on delivering care in a patient-centered, value-based model. In 2015, health care related costs made up 18% of the national gross domestic product and they are expected to increase to 20% by 2025. Estimates project a 5.8% increase in heath care related costs by 2025, reaching nearly $5.5 trillion.[1] This increase is not surprising, especially considering the growing and aging population of the United States, which would inherently lead to increased spending and enrollment in both the Medicare and Medicaid groups.[1]

Musculoskeletal disorders represent a substantial portion of health care costs and are the leading cause of disability in the United States. In 2011, the annual US cost for the treatment of musculoskeletal conditions and lost wages was $874 billion, making up 5.7% of the gross domestic product.[2]

Shoulder disorders make up a substantial portion of this economic burden, with 8.2% of the US adult population reporting chronic shoulder pain in 2008.[3] Just behind the knee, the shoulder was the second most common joint in which patients experienced chronic pain. Studies have also pointed out that, in addition to the direct costs, indirect costs such as missed work secondary to shoulder pathology have resulted in a small number of patients accounting for a large portion of the overall costs.[4,5]

Owing to the increase health care costs and projections for further increases over the next decade, the long-term sustainability of our health care system is in question. As such, there has been a significant increase in focusing on decreasing costs and providing value-based care. Although these economic principles are applicable in a multitude of other markets, they are difficult to apply to health care because of the complexity of the system. The health care system is influenced by patients, providers, hospital systems, insurers, and pharmaceutical or medical technology companies. Each group prioritizes their own interests when it comes to economic success, complicating a consensus.

Value in health care can be defined as patient outcome per dollar spent (direct or indirect) in

---

Disclosure Statement: The authors have no conflicts of interest to disclose.
a Massachusetts General Hospital, Department of Orthopaedics, 55 Fruit Street, Suite 3200, Boston, MA 02114, USA; b Department of Orthopaedics, King Edward VII Memorial Hospital, 7 Point Finger Road, Paget DV 04, Bermuda
* Corresponding author.
E-mail address: bonness54@gmail.com

Orthop Clin N Am 49 (2018) 509–517
https://doi.org/10.1016/j.ocl.2018.05.011

the care provided. Simply, $\frac{outcome}{cost}$ = value. Optimizing value comes as the result of improving outcomes at a lower cost. This consideration is different than focusing solely on reducing costs or limiting treatments without taking patient outcomes into account. The difficulty in this method stems from the greater variation in practice and lack of standardized outcome recording. Bundled opportunities serve as one vehicle to achieve value-based care by decreasing costs and improving outcomes. This article defines and discusses value-based care practices and their applications in the management of shoulder disorders.

VALUE-BASED CARE

Much of what we know about value-based care comes from the work of health care economists Michael Porter and Elizabeth Teisberg. As creators of this health care strategy, they have described 3 principles essential to the system. First, the description of value must be focused on the patient. Therefore, success in the value-based system is not measured by hospital revenues, number of clinic visits, number of cases performed, or relative value units generated by a surgeon. This system shifts the paradigm to improvement of patient outcomes and at a lower cost. Second, they emphasize that care should be focused on specific condition over an entire care cycle. This factor applies to both the measurement of outcomes and the calculation of total costs. With respect to a shoulder practice, value-based care would involve focusing treatments and outcome measurements on specific shoulder conditions, like instability, rotator cuff disease, or arthritis.

Additionally, treatment teams should be organized specifically around the various conditions. This strategy allows for multidisciplinary management to optimize patient outcomes and improve efficiency and, thus, lower overall costs in the long term. Porter and Teisberg[6,7] have termed these organized care teams as integrated practice units. For example, in the management of shoulder instability, these integrated practice units would include orthopedic surgeons, anesthesiologists, physical therapists, and nurses, who all participate from the beginning of a care cycle, collaborating to optimize care for this specific shoulder condition, while accounting for individual patient characteristics (age, medical comorbidities, athletic status).

Finally, crucial to the success of value-based care is the measuring and reporting of results. These results include long-term patient outcomes as well as cost data. Historically, the large outcomes databases included only certain outcomes like readmission rates or mortality. However, it is important to include more specific results, such as patient functional outcomes, pain, patient satisfaction, or condition-specific complications. Complete transparency in outcome data reporting is important, but difficult to achieve. Without these data, however, it is impossible to make determinations as to which treatments are the most cost effective for patients in terms of functional outcomes, pain, durability, and success rate.[8] Interpretation of these data, over the long term, is what leads to the formulation of best practice guidelines for improved patient outcomes, lower cost, and sustainability. With increasing health care costs and the future of the health care system in question, value-based care provides this sustainability by increasing competition and efficiency. Providers, hospitals, and insurers are forced to provide care to achieve the highest outcomes. Transparency in outcomes reporting will allow patients to become knowledgeable consumers in the health care market, seeking the best care at the lowest price. It must be stressed that, because the outcomes and cost data inform on the creation of practice guidelines, continued measurement and refinement of data used to drive the value-driven agenda would ideally create a virtuous cycle of improvement.

From an economic perspective, value-based care practice aims to transition the system from the current zero-sum competition to positive-sum competition. In zero-sum competition, the net value of the system remains constant and hospital systems and insurance companies compete to divide the value among themselves. Often this results in providing the less costly treatments to patients and ultimately decreasing value to the patient. In positive-sum competition, the net value of the system can be increased by using treatments that have been proven to result in improved patient outcomes, thus, lowering the overall cost in the long term. This increased value to the system benefits all parties involved.[6]

Application of the value-based care model is well-suited for the treatment of many orthopedic conditions, and the shoulder is no exception. With an increasing number of shoulder surgeries being performed, increasing health care costs, and an aging population, there exists a great potential for cost savings and increased efficiencies when a value-based strategy is used. Additionally, disorders of the shoulder can be categorized into specific conditions such as instability, rotator cuff pathology, or arthritis and can be studied over a finite care cycle. The potential for multiple providers involved in the care of these conditions (primary care providers, orthopedic surgeons, physical therapists, nurses, etc) lends perfectly to the improvements in efficiency, patient outcomes, and cost reductions in a value-based system. Historically, these multiple care providers have worked independent of one another. Integration of the provider network can improve patient care through collaboration and the formulation of best practice guidelines. Another factor contributing to the potential for improvement in the treatment of shoulder disorders is the wide variability that currently exists in management between providers. This variability exists within multiple aspects of the treatment, from the amount and type of physical therapy performed, advanced imaging obtained, or even surgical procedure performed for the same condition. Variability is a major driver of costs in the current health care sector.[9,10]

Currently, the reported outcomes data for shoulder disorders come from a small number of providers. It is difficult to determine best practice guidelines in a value-based system because these outcomes may not represent those found by most shoulder surgeons. As the market continues to shift to incentivize through value-based outcome measures, providers will be encouraged to report their patient's outcomes and costs. This practice, in turn, will lead to a more large-scale, comprehensive data system to more readily establish best practice guidelines.

Attempting to create a system with uniform universal public reporting of outcomes is a difficult task. Standardization of outcome measures can be challenging, costly, and time consuming, especially when attempting to implement these systems across different clinical settings. Additionally, orthopedic surgeons must consider that outcome measurements may be falsely skewed secondary to unique patient characteristics and, as such, risk adjustments must be made to account for higher risk patients. These risk adjustments add to the complexity of outcome reporting. Additionally, in a system where reimbursement is outcomes based, transparency in outcomes reporting may lead orthopedic surgeons to only operate on healthier patients to improve outcomes and lower risk, if such stratification is not performed accurately. Finally, rare clinical scenarios, whereby inadequate outcome data are available, may not be suitable for risk adjustment and may be best structured in a traditional fee-for-service model.[8,11]

Currently, published large-scale studies in orthopedics use common measures, such as mortality, readmission or reoperation rates, or postoperative complications when reporting outcomes for particular treatments, using hospital-acquired data, which do not accurately measure surgical outcomes. Many registries focus on implant survival and, therefore, have limited focus from a value-based care perspective. Some national registries do report on a variety of outcome scores; however, registry data are observational, subject to confounding variables, and subject to variability in reporting. Analyzing data with this large outcome measure variability can be quite difficult, and patient-centered outcome measures are lacking. With patients taking on more of a consumer role in value-based health care, following satisfaction and patient experience measures will become increasingly important, as they are in other areas of industry. Additionally, organizing and maintaining national registries requires national or governmental funding and organization. Opposition to large-scale outcomes reporting exists among independent providers because the lack of national or government organization and funding makes data recording and reporting expensive, time consuming, and a potential privacy risk for patient health information.[12,13] However, to truly establish best practice guidelines for particular orthopedic procedures, specific patient outcomes such as functional outcomes, pain, or condition-specific complications are required.[14]

LOOKING TO THE FUTURE

The transition to a true value-based care system is undoubtedly challenging and thus will be met with some degree of resistance. Issues including expense, manpower, infrastructure, and fear of transparency all must be overcome. However, as recently described by Lee and colleagues[15] at the University of Utah, the work involved in transitioning health care from volume to value is worth doing. Driven largely by redesign from the Centers for Medicare and Medicaid Services, health care reimbursement is transitioning from a fee-for-service payment system to value-based systems. This system is already the case for bundled payments mandatory for total hip and knee replacements in 67 regions under the Comprehensive Care for Joint Replacement model.[16] Porter and Lee[9] accurately stated that "the clear message is that hospitals, health care centers, and clinicians should no longer be spending time discussing *whether* to participate in bundled payment programs but instead focusing on *how* to do the work necessary to succeed under them," and the work done at the University of Utah is a testament to that statement. They have completely redesigned their management strategy, focused on better quality of care at lower costs, demonstrating significant results. As described elsewhere in this article regarding the fundamentals of the value-based care system, the University of Utah Health Care team attributes its success to 3 specific principles. First, the institution's business model set value improvement as its primary focus. Second, the approach to treatment was organized around specific patient conditions. This step allowed for quality improvements and increased efficiencies for specific conditions. Third, multidisciplinary teams were created to facilitate quality improvements through integrated care and improvements across a care cycle. Care cycles represent the entire continuum of care from the diagnosis of the condition to its resolution. The length of the care cycle can vary significantly depending on the condition. Using these principles, they used a new cost accounting system to improve the accuracy cost analysis across episodes of care delivery. For example, they found costs could be reduced by altering health care delivery patterns that were often only based on clinician preference and did not affect clinical outcome. Although admittedly outcomes reporting included in the work by Lee and colleagues was limited, including mortality and readmission rates, they were still able to show improved clinical outcomes, for example, in the total joint replacement with a decrease in cost of 11%. They are currently working on more comprehensive outcomes data collection, including functional status, pain, and condition-specific complications. Organizational negotiation of bundle payment contracts rewarding improvements in these value outcomes will further promote cost reductions that will benefit all involved parties.[9,15]

Although national and governmental involvement in universal outcomes reporting for organization and funding is frequently necessary, it is the orthopedic shoulder surgeons who should determine which outcome measures should be recorded to best assess and improve on the quality of care delivery. Shoulder surgeons should be encouraged to record and criticize their own outcomes without fear of repercussions in their transparency. It is only then that providers can compare their outcomes to the national averages, and continue or discontinue treatments based on the results. As the number

of providers in the community reporting outcomes increases over time, these small-scale results can be collected and pooled to create a large-scale outcomes database with the power capable affecting best practice management changes. Additionally, as the pool of patients increase across a spectrum of practice types, risk adjustments for comorbidities and specific trends will be identified to allow practice adjustments to be more readily made. Additionally, this task may become easier for the community provider to accomplish with the continued advancement in technology, using new software, tablets, or smartphones for outcomes recording.

CURRENT COST STUDIES IN SHOULDER DISORDERS

Equally important in the value-based care equation are the costs associated with the delivery of care. The true cost calculation includes both direct and indirect costs over the entire episode of care for a given condition. This accounting includes not only the imaging, clinic visits, surgical implants, and hospital fees, but also consideration for the costs of postoperative rehabilitation, costs of the management of complications, and societal costs like missed work.[17]

Studies in the shoulder literature regarding cost are still relative sparse compared with other areas of research. However, with the increased interest in value-based care delivery there has been a significant increase in publications on cost-effectiveness studies over the past several years. Cost-effectiveness studies tend to use generalized outcomes, such as health-related quality of life, when comparing treatment interventions.[18] It can be difficult to make assessments from these studies as they may lack shoulder specific outcome measures, however, quality-adjusted life-year (QALY) calculations for comparative effectiveness research is a powerful tool to inform providers, patients, and payers of the value of their treatment.

Most of the cost studies in the shoulder literature focus on the management of rotator cuff pathology and shoulder arthroplasties owing to the prevalence of procedures performed and high-cost variability associated with their care. From a historic perspective, in 2000, Cordasco and colleagues[19] attempted to describe the management of rotator cuff tears as an outpatient procedure. Patients underwent open rotator cuff repair with a 43% decrease in cost and high patient satisfaction. This study used limited cost analysis and no validated shoulder outcome scores.

The evaluation of surgical techniques of rotator cuff repairs including open versus arthroscopic repair, single-row versus double-row repair, and use of transosseous fixation and platelet-rich plasma have also been investigated from a cost analysis perspective. Churchill and Ghorai[20] compared costs of mini-open versus all-arthroscopic rotator cuff repair at low-, intermediate-, and high-volume centers. Database analysis revealed lower costs associated with mini-open repair compared with all-arthroscopic repair. It was also found that, regardless of the repair technique, high-volume centers cost significantly more than intermediate-volume and low-volume centers.[20] It is possible that these findings may have been related to size of tear, revision surgery, and medical complexity that were not accounted for in their study.

Adla and colleagues[21] also investigated the cost effectiveness of open versus arthroscopic rotator cuff repair. They found no difference in Oxford and Constant shoulder scores at final follow-up. There was no difference between the groups in the cost of time in the operating room, amount of postoperative analgesia, or physical therapy costs.[21] They did note an incremental cost of each arthroscopic rotator cuff repair of $1249 more than open procedures. This finding was primarily related to arthroscopic instrumentation. These investigators, therefore, concluded that open rotator cuff repair was more cost effective than arthroscopic repair.

More recently, Murphy and colleagues[22] investigated the cost effectiveness of open versus arthroscopic rotator cuff repair using data from 273 patients. They found that there were no differences between the arthroscopic and open groups in terms of amount of resources used, the associated cost, or QALYs at any time postoperatively. Despite these findings, there remained uncertainty about which technique was most cost effective.

Huang and colleagues[23] performed a cost-utility analysis comparing single-row versus double-row rotator cuff repair. They found double-row fixation was costlier ($2134.41 compared with $1654.76), but was more effective (4.073 per QALY compared with 4.055 QALY). Additionally, based on their willingness-to-pay threshold of $50,000 per QALY gained, double-row repair was more cost effective.

The management of massive rotator cuff tears is a difficult problem. Dornan and colleagues[24] used a Markov decision model to compare 3 treatment strategies for massive rotator cuff tears in patients with pseudoparalysis without osteoarthritis. The treatment options included arthroscopic rotator cuff repair with the option to arthroscopically revise once, arthroscopic rotator cuff repair with immediate conversion to reverse total shoulder arthroplasty on potential failure, and primary reverse total shoulder arthroplasty. They determined that arthroscopic rotator cuff repair with conversion to reverse total shoulder arthroplasty on potential failure was the most cost-effective strategy. Using the same model, Kang and colleagues[25] compared reverse total shoulder arthroplasty, hemiarthroplasty, arthroscopic debridement with biceps tenodesis, and physical therapy for the management of massive irreparable rotator cuff tears in the elderly. They found reverse total shoulder arthroplasty to be the preferred treatment both in terms of QALYs and cost effectiveness. They also found that, for patients seeking pain relief without functional improvement, arthroscopic debridement and biceps tenodesis can be considered a cost-effective option.

Makhni and colleagues[26] performed an expected-value decision analysis to compare costs and outcomes of arthroscopic rotator cuff repair and reverse total shoulder arthroplasty for large and massive rotator cuff tears. Despite high rates of tendon retearing, arthroscopic repair was found to be the more cost-effective treatment strategy, assuming no adverse effect of the arthroscopic procedure on a subsequent arthroplasty procedure.

Platelet-rich plasma has also been investigated regarding its cost effectiveness in rotator cuff repair. Samuelson and colleagues[27] used a cost-utility analysis to show that the use of platelet-rich plasma to augment rotator cuff repair is not cost effective. Secondary to its high cost, platelet-rich plasma-augmented repairs would not become cost-effective based on their sensitivity analysis until the retear rate was decreased by 9.1%. Similar results regarding the use of platelet-rich plasma were found in a study by Vavken and colleagues.[28]

Multiple cost analysis studies also exist to help answer difficult questions regarding arthroplasty treatment options. Bhat and colleagues[29] used a Markov chain decision tree model to evaluate the cost effectiveness of total shoulder arthroplasty versus hemiarthroplasty for patients 30 to 50 years of age with severe end-stage glenohumeral arthritis, evaluating the costs of management, revision rates, and QALYs. They found that, in this group of patients, total shoulder arthroplasty resulted in lower total costs, decreased rate of revision surgery, greater years of satisfactory or excellent patient outcomes, and greater QALYs. Odum and colleagues[30] evaluated the value of implementing a cost-containment protocol to assess the value of bundled payments in total shoulder arthroplasty. This, in response to the Centers for Medicare and Medicaid Services Bundled Payments for Care Improvement initiative under the Affordable Care Act, investigated expenditures and postacute event rates of fee-for-service versus Bundled Payments for Care Improvement patients. The postacute events included need for inpatient rehabilitation facility, skilled nursing facility, home health admissions, and readmissions. The median expenditure for fee-for-service patients was $21,157 compared with $17,894 with Bundled Payments for Care Improvement patients. This finding was due to control of the postacute care spending with significantly decreased use of rehabilitation facilities and skilled nursing facilities, as well as a lesser 90-day readmission rate.

Cost-utility analysis has also been used to help answer the ongoing debate regarding the optimal surgical intervention for complex proximal humerus fractures in the elderly patient. Using decision tree and Markov modeling for the analysis of data from available published literature, Osterhoff and colleagues[31] compared the cost effectiveness of reverse total shoulder arthroplasty versus hemiarthroplasty in these patients. Their analysis suggested that despite reverse total shoulder arthroplasty being more expensive, it was more cost effective compared with hemiarthroplasty, with an incremental cost-effectiveness ratio of $13,679 (Canadian dollars) per incremental QALY gained. It has been noted previously in similar studies in patients with rotator cuff arthropathy[32,33] that a comparative analysis of reverse total shoulder arthroplasty and hemiarthroplasty is sensitive to the utility lost owing to complications related to the operation, as well as cost of implant. This study was particularly useful given the known increased complication rate and higher patient risk stratification when these procedures are performed for fracture.[34–37]

The cost-effectiveness studies on adhesive capsulitis and shoulder instability are limited. Maund and colleagues[38] performed a systematic review of the available literature and determined that the limited data did not allow for any conclusions regarding the most cost-effective interventions for adhesive capsulitis. Min and colleagues[39] reviewed the existing literature to determine the cost effectiveness of arthroscopic Bankart and open Latarjet procedures in the treatment of primary shoulder instability. These investigators found that, although both the arthroscopic Bankart and open Latarjet procedures were highly cost effective (incremental cost-effectiveness ratio of $4214 and $4681, respectively), the Bankart is more cost effective than the Latarjet. This finding was largely due to the lower health utility state after failed Latarjet, despite a recurrence rate of 8% compared with 14% with arthroscopic Bankart repair. They concluded that the Latarjet remained favorable in certain clinical scenarios, such as critical glenoid bone loss, and surgical treatment decisions should be made on a case-by-case basis.

As the cost analysis literature continues to expand, our understanding of the true value of the procedures performed for various shoulder disorders will hopefully become more clear. A value-based reimbursement model will continue to drive research in this area, promoting a more robustly powered data set on the costs and outcomes of various treatment options.

THE VALUE OF SPECIALIZED CARE

The discussion of the delivery of value in shoulder surgery is not complete without mentioning specialized care in the context of value. We have previously mentioned the transition of volume to value as it relates to reimbursement under a value-based reimbursement model, with increased value delivered benefitting physician reimbursement, in addition to the patent. However, volume can also be an important factor affecting outcome for the patient even in a value-based system.

As is true in other competitive markets, as patients become more like consumers, they will seek out providers providing the best reported outcomes. These providers, in turn, will treat more patients for these conditions, resulting in a larger portion of their practice. This practice will further fuel the value-based care model by increasing volume, expertise, and efficiency, thus, attracting more patients. Orthopedics is already a subspecialized field (ie, spine, hand, arthroplasty).[17] But to what degree does this specialization benefit the patient?

Research in many areas of medicine has shown a strong correlation between physician experience in procedures/condition management and achieving improved outcomes at lower costs.[40] This finding has also been shown to be true in shoulder disorders. Hammond and colleagues[41] found a statistically significant increase in complications for low-volume surgeons when they were compared with high-volume surgeons for shoulder arthroplasties.

Similarly, Weinheimer and colleagues[42] recently reported on surgeon volume as it relates to patient outcomes and cost in shoulder arthroplasty and rotator cuff repair. This systematic review identified 10 studies over a 26-year period. They found outcomes of low-volume surgeons (compared with high-volume surgeons) was associated with longer hospital stays, longer operating room times, increased hospital complications, and higher cost. Criteria for minimum low-volume thresholds were set at 5 arthroplasty cases per year and 12 rotator cuff repairs per year. This finding suggests that controlling volume is critical to optimizing value. However, this practice is currently not the case in shoulder surgery. Hasan and colleagues[43] found that only 3% of shoulder replacement surgeons perform 10 or more such surgeries per year, and 75% of shoulder surgeons perform only 1 or 2 per year. This finding is much different from hip and knee surgery, where cases are more commonly performed by higher volume surgeons.

It has been shown that volume has the greatest impact on outcomes of complex and less commonly performed procedures and is less influential in more commonly performed procedures, as has been well-reported in the cardiothoracic surgery literature.[44–51] This factor is important as it relates to shoulder surgery. The average number of total hip and knee arthroplasties performed in orthopedic residency training programs far exceeds that of total shoulder arthroplasty or rotator cuff repairs.[52–54] Therefore, after residency when orthopedic surgeons perform low volumes of these "less common" procedures, they are more likely to have worse outcomes than in hip and knee surgery. Despite the strong relationship between volume and outcome, modifications can be made through systematic measurement and improvements.[9,55–57]

A prime example of this effort to improve outcomes through outcome measurement and imparting change is the Martini Klinik in Germany. Their surgeons are top performers specializing in prostatectomy for cancer. In 2013, their clinic became the largest and busiest prostate cancer treatment clinic in the world with more than 2200 surgical cases annually.[57] However, the value this clinic delivers to its patients comes not only from the specialization gained through the high volume of cases, but also from the efforts made to systematically improve the care delivered. They formed a "hospital within a hospital" system, integrating all aspects of care delivery. Additionally, and more important, outcomes data are systematically measured to identify which surgeons are underperforming. These underperforming surgeons are then paired with more experienced surgeons to improve outcomes through mentorship. This methodology has led to decreased complication rates, and is a testament to how systematic improvements improve the value of care delivered.[57] Codman wrote, "To effect improvement, the first step is to admit and record the lack of perfection. The next step is to analyze the causes of failure and to determine whether these causes are controllable."[58] Although it is important to acknowledge the effect of surgeon volume on patient outcomes and cost, it is more important to measure outcomes critically and without bias to improve with such measurement.[57]

SUMMARY

The management of shoulder disorders is well-suited for the application of value-based health care with its large expenditure burden and growing outcomes literature. Crucial to its success is the institution of universal outcomes and cost reporting, as well as integration of systematic improvements. By practicing evidenced-based methods for improved outcomes at lower costs, providers can increase both efficiency and margin, while patients experience better care and higher satisfaction. As health care moves toward alternative payment models, this principle will become even more important.

REFERENCES

1. Keehan S, Stone D, Poisal J, et al. National health expenditure projections, 2016-25: price increases, aging push sector to 20 percent of economy. Health Aff 2017;36(3):553–63.
2. United States Bone and Joint Initiative. The burden of musculoskeletal diseases in the United States (BMUS). 3rd edition. Rosemont (IL): 2014. Available at: http://www.boneandjointburden.org/docs/By%20The%20Numbers%20-%20Musculoskeletal%20Conditions%20%28Big%20Picture%29_update%202-24-16.pdf. Accessed February 4, 2018.
3. American Academy of Orthopedic Surgeons. United States bone and joint decade: the burden of musculoskeletal diseases in the United States. Rosemont (IL): American Academy of Orthopaedic Surgeons; 2011.
4. Meislin RJ, Sperling JW, Stitik TP. Persistent shoulder pain: epidemiology, pathophysiology, and diagnosis. Am J Orthop 2005;34(12 Suppl):5–9.
5. Virta L, Joranger P, Brox JI, et al. Costs of shoulder pain and resource use in primary health care: a

cost-of-illness study in Sweden. BMC Musculoskelet Disord 2012;13:17.

6. Porter ME. A strategy for health care reform—toward a value-based system. N Engl J Med 2009;361:109–12.

7. Porter ME, Teisberg EO. Redefining health care: creating value-based competition on results. Boston: Harvard Business School Press; 2006.

8. Porter ME, Teisberg EO. How physicians can change the future of health care. JAMA 2007;297: 1103–11.

9. Porter ME, Lee TH. From volume to value in health care: the work begins. JAMA 2016;316(10):1047–8.

10. Kaplan RS, Haas DA. How not to cut health care costs. Harv Bus Rev 2014;92(11):116–22, 142.

11. Werner RM, Asch DA. The unintended consequences of publicly reporting quality information. JAMA 2005;293:1239–44.

12. Goldstein J. Private practice outcomes: validated outcomes data collection in private practice. Clin Orthop Relat Res 2010;468:2640–5.

13. Wright RW, Baumgarten KM. Shoulder outcomes measures. J Am Acad Orthop Surg 2010;18:436–44.

14. Kennedy A, Bakir C, Brauer CA. Quality indicators in pediatric orthopaedic surgery: a systematic review. Clin Orthop Relat Res 2012;470:1124–32.

15. Lee VS, Kawamoto K, Hess R, et al. Implementation of a value-driven outcomes program to identify high variability in clinical costs and outcomes and association with reduced cost and improved quality. JAMA 2016;316(10):1061–72.

16. Press MJ, Rajkumar R, Conway PH. Medicare's new bundled payments: design, strategy, and evolution. JAMA 2016;315(2):131–2.

17. Black EM, Higgins LD, Warner JJP. Value-based shoulder surgery: practicing outcomes-driven, cost-conscious care. J Shoulder Elbow Surg 2013; 22:1000–9.

18. Lubowitz JH, Provencher MT, Poehling GG. The current issue: clinical shoulder, knee, wrist, hip, and cost-effectiveness analysis. Arthroscopy 2011; 27:1313–6.

19. Cordasco FA, McGinley BJ, Charlton T. Rotator cuff repair as an outpatient procedure. J Shoulder Elbow Surg 2000;9:27–30.

20. Churchill RS, Ghorai JK. Total cost and operating room time comparison of rotator cuff repair techniques at low, intermediate, and high volume centers: mini-open versus all-arthroscopic. J Shoulder Elbow Surg 2010;19:716–21.

21. Adla DN, Rowsell M, Pandey R. Cost-effectiveness of open versus arthroscopic rotator cuff repair. J Shoulder Elbow Surg 2010;19:258–61.

22. Murphy J, Gray A, Cooper C, et al. Costs, quality of life and cost-effectiveness of arthroscopic and open repair for rotator cuff tears. J Shoulder Elbow Surg 2016;98:1648–55.

23. Huang AL, Thavorn K, van Katwyk S, et al. Double-row arthroscopic rotator cuff repair is more cost-effective than single-row repair. J Bone Joint Surg Am 2017;99(20):1730–6.

24. Dornan GJ, Katthagen JC, Tahal DS, et al. Cost-effectiveness of arthroscopic rotator cuff repair versus reverse total shoulder arthroplasty for the treatment of massive rotator cuff tears in patients with pseudoparalysis and non-arthritic shoulders. Arthroscopy 2017;33(4):716–25.

25. Kang JR, Sin AT, Cheung EV. Treatment of massive irreparable rotator cuff tears: a cost-effectiveness analysis. Orthopedics 2017;40(1):e65–76.

26. Makhni EC, Swart E, Steinhaus ME, et al. Cost-effectiveness of reverse total shoulder arthroplasty versus arthroscopic rotator cuff repair for symptomatic large and massive rotator cuff tears. Arthroscopy 2016;32(9):1771–80.

27. Samuelson EM, Odum SM, Fleischli JE. The cost-effectiveness of using platelet-rich plasma during rotator cuff repair: a Markov Model analysis. Arthroscopy 2016;32(7):1237–44.

28. Vavken P, Sadoghi P, Palmer M, et al. Platelet-rich plasma reduces retear rates after arthroscopic repair of small- and medium-sized rotator cuff tears but is not cost-effective. Am J Sports Med 2015; 43(12):3071–6.

29. Bhat SB, Lazarus M, Getz C, et al. Economic decision model suggests total shoulder arthroplasty is superior to hemiarthroplasty in young patients with end-stage shoulder arthritis. Clin Orthop Relat Res 2016;474(11):2482–92.

30. Odum SM, Hamid N, Van Doren BA, et al. Is there value in retrospective 90-day bundle payment models for shoulder arthroplasty procedures? J Shoulder Elbow Surg 2017. https://doi.org/10. 1016/j.jse.2017.10.008.

31. Osterhoff G, O'Hara NN, D'Cruz J, et al. A cost-effectiveness analysis of reverse total shoulder arthroplasty versus hemiarthroplasty for the management of complex proximal humeral fractures in the elderly. Value Health 2017;20(3): 404–11.

32. Coe MP, Greiwe RM, Joshi R, et al. The cost-effectiveness of reverse total shoulder arthroplasty compared with hemiarthroplasty for rotator cuff tear arthropathy. J Shoulder Elbow Surg 2012;21: 1278–88.

33. Renfree KJ, Hattrup SJ, Chang YH. Cost utility analysis of reverse total shoulder arthroplasty. J Shoulder Elbow Surg 2013;22:1656–61.

34. Ferrel JR, Trinh TQ, Fischer RA. Reverse total shoulder arthroplasty versus hemiarthroplasty for proximal humeral fractures: a systematic review. J Orthop Trauma 2015;29:60–8.

35. Namdari S, Horneff JG, Baldwin K. Comparison of hemiarthroplasty and reverse arthroplasty for

treatment of proximal humeral fractures: a systematic review. J Bone Joint Surg Am 2013;95:1701–8.

36. Mata-Fink A, Meinke M, Jones C, et al. Reverse shoulder arthroplasty for treatment of proximal humeral fractures in older adults: a systematic review. J Shoulder Elbow Surg 2013;22:1737–48.

37. Gupta AK, Harris JD, Erickson BJ, et al. Surgical management of complex proximal humerus fractures—a systematic review of 92 studies including 4500 patients. J Orthop Trauma 2015;29:54–9.

38. Maund E, Craig D, Suekarran S, et al. Management of frozen shoulder: a systematic review and cost-effectiveness analysis. Health Technol Assess 2012;16:1–264.

39. Min K, Fedorka C, Solberg MJ, et al. The cost-effectiveness of the arthroscopic Bankart versus open Latarjet in the treatment of primary shoulder instability. J Shoulder Elbow Surg 2018. https://doi.org/10.1016/j. jse.2017.11.013.

40. Kizer KW. The volume-outcome conundrum. N Engl J Med 2003;349:2159–61.

41. Hammond JW, Queale WS, Kim TK, et al. Surgeon experience and clinical and economic outcomes for shoulder arthroplasty. J Bone Joint Surg Am 2003; 85:2318–24.

42. Weinheimer KT, Smuin DM, Dhawan A. Patient outcomes as a function of shoulder surgeon volume: a systematic review. Arthroscopy 2017;33:1273–81.

43. Hasan SS, Leith JM, Smith KI, et al. The distribution of shoulder replacement among surgeons and hospitals is significantly different than that of hip and knee replacement. J Shoulder Elbow Surg 2003; 12:164–9.

44. Shahian DM. Envisioning excellence. Ann Thorac Surg 2016;102:1428–31.

45. Shahian DM, O'Brien SM, Normand S-LT, et al. Association of hospital coronary artery bypass volume with processes of care, mortality, morbidity and The Society of Thoracic Surgeons Composite quality score. J Thorac Cardiovasc Surg 2010;139: 273–82.

46. Shahian DM, Normand S-LT. Low-volume coronary artery bypass surgery: measuring and optimizing performance. J Thorac Cardiovasc Surg 2008;135: 1202–9.

47. Shahian DM. Improving cardiac surgery quality: volume, outcome, process? JAMA 2004;29:246–8.

48. Shahian DM, Normand S-LT. The volume-outcome relationship: from Luft to Leapfrog. Ann Thorac Surg 2003;75:1048–58.

49. Birkmeyer JD, Stukel TA, Siewers AE, et al. Surgeon volume and operative mortality in the United States. N Engl J Med 2003;349:2117–27.

50. Birkmeyer JD, Siewers AE, Finlayson EVA, et al. Hospital volume and surgical mortality in the United States. N Engl J Med 2002;346:1128–37.

51. Welke KF, O'Brien SM, Peterson ED, et al. The complex relationship between pediatric cardiac surgical case volumes and mortality rates in a national clinical database. J Thorac Cardiovasc Surg 2009;137(5):1133–40.

52. Bernard JA, Dattilo JR, Srikumaran U, et al. Reliability and validity of 3 methods of assessing orthopedic resident skill in shoulder surgery. J Surg Educ 2016;73:1020–5.

53. Gil JA, Waryasz GR, Owens BD, et al. Variability of arthroscopy case volume in orthopedic surgery residency. Arthroscopy 2016;32:892–7.

54. Gil JA, Daniels AH, Weiss AP. Variability in surgical case volume of orthopedic surgery residents: 2007-2013. J Am Acad Orthop Surg 2016;24:207–12.

55. Birkmeyer JD, Dimick JB, Berkmeyer NJO. Measuring the quality of surgical care: structure, process or outcomes? J Am Coll Surg 2004;198: 626–32.

56. Porter ME, Deerberg-Wittram J, Marks C. Martini Klinik: prostate cancer care. Harvard Business Review 2014. 1-26:9-714-471, Rev.

57. Warner JJP, Higgins LD. Editorial commentary: volume and outcome: 100 years of perspective on value from E.A. Codman to M.E. Porter. Arthroscopy 2017;33(7):1282–5.

58. Codman EA. The classic: a study in hospital efficiency: as demonstrated by the case report of the first five years of private hospital. Clin Orthop Relat Res 2013;471:1778–83.

The Volume-Value Relationship in Shoulder Arthroplasty

Prem N. Ramkumar, MD, MBA[a],
Heather S. Haeberle, BS[b], Joseph P. Iannotti, MD, PhD[a],
Eric T. Ricchetti, MD[a,*]

KEYWORDS

- Shoulder arthroplasty • Volume • Outcomes • Cost • Value

KEY POINTS

- High-volume surgeons and high-volume hospitals provide superior outcomes including reduced complications, shorter length of stay, and lower mortality rates.
- High-volume surgeons and hospitals may achieve lower costs for shoulder arthroplasty procedures.
- Evidence-based thresholds can be applied to benchmark volumes that yield favorable outcomes from the volume-value relationship in shoulder arthroplasty.

INTRODUCTION

As the US health care system shifts toward a value-based model of reimbursement, the need to optimize outcomes without restricting services is critical.[1–3] Value in health care may be defined as a ratio of benefits gained (including patient outcomes and experience) to the overall cost.[4] Thus, value is increased as outcomes are improved and costs are reduced. Orthopedic surgery is uniquely suited for a value-based model because of the predominance of elective surgery, high procedural costs, and rising volumes.[2,4,5] High-volume surgeons and hospitals have been demonstrated to yield better outcomes delivered at a lower cost, and thus greater value, for several orthopedic procedures including total hip arthroplasty, total knee arthroplasty, spine arthrodesis, and total ankle arthroplasty.[6–14] Improved outcomes in higher volume practices have been attributed to surgeon experience and procedure-specific protocols, although many factors contribute to this complex relationship.[15,16]

Improving value in shoulder arthroplasty has gained increasing importance as procedure volume increases. The procedure volume of shoulder arthroplasty in the United States has grown at a rate of 9.4% annually, with a sharp increase after Food and Drug Administration approval of reverse total shoulder arthroplasty (TSA) in 2003.[17,18] This increase may be attributed to several factors, including the implementation of reverse TSA and its ability to effectively treat problems not otherwise treated with standard shoulder arthroplasty, improved implant design, increased availability, an aging patient population, and more surgeons trained in the procedure.[18,19] Although the hospital length of stay (LOS) decreased significantly from 1993 to 2007, charges for the procedure increased.[18] Data published by Hasan and colleagues[20]

Disclosure Statement: The authors do not have any relevant commercial or financial conflicts of interest or any funding sources to disclose.

[a] Cleveland Clinic, Department of Orthopaedic Surgery, 9500 Euclid Avenue, Cleveland, OH 44195, USA; [b] Baylor College of Medicine, Department of Orthopaedic Surgery, 7200 Cambridge Street, Houston, TX 77030, USA
* Corresponding author. Department of Orthopaedic Surgery, Cleveland Clinic, Orthopaedic and Rheumatologic Institute, 9500 Euclid Avenue, A40, Cleveland, OH 44195.
E-mail address: ricchee@ccf.org

0030-5898/18/© 2018 Elsevier Inc. All rights reserved.

Table 1
Thresholds for annual surgeon and hospital volume

	Surgeon			Hospital				
	Low	Medium	High	Low	Medium	High		
Hammond et al,[29] 2003	<0.9	0.9–4.3	>4.3	<7.1	7.1–14.3	>14.3		
Jain et al,[22] 2004	<2	2–4	>4	<5	5–9	>9		
Lyman et al,[28] 2005	—			<4	4–11.75	>11.75		
Singh et al,[24] 2014	<8	8–17.5	>17.5	<20.5	20.5–26	>26		
Singh & Ramachandran,[27] 2015	—			<5 5–9	10–14	15–24	>24	
Scott et al,[23] 2015	<2	2–5	>5	—				
Ramkumar et al,[26] 2017	<5	5–14	>14	<4	4–14	>14		

analyzing the 1998 New York Statewide Planning and Research Cooperative System database reported that 78.2% of orthopedic surgeons performing shoulder arthroplasty only performed one to two of these procedures annually during the period studied. Thus, it was concluded that shoulder arthroplasty is performed primarily by low-volume providers. Additionally, Somerson and colleagues[21] described the uneven distribution of high-volume shoulder arthroplasty surgeons, arbitrarily defined as those performing at least 11 procedures annually, suggesting a potential disparity in access.

To enhance the value of shoulder arthroplasty, an improvement of outcomes or a decrease in associated costs must occur. There are multiple reports in the literature expanding on the relationship between increased surgeon and hospital procedure volume and increased value for shoulder arthroplasty, by way of improved outcomes or decreased cost. This review article highlights these studies.

VOLUME THRESHOLDS

Among the studies investigating the volume-value relationship in shoulder arthroplasty, there is a lack of consensus in the thresholds used to categorize surgeons and hospitals as low, medium, and high volume. The surgeon and hospital volume thresholds reported in the literature are available in **Table 1**.

Several methods were reported in the determination of thresholds for surgeon volume, with the primary technique using a linear distribution of procedures in each group and creating an equal distribution of surgeons in each group.[22–24] In contrast, Ramkumar and colleagues[25] applied stratum-specific likelihood ratio (SSLR) analysis using a receiver operating characteristics, a technique previously used in the analysis of total knee arthroplasty volume.[26]

The SSLR analysis method generates meaningful volume thresholds using risk stratification for any given dependent variable, from readmission rates to patient-reported outcome measures (PROMs) to revision rate, by providing cutoffs that are supported by a significant difference between adjacent groups.[26] Using these evidence-based thresholds, surgeons were stratified into low (<5), medium (5–14), and high (>14) volume. The upper threshold for low-volume surgeons ranged from 0.9 to 8 cases annually. The lower threshold for annual caseload for high-volume surgeons ranged from 4 to 17.5.

Similarly, there is a lack of consensus regarding the appropriate thresholds in defining low- and high-volume hospitals, with several studies dividing hospitals linearly to allocate an equal proportion of procedures or surgeons in each category.[22,24,27] Lyman and colleagues[28] suggested that meaningful thresholds may be defined as low-volume hospitals performing shoulder arthroplasty procedures less than once per quarter and high-volume hospitals more than once per month. Ramkumar and colleagues[26] repeated the SSLR analysis for both annual hospital volume to generate statistically significant thresholds in terms of LOS and cost, which produced three strata, as follows: low (<4), medium (4–14), and high (>14) volume strata. The upper threshold for low-volume hospitals ranged from 4 to 20.5 annual cases. The minimum cutoff for high-volume hospitals ranged from 9 to 26 annual procedures.

There is currently no consensus regarding the most appropriate method of determining volume thresholds, or the cutoff values defining these thresholds, in shoulder arthroplasty. Standardized, evidence-based thresholds using SSLR analysis from larger scale population data for surgeon and hospital volume may be needed to fully evaluate the volume-value relationship in shoulder arthroplasty across various different study cohorts.

SURGEON VOLUME

Several studies investigating the relationship between surgeon volume and value have been published, although there remains discrepancy in the thresholds used to categorize low-, medium-, and high-volume surgeons.[22–24,26,29] The relationship between higher surgeon volume and its effect on outcomes and costs is described in **Table 2**.

Outcomes

Overall, surgical outcomes are improved with increasing surgeon volume. Patients undergoing TSA performed by a low-volume surgeon were 1.7 to 2.5 times more likely to experience postoperative complications and 4.4 times more likely to die during the hospital admission.[22,29] LOS, an outcome with a direct economic impact, was greater for low-volume surgeons, with the difference between low- and high-volume surgeons ranging from 7 hours to 1.4 days.[22,24,26,29] Additional outcomes reported in the literature include an increasing rate of nonroutine discharge and increased blood loss for low-volume surgeons as compared with the high-volume cohort.[22,24]

Several possible explanations exist regarding the improvement of outcomes with increasing surgeon volume. Ramkumar and colleagues[26] suggests that higher volume surgeons may have a greater level of training and experience. This assertion is supported by the fact that surgeons who have completed an American Shoulder and Elbow Surgeons fellowship have a higher surgical volume, with a mean of 32.1 annual shoulder arthroplasties, compared with a mean of 22.6 shoulder arthroplasties by surgeons without American Shoulder and Elbow Surgeons fellowship training.[21] Similarly, Singh and colleagues[24] suggested that this relationship between increased surgeon volume and improved outcomes after shoulder arthroplasty may be partially attributed to the learning curve associated with reverse TSA, aligning with the idea that "practice makes perfect."[30,31] In the literature, the documented threshold of annual cases required to surpass a baseline level of proficiency for reverse TSA ranges from 7 to 40, a caseload that high-volume surgeons are likely reach.[32–34] This principle of specialization may be possible within a single institution, in which cases may be referred to specific surgeons who most frequently perform the procedure.[26] An additional explanation for this relationship may be the idea of "selective referral," in which patients are referred to surgeons with greater comfort in both routine and complex cases, only furthering surgeon volume.[31,35] Luft and colleagues[31] suggests that the concept of "practice makes perfect" may have a greater impact on outcomes of more routine procedures that are unlikely to require referrals, whereas the practice of "selective referral" is more predominant in complex procedures.

A shorter LOS in the high-volume surgeon group may be attributed to pre-existing discharge plans and rehabilitation protocol, and the surgeon familiarity with the recovery from the procedure.[29] Procedure-specific protocols may involve an approach using a multidisciplinary team familiar with the operation, incorporating patient education regarding postoperative care and discharge, standardized orders, regional anesthesia and scheduled narcotics when appropriate, patients grouped in the wards by procedure type, and early use of physical therapy.[16,36–38]

Cost

Higher volume surgeons performed shoulder arthroplasties with reduced costs, thus reaching greater value.[23,26,29] The total cost of hospitalization was lower for patients with high-volume surgeons as compared with low-volume surgeons, with the reduction ranging from $1000

	Surgical Outcomes	Cost Effects
Table 2 Trends of outcomes and costs with increasing surgeon volume		
Hammond et al,[29] 2003	Complications ↓ LOS ↓	Cost ↓[a]
Jain et al,[22] 2004	Hospital mortality ↓ Complications ↓ Nonroutine discharge ↓ LOS ↓	
Singh et al,[24] 2014	Blood loss ↓ Operative time ↓ LOS ↓	
Scott et al,[23] 2015		Cost ↓
Ramkumar et al,[26] 2017	LOS ↓	Cost ↓

[a] Not statistically significant.

to $3700.[26,29] Scott and colleagues[23] demonstrated an average increase in cost attributable to complications and nonroutine discharge from $1692 per case for high-volume providers to $2021 per case for low-volume providers, with a relative reduction of $329 in additional costs per case from a lower rate of adverse events for high-volume surgeons. Overall, the reduction in cost per case for high-volume surgeons may be attributed to the shorter LOS, lower complication rate, lower likelihood of nonroutine discharge, and shorter operative time.

HOSPITAL VOLUME

The relationship between hospital volume and value in shoulder arthroplasty has been described in the literature, although the thresholds used to classify low-, medium-, and high-volume hospitals are inconsistent.[22,24,26–29] The association between increased hospital volume and its effect on surgical outcomes and cost are described in **Table 3**.

Outcomes

Generally, patients treated at higher volume hospitals experience superior surgical outcomes.[22,24,26–29] Patients undergoing shoulder arthroplasty at low-volume hospitals were 1.25

to 2.5 times more likely to experience complications and 2.1 times more likely to die than patients at high-volume hospitals.[22,28,29] Similarly, patients at low-volume hospitals had a significantly higher revision rate (0.5%), compared with those at high-volume hospitals (0.3%).[27] Several studies have demonstrated that patients at low-volume hospitals are up to 1.7 times more likely to experience an increased LOS, ranging from an additional 7.2 hours to 1.1 days[22,26–29], although the 2014 study by Singh and colleagues[24] did not report a difference in LOS. Additional surgical outcomes reported in the literature include an increasing rate of nonroutine discharge, more frequent readmissions, and greater blood loss or need for transfusions for patients at low-volume hospitals as compared with high-volume hospitals.[22,24,27,28] The increased need for blood transfusions at low-volume hospitals may be attributed to increased blood loss, although it is possible that low-volume hospitals may have set a lower threshold for transfusion.[27]

There are several possible explanations for the relationship between improved outcomes and increased hospital volume as described. The 2015 study by Singh and Ramachandran[27] reported that low-volume hospitals are more likely to be located in rural areas, presenting a possible disparity in access to rehabilitation

Table 3 Trends of outcomes and costs with increasing hospital volume		
	Surgical Outcomes	**Cost Effects**
Hammond et al,[29] 2003	Complications ↓[a] LOS ↓	Cost ↓[a]
Jain et al,[22] 2004	Hospital mortality ↓ Complications ↓ Nonroutine discharge ↓ LOS ↓	
Lyman et al,[28] 2005	Readmission ↓ Revision ↓[a] Complications ↓[a] 60-day mortality ↓[a] LOS ↓	Cost –
Singh et al,[24] 2014	Blood loss ↓ Operative time ↓ LOS –	
Singh & Ramachandran,[27] 2015	Nonroutine discharge ↓ Postarthroplasty fracture ↓ Blood transfusion ↓ Revision ↓ LOS ↓	
Ramkumar et al,[26] 2017	LOS ↓	Cost ↓

[a] Not statistically significant.

facilities, and social support and insurance coverage. These factors may have an impact on discharge planning, because LOS may be prolonged in patients without access to rehabilitation facilities. Additionally, hospitals performing a high volume of shoulder arthroplasties may have an organized discharge process with a streamlined transition to care, and care teams are likely to be more familiar with the procedure.[27] Singh and Ramachandran[27] demonstrated that high-volume hospitals were likely to treat patients with a greater comorbidity index, yet maintained a shorter LOS with greater discharge to home, suggesting that these higher volume institutions may have more efficient resource utilization. The hospitals of high-volume surgeons are likely to be high-volume hospitals, thus also conferring the previously discussed benefits of high surgeon caseloads on these hospitals.

Cost

Higher volume hospitals may achieve reduced cost for shoulder arthroplasty, although this relationship was inconsistent.[26,28,29] Hammond and colleagues[29] demonstrated a 1.25 times greater risk of increased cost for patients undergoing shoulder arthroplasty at low-volume institutions, although this relationship was not significant. Ramkumar and coworkers[26] reported a significant reduction in costs by $3300 for high-volume institutions as compared with low-volume hospitals. In the study published by Lyman and colleagues,[28] costs were lowest for the medium-volume hospitals, and there was no significant difference between low- and high-volume institutions, although these differences were attributed to the trends of LOS in this cohort. Additionally, the minimum threshold for an institution to be characterized as high volume was lower for the Lyman and colleagues[28] study than the Hammond and colleagues[29] and Ramkumar and colleagues[28] studies, suggesting that the cohort stratification may be insufficient for capturing a potential relationship between hospital volume and cost.

A potential relationship between reduced costs and increasing surgical volume may be explained by the concept of economies of scale.[26] This principle suggests that high-volume institutions are able to realize lower costs by reducing fixed per-unit costs (ie, implants) and potentially lessening variable costs.[39–41] For example, low-volume hospitals are likely to pay a greater cost for orthopedic implants.[42,43] Additionally, variable costs may be reduced by standardizing the care of a patient among the multiple teams providing care, including

operating room and nursing staff.[26] The implementation of specialized care teams that function as an integrated practice may provide another method by which high-volume hospitals demonstrate reduced costs.[5] Similarly, high-volume institutions may be able to achieve greater value with the availability of multiple operating rooms, because up to one-third of the time that a patient spends in the operating room for shoulder arthroplasty is nonsurgical, translating to approximately 1 hour per case.[44] Hospitals with dedicated orthopedic operating rooms may also have the potential to achieve improved efficiency, which can also reduce costs.[45]

SUMMARY

With the ever-increasing pressure to improve the value of care delivered in orthopedic surgery, the relationship between increasing volume and enhanced value presents a unique opportunity in shoulder arthroplasty. The literature supports a relationship between increasing surgeon and hospital volume with improved surgical outcomes and reduced cost, and thus increased value, although the primary drivers of this relationship have not been fully defined. Only one study to date has attempted to apply evidence-based cut-offs to establish the significant thresholds that define low-, medium-, and high-volume hospitals and surgeons in shoulder arthroplasty.[26] Several studies demonstrated a stronger relationship of value with surgeon volume as compared with hospital volume, indicating that surgeon volume may be the driving force in this relationship.[24,29] To date, the studies investigating the volume-value relationship in shoulder arthroplasty have been retrospective and do not include PROMs, indicating a potential direction of further study in this field.

REFERENCES

1. Porter ME. A strategy for health care reform: toward a value-based system. N Engl J Med 2009; 361(2):109–12.
2. Shervin N, Rubash HE, Katz JN. Orthopaedic procedure volume and patient outcomes. Clin Orthop Relat Res 2007;457:35–41.
3. Hamid KS, Nwachukwu BU, Ellis SJ. Competing in value-based health care: keys to winning the foot race. Foot Ankle Int 2014;35(5):519–28.
4. Bozic KJ, Wright JG. Value-based healthcare and orthopaedic surgery: editorial comment. Clin Orthop Relat Res 2012;470(4):1004–5.
5. Black EM, Higgins LD, Warner JJP. Value-based shoulder surgery: practicing outcomes-driven,

cost-conscious care. J Shoulder Elbow Surg 2013; 22(7):1000–9.

6. Gutierrez B, Culler SD, Freund DA. Does hospital procedure-specific volume affect treatment costs? A National Study of Knee Replacement Surgery. Available at: https://www-ncbi-nlm-nih-gov.ezproxyhost.library.tmc.edu/pmc/articles/PMC1070273/pdf/hsresearch00027-0063.pdf. Accessed November 12, 2017.

7. Paul JC, Lonner BS, Vira S, et al. High-volume hospitals and surgeons experience fewer early reoperation events after adolescent idiopathic scoliosis surgery. Spine Deform 2015;3(5):496–501.

8. Ravi B, Jenkinson R, Austin PC, et al. Relation between surgeon volume and risk of complications after total hip arthroplasty: propensity score matched cohort study. BMJ 2014;348:g3284.

9. Basques BA, Bitterman A, Campbell KJ, et al. Influence of surgeon volume on inpatient complications, cost, and length of stay following total ankle arthroplasty. Foot Ankle Int 2016;37(10): 1046–51.

10. Norton EC, Garfinkel SA, McQuay LJ, et al. The effect of hospital volume on the in-hospital complication rate in knee replacement patients. Health Serv Res 1998;33(5 Pt 1):1191–210. Available at: http://www.ncbi.nlm.nih.gov/pubmed/9865217. Accessed November 12, 2017.

11. Kreder HJ, Deyo RA, Koepsell T, et al. Relationship between the volume of total hip replacements performed by providers and the rates of postoperative complications in the state of Washington. J Bone Joint Surg Am 1997;79(4):485–94. Available at: http://www.ncbi.nlm.nih.gov/pubmed/9111392. Accessed November 12, 2017.

12. Singh JA, Kwoh CK, Boudreau RM, et al. Hospital volume and surgical outcomes after elective hip/knee arthroplasty: a risk adjusted analysis of a large regional database. Arthritis Rheum 2011. https://doi.org/10.1002/art.30390.

13. Taylor HD, Dennis DA, Crane HS, et al. Relationship between mortality rates and hospital patient volume for Medicare patients undergoing major orthopaedic surgery of the hip, knee, spine, and femur. J Arthroplasty 1997;12(3):235–42.

14. Munoz E, Boiardo R, Mulloy K, et al. Economies of scale, physician volume for orthopedic surgical patients, and the DRG prospective payment system. Orthopedics 1990;13(1):39–44. Available at: https://search-proquest-com.ezproxyhost.library.tmc.edu/docview/962451592/fulltextPDF/CF018073B6C4895PQ/1?accountid=7034. Accessed January 15, 2018.

15. Tessier JE, Rupp G, Gera JT, et al. Physicians with defined clear care pathways have better discharge disposition and lower cost. J Arthroplasty 2016; 31(9):54–8.

16. Stambough JB, Nunley RM, Curry MC, et al. Rapid recovery protocols for primary total hip arthroplasty can safely reduce length of stay without increasing readmissions. J Arthroplasty 2015;30(4):521–6.

17. Kim SH, Wise BL, Zhang Y, et al. Increasing incidence of shoulder arthroplasty in the United States. J Bone Joint Surg Am 2011;93(24):2249–54.

18. Day JS, Lau E, Ong KL, et al. Prevalence and projections of total shoulder and elbow arthroplasty in the United States to 2015. J Shoulder Elbow Surg 2010;19(8):1115–20.

19. Brolin TJ, Throckmorton TW. Outpatient shoulder arthroplasty. Orthop Clin North Am 2018;49(1): 73–9.

20. Hasan SS, Leith JM, Smith KL, et al. The distribution of shoulder replacement among surgeons and hospitals is significantly different than that of hip or knee replacement. J Shoulder Elbow Surg 2003; 12(2):164–9.

21. Somerson JS, Stein BA, Wirth MA. Distribution of high-volume shoulder arthroplasty surgeons in the United States. J Bone Joint Surg Am 2016; 98(18):e77.

22. Jain N, Pietrobon R, Hocker S, et al. The relationship between surgeon and hospital volume and outcomes for shoulder arthroplasty. J Bone Joint Surg Am 2004;86-A(3):496–505.

23. Scott DJ, Sherman S, Dhawan A, et al. Quantifying the economic impact of provider volume through adverse events: the case of sports medicine. Orthop J Sports Med 2015;3(3). 2325967115574476.

24. Singh A, Yian EH, Dillon MT, et al. The effect of surgeon and hospital volume on shoulder arthroplasty perioperative quality metrics. J Shoulder Elbow Surg 2014;23(8):1187–94.

25. Wilson S, Marx RG, Pan T-J, et al. Meaningful thresholds for the volume-outcome relationship in total knee arthroplasty. J Bone Joint Surg Am 2016;98(20):1683–90.

26. Ramkumar PN, Navarro SM, Haeberle HS, et al. Evidence-based thresholds for the volume-value relationship in shoulder arthroplasty: outcomes and economies of scale. J Shoulder Elbow Surg 2017; 26(8):1399–406.

27. Singh JA, Ramachandran R. Does hospital volume predict outcomes and complications after total shoulder arthroplasty in the US? Arthritis Care Res (Hoboken) 2015;67(6):885–90.

28. Lyman S, Jones EC, Bach PB, et al. The association between hospital volume and total shoulder arthroplasty outcomes. Clin Orthop Relat Res 2005;(432): 132–7.

29. Hammond JW, Queale WS, Kim TK, et al. Surgeon experience and clinical and economic outcomes for shoulder arthroplasty. J Bone Joint Surg Am 2003; 85-A(12):2318–24.

30. Luft HS, Bunker JP, Enthoven AC. Should operations be regionalized? The empirical relation between surgical volume and mortality. N Engl J Med 1979;301(25):1364–9.

31. Luft HS, Hunt SS, Maerki SC. The volume-outcome relationship: practice-makes-perfect or selective-referral patterns? Health Serv Res 1987;22(2): 157–82.

32. Wierks C, Skolasky RL, Ji JH, et al. Reverse total shoulder replacement: intraoperative and early postoperative complications. Clin Orthop Relat Res 2009;467(1):225–34.

33. Riedel BB, Mildren ME, Jobe CM, et al. Evaluation of the learning curve for reverse shoulder arthroplasty. Orthopedics 2010;33(4). https://doi.org/10.3928/01477447-20100225-09.

34. Kempton LB, Ankerson E, Michael Wiater J. A complication-based learning curve from 200 reverse shoulder arthroplasties. Clin Orthop Relat Res 2011;469:2496–504.

35. Berglund DD, Samuel R, Levy JC. American shoulder and elbow surgeons membership and its association with primary and revision shoulder arthroplasty volume. JSES Open Access 2017;1(2): 51–4.

36. Walter FL, Bass N, Bock G, et al. Success of clinical pathways for total joint arthroplasty in a community hospital. Clin Orthop Relat Res 2007;457(457): 133–7.

37. Peters CL, Shirley B, Erickson J. The effect of a new multimodal perioperative anesthetic regimen on postoperative pain, side effects, rehabilitation, and length of hospital stay after total joint arthroplasty. J Arthroplasty 2006;21(6 Suppl.):132–8.

38. Larsen K, Hansen TB, Thomsen PB, et al. Cost-effectiveness of accelerated perioperative care and rehabilitation after total hip and knee arthroplasty. J Bone Joint Surg Am 2009;91(4):761–72.

39. Bernoff J. Economies of scale in a personalized world. Harvard Business Review 2008. Available at: https://hbr.org/2008/04/economies-of-scale-in-the-very.html. Accessed November 12, 2017.

40. McGrath ME, Hoole RW. Manufacturing's new economies of scale. Harvard Business Review 1992. Available at: https://hbr.org/1992/05/manufacturings-new-economies-of-scale. Accessed November 12, 2017.

41. Gaynor M, Seider H, Vogt WB. The volume-outcome effect, scale economies, and learning-by-doing. Am Econ Rev 2005;95:243–7.

42. Martineau P, Filion KB, Huk OL, et al. Primary hip arthroplasty costs are greater in low-volume than in high-volume Canadian hospitals. Clin Orthop Relat Res 2005;(437):152–6.

43. Bosco JA, Alvarado CM, Slover JD, et al. Decreasing total joint implant costs and physician specific cost variation through negotiation. J Arthroplasty 2014;29(4):678–80.

44. Padegimas EM, Hendy BA, Lawrence C, et al. An analysis of surgical and nonsurgical operating room times in high-volume shoulder arthroplasty. J Shoulder Elbow Surg 2017;26(6):1058–63.

45. Small TJ, Gad BV, Klika AK, et al. Dedicated orthopedic operating room unit improves operating room efficiency. J Arthroplasty 2013;28(7):1066–71.e2.

Foot and Ankle

Patient Safety
Driving After Foot and Ankle Surgery

John J. Carroll, MD*, William D. McClain, MD,
Thomas C. Dowd, MD

KEYWORDS

• Driving • Surgery • Braking • Lower extremity • Foot and ankle • Patient safety

---

KEY POINTS

• It is important for orthopedic surgeons to inform their foot and ankle postsurgical patients when it is unsafe to return to driving. Several studies have examined the impact of surgery and immobilization on braking time.
• Orthopedic surgeons should not inform patients that it is definitely safe to return to driving after surgery. The return to driving is multifactorial, depending on the particular procedure performed, the timing of that procedure, immobilization, comorbidities, medications, and personal driving capabilities and habits.
• The decision to return should be informed by clinical considerations as well as state laws and insurance policy limitations.

BACKGROUND

Driving after surgery is regularly associated with the ability to stop the vehicle. Brake reaction time (BRT) is the amount of time necessary to react to a stimulus and depress the brake pedal. BRT is an important component of driving behavior and is of interest in research and in litigation with accidents. In 2000, Green[1] described a series of steps that constituted the process of emergency braking, from stimulation or situation to result (car braking). The first one is mental processing time, which includes sensation, perception, and response selection and programming. For example, one must sense an object in the road, determine the meaning of the sensation, choose which response to make, and then mentally program the movement. The second step is movement time. The final step is device response time, or the time is takes for the physical device (vehicle) to respond to the driver's input.[1] The US Federal Highway Administration defines the threshold for safe total brake response time (TBRT) as 700 milliseconds (ms).[2] TBRT is the sum of the reaction time, movement time, and device response time. It is sometimes difficult to compare and contrast studies because there is variability regarding terms and measures of time that are used to evaluate braking time and reaction. Situation-type and driver-related variables are key when evaluating BRT.[3] These driver-related variables are particularly important in the postoperative period when age, overall health, immobilization, and procedure performed play a role in a patient's mental processing and movement time.

Foot and ankle surgeons are interested in the answer to the common question of when a patient can return to driving following surgery; patients are no less interested. Although many articles are devoted to the impact of orthopedic surgery on driving, the purpose of this article is

---

Disclosure Statement: No disclosures.
Department of Orthopaedic Surgery, SAUSHEC Orthopaedic Residency Program Position, 3551 Roger Brooke Drive, Fort Sam Houston, TX 78234, USA
* Corresponding author.
E-mail address: John.j.carroll6.mil@mail.mil

Orthop Clin N Am 49 (2018) 527–539
https://doi.org/10.1016/j.ocl.2018.06.002
0030-5898/18/Published by Elsevier Inc.

to specifically review the available evidence regarding driving and foot and ankle surgery.[4–8]

MEDICOLEGAL

It is important for physicians to be aware of their medical and legal responsibilities as perceived in the court of law. In the United States, most states do not have regulations about driving in a lower extremity cast, removable lower extremity immobilization device, or after foot and ankle surgery. Sansosti and colleagues[9] reviewed the US driving laws relative to foot and ankle patients for all 50 states. In their study, the District of Columbia, Connecticut, Maine, and Vermont were the only states identified with any information about driving with a lower extremity cast or immobilization device. Even within these 3 sets of state regulations, the information and wording were vague. Maine was the most specific and included the wording "driving may need to be temporarily prohibited due to an immobilizing cast...if it impedes safe operation of a motor vehicle." The words "may" and "if" still left much to the interpretation of the driver. Other states indicated that "any health problems can affect your driving," and that the "foot should be able to pivot smoothly from brake to accelerator while the heel is kept on the floor." Pennsylvania was the only state that required a medical evaluation and clearance to apply for a driver's permit.

Even though no states have laws specifically referring to cast, brace, or postoperative period, all states have offenses for carelessness, recklessness, and negligence. The definitions for these 3 offenses are not specific and can be interpreted to mean different things by law enforcement officials. One might argue that driving with a lower extremity cast or brace on or driving in the postoperative period falls under carelessness, recklessness, or negligence. Driving while using narcotic pain medications will result in "driving under the influence charge" in most states.

Very few states require physicians to report patients with impaired driving function, but other states do have ways for physicians to do so if they wish. Oregon and Pennsylvania specifically require physicians to report patients with impaired driving ability. In Oregon, physicians "must report patients if cognitive and functional impairments become severe and uncontrollable." In Pennsylvania, physicians must report any patient 15 and older who has a condition that could "impair his/her ability to safely operate a motor vehicle." Most states grant immunity to physicians with respect to reporting potentially impaired drivers, but Alaska, Arkansas, the District of Columbia, Nevada, New Hampshire, New Jersey, New Mexico, New York, South Dakota, Texas, Virginia, and Washington do not.[9] Physicians may have liability if they fail to correctly advise patients not to drive.[10]

Several studies have looked into the medical and legal implications of returning to drive in the United Kingdom. Although the specific rules and laws may differ from the United States, the review papers offer useful advice for physicians to provide patients on returning to drive.[11,12] When a patient is likely fit to return to driving, he or she should first practice with the pedals and hand controls in a stationary car. Next, he or she should take the car for a short drive while accompanied by another driver who could take over should the patient feel unable to continue. Finally, the patient may then progress to driving unaccompanied. The important thing is to slowly build up to a full return to driving alone.

INSURANCE

Insurance companies typically do not publically detail when a patient can or cannot return to driving after surgery, and there have been no studies up until this point surveying insurance companies in the United States. Several studies from the United Kingdom have surveyed insurance companies for their recommendations following orthopedic surgery, and the consensus from these studies is that the ability to return to driving depends on the patient even though the physician's opinion plays a role.[13] The patient is ultimately responsible, and the key is that the patient is in control of the vehicle. If stopped by the police, the patient needs to demonstrate that he or she was in control of the vehicle.[12] A 1996 study from the United Kingdom sought the opinion of major insurance companies for returning to drive after orthopedic surgery. This study indicated that insurers could refuse insurance coverage when a driver had an accident while still recovering from an earlier injury or operation, but insurers did say that coverage typically would be maintained if patients followed the physician's advice.[11] In 2003, Von Arx and colleagues[14] had a poor survey response of the insurance companies in the United Kingdom, but the consensus was that patients should follow the advice of the physicians even though all cases would be evaluated individually.

INJURY

Lower extremity trauma requiring operative fixation is common and impacts a patient's ability to drive. There have been studies describing returning to drive after operative management of ankle fractures, calcaneus fractures, tibial plafond fractures, Achilles tendon injuries, and traumatic amputations. Egol and colleagues[15] looked at 31 operatively treated right ankle fractures (isolated malleolar, bimalleolar, or trimalleolar) and compared total braking time (initial reaction time plus foot movement plus total braking time) with 11 healthy volunteers. All 31 patients were allowed to weight bear at 6 weeks and were measured in a simulator at 6 weeks, 9 weeks, and 12 weeks postoperatively. At 9 weeks postoperatively, there was no difference in total braking time. A similar study by Yousri and Jackson[16] determined that patients with operatively treated right ankle fractures were able to generate a brake force equal to the contralateral lower extremity within 3 weeks after starting to fully weight bear out of plaster.

A separate study by Egol and colleagues[17] looked at all right lower extremity trauma and separated long bone fractures (tibia and femur) from articular fractures (calcaneus, pilon, plateau, and acetabulum). This study did not deal solely with foot and ankle trauma, but it used a simulator to determine that brake travel time equaled the uninjured, albeit atypical, left side at 6 weeks after being allowed to fully weight bear. Those patients with articular fractures required additional time to recover before return to full weight bearing when compared with nonarticular fractures and, as a result, required additional time before return to driving.[17] A 2000 survey of 66 orthopedic surgeons in the United Kingdom looked into when patients might be able to return to drive after operative management of upper and lower extremity fractures. With regard to the lower extremity fractures, there was a consensus that if a patient had an external fixator or lower extremity splint, they should not be driving.[18]

Achilles tendon ruptures create soft tissue trauma that typically requires prolonged immobilization and therapy after surgery. In 2004, Jennings and colleagues[19] described a novel technique for repairing Achilles tendon ruptures using polyester tape and patients were allowed to weight bear at 6 weeks and drive at an average of 49 days. There was no assessment of strength or movement time in this study, but they reported no complications with regard to the return to driving.

Lower extremity amputations can be the result of trauma, and these injuries pose significant challenges when attempting to return to driving. Pauley and Devlin[20] looked at 10 patients with traumatic transtibial amputations (5 right and 5 left) and matched them with age-related controls. Foot pedal reaction time and movement time were recorded for each with simple and dual-task scenarios. This study did not talk specifically about timing to return to driving but conducted the testing at least 12 months after prosthetic fitting for all subjects. This study found that patients with transtibial amputations had increased reaction time, movement time, and total response time when compared with controls ($P<.001$). When asked to complete dual tasks, amputees demonstrated nearly equal slowing of reaction time with their uninjured limb and prosthetic limb. This likely was secondary to deconditioning and neural re-organization following the traumatic injury. This study demonstrated that there are significant challenges with returning to driving after a traumatic transtibial amputation and that even the noninjured limb may have deficits with regard to speed and movement compared with a healthy control.

ELECTIVE

The question about when patients can return to driving also comes up after elective foot and ankle procedures. Hallux valgus is a common condition often treated via first metatarsal osteotomy. McDonald and colleagues[21] looked at time to return to driving after hallux valgus surgery. Sixty patients underwent right first metatarsal osteotomy (36 proximal, 24 distal) by 1 of 4 providers at the same facility and their BRT was compared with 20 healthy volunteer controls. A passing BRT was set at less than 0.85 seconds, which was the slowest time from the control group and within the accepted range of 0.5 to 1.25 seconds.[1,15] At 6 weeks postoperatively, 89% of patients had passing BRT and at 8 weeks postoperatively, 100% had passing BRT.[21] Holt and colleagues[22] completed a similar study looking brake response in 28 patients undergoing right first metatarsal osteotomy. A chevron, Scarf, or proximal first osteotomy performed by the same investigators and BRT were measured at 2 and 6 weeks postoperatively. At 6 weeks, all patients had significant improvement in BRT compared with preoperatively ($P = .047$), although still slower than control subjects. Only 7 of 28 patients were able to complete the test at 2 weeks secondary to postoperative pain.

Elective procedures of the ankle and hindfoot have been studied as well with regard to return to driving. Ankle arthroscopy is a procedure being performed with increasing frequency. Liebensteiner and colleagues[23] evaluated 19 patients undergoing right ankle arthroscopy. BRT was evaluated preoperatively, in addition to 2 days, 2 weeks, 6 weeks, and 12 weeks postoperatively. The average BRT was 606 ms preoperatively and this increased to 821 ms at 2 days postoperatively ($P<.001$). This returned to an average of 606 ms at 2 weeks postoperatively. Based on this study, patients should not return to driving before 2 weeks following a right ankle arthroscopy. Two studies have looked at BRT following right ankle arthrodesis. Jeng and colleagues[24] investigated 10 patients who underwent a right ankle arthrodesis. These subjects were evaluated with a driving simulator at least 1 year after surgery, provided there was radiographic evidence of fusion and a pain-free ankle. Their results were compared with 10 age-matched controls. The mean BRT for the ankle fusion group (0.42 s) was significantly slower than the control group (0.33 s) ($P = .03$), but there was no difference between patients with ankle fusion and controls with regard to brake force, peak pressure, or contact area. A separate study was a comparative case series looking at 12 patients undergoing ankle arthrodesis and 12 undergoing midfoot or hindfoot arthrodesis (6 talonavicular, 2 subtalar, 1 triple, 1 calcaneocuboidal) compared with a series of controls. All patients were more than 6 months from surgery. Movement time (MT) ($P = .034$) and TBRT ($P = .026$) were significantly longer in patients undergoing ankle arthrodesis compared with those with midfoot/hindfoot arthrodeses and controls. Also, significantly more patients undergoing ankle arthrodesis had TBRT greater than the safe driving threshold of 700 ms ($P = .028$) when compared with the other 2 groups. There was no significant difference in MT or TBRT in patients with the midfoot/hindfoot arthrodeses compared with the controls.[2]

A final group of elective procedures that have been studied with return to driving is lower extremity amputations. Lower extremity amputations can be related to trauma, as was previously discussed, but also can be related to peripheral vascular disease and nonhealing wounds. A 2012 study sampled 90 patients who underwent unilateral or bilateral lower extremity amputations and investigated their return to driving and riding motorcycles. This study includes transtibial and transfemoral amputations, but 77.8% of the study patients had

either unilateral or bilateral transtibial amputations, with 75.5% of all the patients undergoing the procedures for diabetic foot complications and 6.7% undergoing them for peripheral vascular disease. The remaining procedures were performed for trauma and tumor. Approximately 46% of patients were able to return to driving, and factors associated with return to driving included being male ($P<.05$) and wearing a prosthesis ($P<.001$). There was no difference between right and left lower extremity amputations and the median time to return was 6 months.[25] A separate study explored this same question several years earlier in 2006. A total of 123 patients undergoing either unilateral or bilateral transtibial or transfemoral amputations were evaluated for return to driving postoperatively. Approximately 75% of the patients underwent either unilateral or bilateral transtibial amputations, with 73.2% of all the patients undergoing their procedures for peripheral vascular disease and the remainder for trauma, tumor, or lymphedema. Patients returned to driving at a rate of approximately 80% at an average of 3.8 months postoperatively. Factors significantly associated with decreased likelihood for return to driving included female sex ($P<.01$), age older than 55 ($P<.05$), right-sided amputation ($P<.05$), and pre-amputation driving frequency of less than every other day ($P<.05$). Those with right-sided amputations more commonly required vehicle modifications ($P<.001$).[26]

IMMOBILIZATION

Immobilization is common after lower extremity injury or foot and ankle surgery. There are a number of available studies on both healthy patients with immobilization devices as well as postsurgical patients that have evaluated how immobilization of the lower extremities affects braking time.

Studies on healthy volunteers with lower extremity immobilization devices have looked into the impact on aspects of driving. In 2009, Tremblay and colleagues[27] examined the effect of immobilization of the right lower extremity on driving performance during simulated driving by healthy volunteers. They compared a regular running shoe, walking cast, and Aircast walker (CAM) on the right lower extremity and measured maximum force applied to the brake pedal, BRT, and total braking time with and without a distractor. The maximum braking force in patients wearing the walking casts was significantly lower than in patients wearing a running shoe or CAM ($P = .003$). The mean braking time was significantly lower for those wearing running shoes compared with walking cast or CAM ($P<.001$). Although statistically significant differences existed, investigators were not sure of the clinical significance and impact on driving. A follow-up study to this in 2015 in the *Journal of Foot and Ankle Surgery* by Murray and colleagues[28] evaluated the effects of the short leg cast or CAM on the right lower extremity in patients in a real driving situations. Outcomes measured included foot MT, BRT, and total braking time with and without a distractor. They observed a statistically significant increase in foot MT, BRT, and total braking time when comparing walking cast or CAM with running shoes ($P<.01$). They concluded that immobilization increases emergency braking time and must be taken into consideration when counseling on returning to driving, but that it is not the only thing that matters.

Several additional studies investigated similar research questions. In 2010, a study from the authors' institution examined the effect of right lower limb immobilization and left-foot adapter devices on brake response time during simulated driving (Fig. 1). Thirty-five healthy volunteers were assessed with normal footwear, CAM boot, short leg cast, and with a left-foot driving adapter. The mean TBRT was significantly increased in all groups in comparison with the control group. The mean reaction time was significantly increased for the short leg cast and CAM boot as compared with the reaction time in the control group. Mean braking time was significantly increased in the CAM and left-foot driving adapter group as compared with braking time in the control group. Ultimately, they recommended that no patient

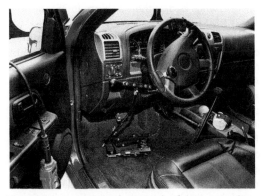

Fig. 1. Representative photograph of driving simulator for assessment of braking time. (*Courtesy of* G. Balfour, Brooke Army Medical Center, San Antonio, TX.)

should be allowed to drive when immobilized in a short leg cast, CAM boot, or with a left-foot driving adaptor.[29] A study by Sansosti and colleagues[30] assessed the effect of lower extremity immobilization on emergency braking response in 25 healthy participants. This was a young group of patients (25 ± 3.2 years) who were evaluated with different forms of immobilization to include a regular shoe, surgical shoe, or walking boot. Outcomes included mean emergency brake response time, frequency of abnormally delayed brake responses, and frequency of inaccurate brake responses were measured. The investigators found that compared with the regular shoes, these healthy young patients with either form of immobilization demonstrated significantly longer mean brake response time and frequency of abnormally delayed brake responses ($P<.001$). Those with walking boots compared with those with normal shoes also had a significantly increased number of inaccurate or inadvertent brake responses ($P<.001$). A smaller study looking at healthy volunteers was performed by Nunn and colleagues.[31] Two subjects, one trained police officer and one medical physician, were assessed while driving with below-knee casts on the right or left leg with and without a cast boot. They concluded, on the basis of the performance of the participants, that patients with below-knee casts were not suited to drive vehicles with a manual transmission, and recommended allowing driving only in automatic cars in patients with left-sided casts.

Two additional studies investigated the effect of immobilization on driving in healthy volunteers. Waton and colleagues[32] evaluated the effect of restriction of the right leg at the knee, ankle, or both on driver's braking times. They placed patients in an above-knee plaster cast, below-knee cast, or knee brace with restriction on motion. They demonstrated that total BRT was significantly longer in subjects wearing an above-knee plaster cast or knee brace fixed at $0°$ compared with braking without immobilization ($P<.001$). They also found that thinking time, or the time between a lead car braking and the commencement of the release of the accelerator was significantly increased ($P<.001$). They suggested that any patient wearing a lower limb plaster cast or knee brace be prevented from driving. Hofmann and colleagues[33] reviewed the effect of 4 commonly prescribed ankle braces (Kallassy, CaligaLoc, Air Stirrup, and ASO) on driving performance in healthy volunteers and found that all 4 braces resulted in a statistically significant increase in foot transfer time compared with measurements without a brace ($P<.001$). Three of the 4 braces resulted in a significantly prolonged BRT. A limitation with this study, as with the other studies evaluating healthy volunteers, is the unclear impact of ankle pathology on the results.

In addition to evaluating healthy volunteers, Dammerer and colleagues[34] evaluated postoperative patients. Dammerer and colleagues[34] studied the effect of surgical shoes on brake response time after first metatarsal osteotomy. They collected 42 patients who underwent right-sided first metatarsal osteotomy and tested brake response time 1 day preoperatively, as well as at 2 and 6 weeks postoperatively with hallux valgus shoes and forefoot relief shoes. BRT was significantly slower ($P<.001$) postoperatively at both 2 and 6 weeks with both forms of immobilization. By the 8-week examination, all patients had returned to wearing regular shoes. The investigators recommended that patients not return to driving for a minimum of 6 weeks after right-sided first metatarsal osteotomy.

OPIOIDS

Opioid medications are a common adjunct to pain control in postsurgical patients as well as patients with recent lower extremity injuries. Common adverse effects of opioid-based analgesics include nausea, sedation, mental clouding, dizziness, and mental impairment. Most literature supports the idea that there is an association between the use of opioid pain medications and motor vehicle accidents. This is attributed to the fact that numerous studies have implicated these medications in reducing patients' potential to process visual information, which affects driving-related functions. Studies, such as that by Byas-Smith and colleagues,[35] demonstrated that nonmedicated drivers scored significantly better on a test measuring the speed by which visual information is processed and then translated into motor activity, and a study by Verster and colleagues[36] found an association between opioid analgesic dose and increased weaving support this idea. One study in particular by Dubois and colleagues[37] attempted to isolate the effect of opioid pain medication on drivers involved in fatal crashes. They felt that many studies involving the use of opioids and motor vehicle crashes were confounded by the fact that users of opioid pain medications are often under the influence of other substances, such as benzodiazepines or alcohol. Using a case-control methodology,

they compared drivers on an isolated opioid (cases) involved in fatal crashes who had a previous record of unsafe driving actions (lane violations, speeding, failure to yield, improper turn, erratic driving) with drivers without a history of unsafe driving actions (controls). Additionally, they excluded drivers with confirmed elevated blood-alcohol content, urine drug screen positive for more than 2 opioid pain medications, and patients younger than 20 years old, as they did not have sufficient time to acquire a driving history. They then calculated odds ratios (ORs) of unsafe driving actions after controlling for age, sex, other medications, and driving record. Female drivers who tested positive for opioids had increased odds of performing an unsafe driving action from age 25 to 55 when compared with those drivers who tested negative (OR 1.35, 1.30). For male drivers, this effect was true from age 25 to 65 (OR 1.39, 1.67). This study did not determine an increased risk for unsafe driving actions preceding a fatal crash in older patients. The surgeon must consider use of narcotics postoperatively when counseling patients about return to driving with its associated medicolegal implications.

OBESITY

Obesity is another patient-specific characteristic that should be considered by the foot and ankle surgeon when considering allowing a patient to return to drive. Zhu and colleagues[38] examined the role of body mass index (BMI) and other factors in driver deaths within 30 days after motor vehicle accidents. They used logistic regression and adjusted for confounding factors to analyze associations between BMI and driver fatality and the associations among BMI, gender, age, seatbelt use, type of collision, airbag deployment, and change in velocity during a crash. Male drivers who had either a high (>35) or low (<22) BMI had a significantly increased risk for death compared with those who had an intermediate BMI. A similar association, which did not reach significance, was found in women. Another study, by Mock and colleagues,[39] sought to investigate the effect of increased body weight on the risk of death and serious injury to occupants in motor vehicle crashes. The found that increased body weight was associated with increased risk of mortality and severe injury. ORs were increased for death with each kilogram increase in body weight (1.013) and sustaining an injury with Injury Severity Score greater than 9 for each kilogram increase in body weight (1.008) after adjustment for confounding variables. They felt that increased association of BMI with mortality is in part due to increased comorbid factors in these patients as well as the possibility of increased injury severity in overweight occupants. Another large cohort study of more than 10,000 patients investigating the risk between motor vehicle driver injury and BMI demonstrated similar findings. There was an increased hazard ratio in participants in the highest (>28) and lowest (<23) quartiles for BMI.[40] Ultimately, although the suggestion of most of these studies had more to do with the implications for traffic safety and motor vehicle design, the foot and ankle surgeon should be aware that the obese patient is at a higher risk of adverse outcomes when operating a motor vehicle, either before injury or after surgical intervention.

OBSTRUCTIVE SLEEP APNEA

In conjunction with obesity, obstructive sleep apnea is another common patient factor that has been studied and found to contribute to risk of motor vehicle crash. Ellen and colleagues,[41] in a systematic review of the risk of motor vehicle crash in persons with sleep apnea, identified 40 pertinent studies on the topic. Most studies found a statistically significant increased risk of motor vehicle accident in patients with obstructive sleep apnea, some as high as 2 to 3 times increased risk. This association was not affected by the methodological quality of studies. With regard to the severity of the disease, approximately half of the studies found a statistically significant increased risk of accident with increasing severity of disease. Treatment of obstructive sleep apnea consistently improved driver performance, including crash rates, across all studies. Foot and ankle surgeons should be aware of all patient medical comorbidities and educate their patients with sleep apnea about the importance of adhering to treatment, especially in the post-operative period, for driving safety.

AGE

As patients age, additional considerations must be taken by foot and ankle surgeons when assessing their ability to return to drive. Carr et al produced a comprehensive review on assessing and counseling elderly drivers that has many key points.[42] Motor vehicle crashes are the leading cause of injury-related death in 65 to 74-year-olds and second leading cause in 75 to 84-year-olds. Older people are more likely to die than younger people when they get into a

car crash.[43,44] As people age, they tend to drive less, and may begin to feel limited by reaction times, health problems, and medication side effects. These effects and limitations can be exacerbated in the post-operative period. In the post-operative period, there may be decreased range of motion, strength, proprioception, and reaction time. These limitations may be as a result of the surgery, anesthesia, pain, or extremity immobilization. Carr et al recommended that when patients do return to driving, they should practice first in familiar, traffic-free roads prior to returning to roads with higher activity. Age plays a very important role in the baseline risk of driving and is an additional consideration that foot and ankle surgeons must account for when determining when patients may return to driving following surgery.[42,45]

DISTRACTED

Literature on distracted driving has become more available in recent years in response to advances in mobile technology. *Driver Electronic Device Use* in 2015 estimated that 9% of people who drive during the day do so while dialing or talking on a cell phone or sending and receiving text messages.[46] However, other studies have indicated that the prevalence of cell phone use while driving may be much higher.[47] One study by Redelmeier and Tibshirani[48] studied 699 drivers who had cellular telephones and were involved in motor vehicle collisions resulting in substantial property damage without personal injury. The risk of a collision when using a cellular telephone was 4 times higher than the risk when a cellular telephone was not being used. An interesting note made during that study was that units that allowed the hands to be free offered no safety advantage over handheld units.[48] Klauer and colleagues[49] reviewed the risk of road crashes among novice and experienced drivers. They collected data from 2 separate studies of newly licensed drivers and experienced drivers and identified ORs for risk of a crash or near-crash while driving. Their analysis showed that the performance of secondary tasks, such as dialing or reaching for a cell phone, texting, reaching for an object other than a cell phone, looking at roadside objects, and eating were associated with significantly increased risk of a crash among novice drivers. Among experienced drivers, only dialing a cell phone was associated with an increased risk of crash or near-crash. Commentary by Kahn and colleagues[50] reviewing data from the National

Table 1
Brake times and results in primary studies

Study	Authors	Listed Normal Brake Time	Brake Reaction Time Results	Conclusions
Driving ability after right-sided ankle arthroscopy—a prospective study	Liebensteiner et al,[23] 2015	None	BRT: 606 ± 148 ms preoperatively, 821 ± 351 ms 2 d postoperatively, 606 ± 180 ms at 2 wk, 596 ± 142 ms at 6 wk, 603 ± 142 ms at 12 wk.	Patients should not return to driving for 2 wk after right-sided ankle arthroscopy.
Driving after hallux valgus surgery	McDonald et al,[21] 2017	BRT 850 ms	BRT: Average passing score at 6 wk 640 ms, those who failed retested by 8 wk with average score of 670 ms.	Most patients can return to driving 8 wk after first metatarsal osteotomy. Some may be okay to return sooner.
Driving and emergency braking may be impaired after tibiotalar joint arthrodesis: conclusions after a case series	Schwienbacher et al,[2] 2015	TBRT 700 ms	Assessed >6 mo from surgery; TBRT control 475.7 ± 63.5 ms, OFJA 596.2 ± 141.4 ms, tibiotalar joint arthrodesis 729.7 ± 332.9 ms; BRT control 193.3 ± 24.3 ms, OFJA 223.8 ± 74 ms, TTJA 250.2 ± 120.3 ms.	Significantly more patients exceeded safe driving threshold following tibiotalar joint arthrodesis in comparison with controls. OFJA not significantly different from controls.
Emergency brake response time after first metatarsal osteotomy	Holt et al,[22] 2008	TBRT 750 ms	TBRT control 573 ± 91 ms, study group preoperative 806 ± 244 ms, 2 wk after surgery 850 ± 175 ms, 6 wk after surgery 684 ± 148 ms; reaction time control 407 ± 84 ms, study group preoperative 515 ± 131 ms, 2 wk after surgery 550 ± 102 ms, 6 wk after surgery 449 ± 93 ms.	By 6 wk after surgery, emergency braking time in patients who had first metatarsal osteotomy was similar to that of healthy patients.
The effect of immobilization devices and left-foot adapter on brake response time	Orr et al,[29] 2010	Brake time 1000 ms	TBRT: CAM Boot 675 ± 136 ms, SLC 640 ± 144 ms, left-foot driving adapter 639 ± 133 ms, reaction time CAM 417 ± 77 ms, SLC 404 ± 92 ms, LFA 354 ± 70 ms.	Total brake response time while wearing a controlled-ankle-motion boot or a short leg cast or while using a left-foot driving adapter is significantly increased compared with normal footwear.

Title	Author	BRT	Results	Conclusions
Effect of variable lower extremity immobilization devices on emergency brake response driving outcomes	Sansosti et al,[30] 2016	BRT 700 ms	BRT: surgical shoe 611 ms, walking boot 736 ms, control 575 ms.	Surgical shoe and walking boot demonstrated slower mean brake response times and more frequent abnormally delayed brake responses compared with control shoe. The walking boot demonstrated more frequent inaccurate brake responses, whereas the walking boot did not.
Effects of orthopedic immobilization of the right lower limb on driving performance: an experimental study during simulated driving by health volunteers	Tremblay et al,[27] 2009	None	Mean BRT without distractor: running shoe 548 ± 43 ms, walking cast 571 ± 51 ms, Aircast walker 581 ± 46 ms; mean BRT with distractor running shoe 602 ± 46 ms, walking cast 625 ± 57 ms, Aircast walker 642 ± 53 ms.	Immobilization of right leg affects braking force as well as BRT and total braking time during emergency braking by healthy volunteers.
Effects of right lower limb orthopedic immobilization on braking function: an on-the-road experimental study with health volunteers	Murray et al,[28] 2015	None	Average BRT without distractor: running shoe 399 ms, Aircast walker 444 ms, walking cast 459 ms; average BRT with distractor: running shoe 429 ms, Aircast walker 481 ms, walking cast 474 ms.	Wearing an immobilization device on right lower limb minimally lengthens emergency braking time in healthy drivers under actual driving conditions.
How do ankle braces affect braking performance? An experimental driving simulation study with healthy volunteers	Hofmann et al,[33] 2015	BRT 600 ms	BRT no brace 410 ± 39 ms, with brace Kallasy 429 ± 45 ms, CaligaLoc 450 ± 307 ms, Air Stirrup 440 ± 43 ms, ASO 441 ± 49 ms.	Ankle braces lead to impaired braking performance.
Effect of surgical shoes on brake response time after first metatarsal osteotomy—a prospective cohort study	Dammerer et al,[34] 2016	700–1500 ms	Average BRT, HVS 2 wk 804 ± 275 ms, FRS 2 wk 841 ± 245 ms, HVS 6 wk 750 ± 200 ms, FRS 6 wk 811 ± 211 ms.	Recommend avoiding driving for a minimum of 6 wk postoperatively when using a surgical shoe after bunionectomy.
Lower extremity function for driving an automobile after operative treatment of ankle fracture	Egol et al,[15] 2003	None	BRT: 777 ± 111 ms in control, 870 ± 143 ms at 6 wk, 854 ± 120 ms at 9 wk, 870 ± 131 ms at 12 wk; total braking time 1079 ± 165 ms in controls, 1330 ± 436 ms at 6 wk, 1172 ± 224 ms at 9 wk, 1160 ± 203 ms at 12 wk.	Total braking time returns to normal 9 wk after undergoing surgical fixation of displaced right ankle fracture.

(continued on next page)

Study	Authors	Listed Normal Brake Time	Brake Reaction Time Results	Conclusions
Influence of a concurrent cognitive task on foot pedal reaction time following traumatic, unilateral transtibial amputation	Pauley & Devlin,[20] 2011	None	All subjects >12 mo from surgery. Reaction Time: Simple task control 239 ± 34 ms. With dual task and study subject, 260 ± 54 ms intact leg, 255 ± 55 ms prosthetic leg. With dual task, control 317 ± 63 ms. With dual task in study subjects, intact leg 438 ± 107 ms, prosthetic leg 426 ± 110 ms.	Slowing of BRT in both intact leg and prosthetic leg following transtibial amputation.
Driving brake reaction time following right ankle arthrodesis	Jeng et al,[24] 2011	640–700 ms	All study subjects at least 12 mo postoperative. BRT tight ankle arthrodesis 420 ± 140 ms, controls 330 ± 60 ms.	BRT significantly slower in fusion group but still below accepted normal range.
The effect of opioids on driving and psychomotor performance in patients with chronic pain	Byas-Smith et al,[35] 2005	None	Opioid group: reaction time (first half of test) 389.9 ± 55.7 ms, (second half) 358.6 ± 62.0 ms, nonopioid (chronic pain not on medication) (first half) 394.6 ± 77 ms, (second half) 379.6 ± 8 ms, healthy (no chronic pain or medication): (first half) 406.9 ± 87 ms, (second half) 367.2 ± 69 ms.	Patients taking opioids or with chronic pain with comparable driving ability to healthy patients.
Effects of an opioid (oxycodone/paracetamol) and an NSAID (bromfenac) on driving ability, memory functioning, psychomotor performance, pupil size, and mood	Verster et al,[36] 2006	None	Reaction time: placebo 517 ± 19 ms, bromfenac (25 mg) 520 ± 21 ms, bromfenac (50 mg) 520 ± 20 ms, oxycodone/paracetamol (5/325 mg) 537 ± 28 ms, oxycodone/paracetamol (10/650 mg) 550 ± 22 ms.	No significant impairment with bromfenac or oxycodone/paracetamol at varying doses.

BRT: United States 700 ms, Australia 750 ms, Germany 1500 ms.

Abbreviations: BRT, brake reaction time; FRS, forefoot relief shoe; HVS, hallux valgus shoe; LFA, left foot adapter; NSAID, nonsteroidal anti-inflammatory drug; OFJA, other foot joint arthrodesis; SLC, short leg cast; TBRT, total brake response time.

Highway Traffic Safety Administration noted that for drivers 15 to 19 years old involved in a fatal crash, 21% were distracted by use of a cell phone. The foot and ankle surgeon should have an awareness of patient factors associated with higher risk when considering allowing a patient to return to driving.

SUMMARY

Current medicolegal requirements and insurance recommendations leave much to the interpretation of the patient or driver and surgeon. Studies looking into returning to drive after surgery as well as with immobilization devices can guide surgeons in their recommendations to patients. Table 1 summarizes the available literature regarding braking time. Box 1 provides recommendations regarding driving after orthopedic foot and ankle surgery. BRT returns to normal 9 weeks after operative management of a right ankle fracture and typically 6 weeks after being allowed to weight bear following operative management of articular fractures (tibial plafond, calcaneus). Patients undergoing surgery for hallux valgus should wait to return to driving for at least 6 to 8 weeks postoperatively. Patients should not return to driving until at least 2 weeks after a right ankle arthroscopy and a right ankle arthrodesis may have lasting effects with prolonged BRT. Lower extremity amputations for trauma and peripheral vascular disease/wound-healing problems require extensive rehabilitation and often car modifications before returning to driving. Patients should not drive with right lower extremity immobilization.

Box 1
Recommendations regarding patients being unsafe to return to driving after orthopedic foot and ankle surgery

- For 9 weeks after operative fixation of right ankle fracture
- For 6 to 8 weeks after surgery for right hallux valgus
- For 2 weeks after right ankle arthroscopy
- While the right lower extremity is immobilized
- Right ankle arthrodesis may have lasting impact on brake reaction time
- Amputations require extensive rehabilitation and car modifications before driving
- Opioids, obesity, obstructive sleep apnea, age, and distractions are risk factors that should be considered

---

Opioid use, obesity, obstructive sleep apnea, increasing age, and distractions all place drivers at increased risk for accidents and are variables that must be assessed in the postoperative period when counseling patients on when to return to driving.

REFERENCES

1. Green M. "How long does it take to stop?" Methodological analysis of driver perception-brake times. Transport Hum Factors 2000;2(3):195–216.
2. Schwienbacher S, Aghayev E, Hofmann UK, et al. Driving and emergency braking may be impaired after tibiotalar joint arthrodesis: conclusions after a case series. Int Orthop 2015;39(7):1335–41.
3. Summala H. Brake reaction times and driver behavior analysis. Transport Hum Factors 2009; 2(3):1–11.
4. Roberts C, Protzer L. Doctor, can I drive?": the need for a rational approach to return to driving after musculoskeletal injury. Injury 2016;47(3):513–5.
5. Goodwin D, Baecher N, Pitta M, et al. Driving after orthopedic surgery. Orthopedics 2013;36(5):469–74.
6. Marecek GS, Schafer MF. Driving after orthopaedic surgery. J Am Acad Orthop Surg 2013;21(11):696–706.
7. Rod Fleury T, Favrat B, Belaieff W, et al. Resuming motor vehicle driving following orthopaedic surgery or limb trauma. Swiss Med Wkly 2012;142:w13716.
8. DiSilvestro KJ, Santoro AJ, Tjoumakaris FP, et al. When can I drive after orthopaedic surgery? A systematic review. Clin Orthop Relat Res 2016;474(12):2557–70.
9. Sansosti LE, Greene T, Hasenstein T, et al. U.S. state driving regulations relevant to foot and ankle surgeons. J Foot Ankle Surg 2017;56(3):522–42.
10. Cooper JM. Clinical decision making: doctor, when can I drive? Am J Orthop (Belle Mead NJ) 2007; 36(2):78–80.
11. Giddins GEB, Hammerton A. "Doctor, when can I drive?": a medical and legal view of the implications of advice on driving after injury or operation. Injury 1996;27(7):495–7.
12. Nunez VA, Giddins GEB. "Doctor, when can I drive?": an update on the medico-legal aspects of driving following an injury or operation. Injury 2004;35(9):888–90.
13. MacLeod K, Lingham A, Chatha H, et al. "When can I return to driving?" A review of the current literature on returning to driving after lower limb injury or arthroplasty. Bone Joint J 2013;95(B):290–4.
14. Von Arx OA, Langdown AJ, Brooks RA, et al. Driving whilst plastered: Is it safe, is it legal? A survey of advice to patients given by orthopaedic

surgeons, insurance companies and the police. Injury 2004;35(9):883–7.

15. Egol KA, Sheikhazadeh A, Mogatederi S, et al. Lower-extremity function for driving an automobile after operative treatment of ankle fracture. J Bone Joint Surg Am 2003;85-A(7):1185–9.

16. Yousri T, Jackson M. Ankle fractures: when can I drive doctor? A simulation study. Injury 2015;46(2): 399–404.

17. Egol KA, Sheikhazadeh A, Koval KJ. Braking function after complex lower extremity trauma. Crit Care 2008;65(6):10–3.

18. Rees JL, Sharp RJ. Safety to drive after common limb fractures. Injury 2002;33(1):51–4.

19. Jennings AG, Sefton GK, Newman RJ. Repair of acute rupture of the Achilles tendon: a new technique using polyester tape without external splintage. Ann R Coll Surg Engl 2004;86(6):445–8.

20. Pauley T, Devlin M. Influence of a concurrent cognitive task on foot pedal reaction time following traumatic, unilateral transtibial amputation. J Rehabil Med 2011;43(11):1020–6.

21. McDonald E, Shakked R, Daniel J, et al. Driving after hallux valgus surgery. Foot Ankle Int 2017;38(9): 982–6.

22. Holt G, Kay M, McGrory R, et al. Emergency brake response time after first metatarsal osteotomy. J Bone Joint Surg Am 2008;90(8):1660–4.

23. Liebensteiner MC, Braito M, Giesinger JM, et al. Driving ability after right-sided ankle arthroscopy—a prospective study. Injury 2015;47(3): 762–5.

24. Jeng CL, Lin JS, Amoyal K, et al. Driving brake reaction time following right ankle arthrodesis. Foot Ankle Int 2011;32(9):896–9.

25. Patrick Engkasan J, Mohd Ehsan F, Yang Chung T. Ability to return to driving after major lower limb amputation. J Rehabil Med 2012;44(1):19–23.

26. Boulias C, Meikle B, Pauley T, et al. Return to driving after lower-extremity amputation. Arch Phys Med Rehabil 2006;87(9):1183–8.

27. Tremblay M-A, Corriveau H, Boissy P, et al. Effects of orthopaedic immobilization of the right lower limb on driving performance: an experimental study during simulated driving by healthy volunteers. J Bone Joint Surg Am 2009;91:2860–6.

28. Murray JC, Tremblay MA, Corriveau H, et al. Effects of right lower limb orthopedic immobilization on braking function: an on-the-road experimental study with healthy volunteers. J Foot Ankle Surg 2015;54(4):554–8.

29. Orr MJ, Dowd CT, Rush CJK, et al. The effect of immobilization devices and left-foot adapter on brake-response time. J Bone Joint Surg Am 2010; 92(18):2871–7.

30. Sansosti LE, Rocha ZM, Lawrence MW, et al. Effect of variable lower extremity immobilization devices

on emergency brake response driving outcomes. J Foot Ankle Surg 2016;55(5):999–1002.

31. Nunn T, Baird C, Robertson D, et al. Fitness to drive in a below knee plaster? An evidence based response. Injury 2007;38(11):1305–7.

32. Waton A, Kakwani R, Cooke NJ, et al. Immobilisation of the knee and ankle and its impact on drivers' braking times: a driving simulator study. J Bone Joint Surg Br 2011;93(7):928–31.

33. Hofmann UK, Thumm S, Jordan M, et al. How do ankle braces affect braking performance? An experimental driving simulation study with healthy volunteers. J Rehabil Med 2015;47(10):963–9.

34. Dammerer D, Braito M, Biedermann R, et al. Effect of surgical shoes on brake response time after first metatarsal osteotomy–a prospective cohort study. J Orthop Surg Res 2016;11:14.

35. Byas-Smith MG, Chapman SL, Reed B, et al. The effect of opioids on driving and psychomotor performance in patients with chronic pain. Clin J Pain 2005;21(4):345–52.

36. Verster JC, Veldhuijzen DS, Volkerts ER. Effects of an opioid (oxycodone/paracetamol) and an NSAID (bromfenac) on driving ability, memory functioning, psychomotor performance, pupil size, and mood. Clin J Pain 2006;22(5):499–504.

37. Dubois S, Bédard M, Weaver B. The association between opioid analgesics and unsafe driving actions preceding fatal crashes. Accid Anal Prev 2010;42(1): 30–7.

38. Zhu S, Layde PM, Guse CE, et al. Obesity and risk for death due to motor vehicle crashes. Am J Public Health 2006;96(4):734–9.

39. Mock CN, Grossman DC, Kaufman RP, et al. The relationship between body weight and risk of death and serious injury in motor vehicle crashes. Accid Anal Prev 2002;34(2):221–8.

40. Whitlock G, Norton R, Clark T, et al. Is body mass index a risk factor for motor vehicle driver injury? A cohort study with prospective and retrospective outcomes. Int J Epidemiol 2003;32(1): 147–9.

41. Ellen RL, Marshall SC, Palayew M, et al. Systematic review of motor vehicle crash risk in persons with sleep apnea. J Clin Sleep Med 2006;2(2): 193–200.

42. Carr DB, Schwartzberg JG, Manning L, et al. Physician's Guide to Assessing and Counseling Older Drivers. 2nd edition. Washington, DC: NHTSA; 2010.

43. McGwin G Jr, Sims RV, Pulley L, et al. Relations among chronic medical conditions, medications, and automobile crashes in the elderly: a population based case-control study. Am J Epidemiol 2000; 152(5):424–31.

44. Kent R, Henary B. On the fatal crash experience of older drivers. Annu Proc Assoc Adv Automot Med 2005;49(1993):371–91.

45. Chen V, Chacko AT, Costello FV, et al. Driving after musculoskeletal injury. J Bone Joint Surg Am 2008; 90(12):2791–7. https://doi.org/10.2106/JBJS.H. 00431.

46. Pickrell TM, Li H. Driver electronic device use in 2016 (Traffic Safety Facts Research Note. Report No. DOT HS 812 426). Washington, DC: National Highway Traffic Safety Administration; 2017.

47. Centers for Disease Control and Prevention (CDC). Mobile device use while driving–United States and seven European countries. MMWR Morb Mortal Wkly Rep 2011;62(10):177–82.

48. Redelmeier DA, Tibshirani RJ. Association between cellular-telephone calls and motor vehicle collisions. N Engl J Med 1997;336(7): 453–8.

49. Klauer SG, Guo F, Simons-Morton BG, et al. Distracted driving and risk of road crashes among novice and experienced drivers. N Engl J Med 2014;307(1):54–9.

50. Kahn C, Cisneros V, Lotfipour S, et al. Distracted driving, a major preventable cause of motor vehicle collisions: "just hang up and drive". West J Emerg Med 2015;16(7). https://doi.org/10.5811/westjem. 2011.5.6700.

Optimizing Outpatient Total Ankle Replacement from Clinic to Pain Management

Michel A. Taylor, MD, MSc, FRCSC[a],
Selene G. Parekh, MD, MBA[a,b,c,*]

KEYWORDS

- Total ankle arthroplasty • Cost savings • Outpatient surgery • Joint replacement

---

KEY POINTS

- Recent health care policy changes, such as bundle payments and outcome-based reimbursement, aim to reduce costs by improving the efficiency with which healthcare is delivered. This must be done while ensuring excellent patient outcomes and satisfaction.
- Many orthopedic specialties have converted inpatient procedures with historically long admissions to "fast tracked" outpatient surgery without compromising patient safety, satisfaction, and outcomes. These "fast tracked" programs are multimodal and multidisciplinary and focus on preoperative, perioperative, and postoperative optimization and have been successful in significantly reducing length of stay in total hip arthroplasty and total knee arthroplasty patients.
- The ability to institute an effective outpatient total ankle program depends on appropriate patient selection, surgeon experience with total ankle replacement, addressing preoperative patient expectations, the involvement of an experienced multidisciplinary care team including experienced anesthesiologists, nurse navigators, recovery room nursing staff, and physical therapists, and most importantly, such a program requires complete institutional logistical support.

INTRODUCTION

End-stage ankle arthritis (ESAA) is a disabling condition with patient morbidity that approaches congestive heart failure and end-stage kidney disease.[1] Historically, the operative treatment gold standard for ESAA has been ankle arthrodesis. Although a significant percentage of patients experience pain relief and high functional outcomes, postoperative stiffness and adjacent joint arthritis can decrease patient satisfaction and postoperative function.[2,3] Total ankle arthroplasty (TAA) was introduced in the 1970s[4,5] and provided surgeons and patients with an alternative to

ankle arthrodesis when treating ESAA. TAA allows for increased range of motion at the tibiotalar joint, which leads to improved postoperative function.[6] In addition, as a result of increased ankle motion, the rate of symptomatic adjacent joint arthrosis is potentially decreased. First-generation TAA implants were associated with high failure and complication rates in addition to inferior outcomes when compared with ankle arthrodesis,[7] and as a result, TAA was not widely adopted. With time, both the surgical technique and the component design have greatly improved, and as a result, TAA has become an important surgical option in the management of ESAA[7] and its

---

[a] Department of Orthopaedic Surgery, Duke University Medical Center, 2301 Erwin Road, Durham, NC 27710, USA; [b] Duke Fuqua School of Business, 100 Fuqua Drive, Durham, NC 27708, USA; [c] North Carolina Orthopedic Clinic, 3609 Southwest Durham Drive, Durham, NC 27707, USA
* Corresponding author. North Carolina Orthopedic Clinic, 3609 Southwest Durham Drive, Durham, NC 27707.
E-mail address: selene.parekh@gmail.com

Orthop Clin N Am 49 (2018) 541–551
https://doi.org/10.1016/j.ocl.2018.06.003
0030-5898/18/© 2018 Elsevier Inc. All rights reserved.

popularity has grown accordingly: between 1998 and 2010, the use of TAA for ESAA has increased 7-fold.[8]

Over the last decade, the demand for health care cost accountability has grown significantly. Recent health care policy changes, such as bundle payments and outcome-based reimbursement, aim to reduce costs by improving the efficiency with which health care is delivered. Policy changes designed to improve cost savings must be implementing without compromising patient care, outcomes or satisfaction. A major area of potential cost savings is hospital admissions following surgical procedures. There is a mounting body of literature that has shown that by decreasing hospital length of stay (LOS), significant cost saving can be achieved.[9–11] Currently, following TAA, patients are typically admitted for 1 to 3 days for pain control, physical therapy, and mobilization.[8,12–14] Reducing this LOS to same day outpatient surgery would represent a significant avenue for cost savings. Although there currently is a lack of research specifically relating to foot and ankle surgery, there have been recent studies that have shown promise relating to outpatient foot and ankle surgery, and more specifically, TAA.[14,15]

Outpatient TAA can be achieved by optimizing patient selection, surgeon experience, surgical technique, use of effective intraoperative pain management, and efficient communication and coordination with physical and occupational therapists. A study by Mulligan and Parekh[14] compared complication, readmission, and reoperation rates between outpatient, overnight, and extended admissions following TAA. They also compared narcotic prescription refills and patient reported visual analogue scores (VAS) postoperatively. They found that outpatient and overnight patients had significantly less complications compared with extended stay patients without finding a difference in postoperative readmission, reoperation, pain scores, or narcotic prescription refills. A study by Gonzalez and colleagues,[12] looking at cost comparison between inpatient and outpatient TAA surgery, found cost savings of approximately 13.4% or $2500 per outpatient case as well as a decrease in average LOS by 2.5 days. Of note, the investigators admitted this was likely a conservative estimate. These results have also been substantiated by significant cost savings in other total joint specialties.[16–19] A study comparing outpatient and inpatient surgery in unicompartmental knee arthroplasty (UKA) found that the cost of outpatient UKA

was approximately 20 thousand dollars less per patient when compared with inpatient admissions.[20]

Many orthopedic specialties have converted inpatient procedures with historically long admissions to "fast tracked" outpatient surgery without compromising patient safety, satisfaction, and outcomes.[18,19] These "fast track" programs are multimodal and multidisciplinary and focus on preoperative, perioperative, and postoperative optimization and have been successful in significantly reducing LOS in total hip arthroplasty (THA) and total knee arthroplasty (TKA) patients.[21] The success of the programs has been attributed to multidisciplinary care coordination, standardized perioperative protocols, discharge planning, and careful patient selection. Currently, certain high-volume centers are performing short-stay admission following TAA, but same day discharge is rarely done.[14]

PATIENT SELECTION

In TAA, like in all joint reconstructive procedures, a successful outcome depends on proper patient selection. Historically, the ideal TAA patient has been an older (>65), lower demand, and nonobese patient.[22–24] However, recent reports have shown that patients undergoing TAA who are under the age of 50 can also expect excellent postoperative results.[6,25] The surgical indications have dramatically changed over the last decade and will likely continue to expand. Following a thorough assessment of the patient and their suitability for TAA, patients can be stratified to inpatient, short stay, or outpatient surgery. This decision should include input from the patient and their family, the surgeon, the anesthesiologist, and preoperative medical consultants. There is a paucity of available data in the TAA literature to guide patient selection for outpatient TAA. There is currently no TAA-specific tool to predict which patients will be discharged on the same day; however, there have been various scoring-based strategies used in the THA and TKA literature.[26,27] Patient suitability for outpatient TAA should include patient and family preference, the ability of the patient to care for themselves following discharge, medical comorbidities precluding fast track pathway, and the number of associated procedures that will be performed. A study looking at outpatient THA and TKA found that in preoperatively unselected patients, 15% of patients were able to be discharged home the same day; they also found that female sex and surgery later in the day increased the odds of not being discharged the same day.[28] In a separate study looking at ankle fracture fixation, they found that women consistently experienced higher postoperative pain scores,[29] a potentially important finding when trying to assess a patient's suitability for major foot ankle surgery in the outpatient setting. In another study assessing predictive factors for accelerated discharge following TKA and THA, the investigators found that younger age, better preoperative mobility, and a supportive home situation were the main predictors for an early discharge from hospital.[30]

The importance of a supportive home environment should not be underestimated. A study looking at partner factors, which affected postoperative recovery, found that patients who had spouses that did not experience negative emotions, who had been employed in health care or the social services, and who felt that nurses had spent enough time explaining matters relating to the patient's care and treatment, were more likely to experience higher quality of recovery.[31] The Outpatient Arthroplasty Risk Assessment (OARA) score has been used in THA and TKA to predict safe early discharge. It comprises 9 areas of comorbidity containing specific conditions wherein a higher score suggests more comorbidities and predicts a longer LOS. A study looking at early discharge following TKA and THA using this scoring system found that early discharge was more common in men, younger patients, and those with a lower body mass index (BMI). In addition, patients who scored lower on the OARA (ie, a score <59) were 2 times more likely to be discharged early. In addition, patients with American Society of Anesthesiologists (ASA) scores less or equal to 2 were 1.7 times more likely to be discharged early than patients with higher ASA-PS scores.[32] An adapted scoring system specific to TAA could represent a valuable tool when trying to establish an outpatient foot and ankle surgery program.

In terms of specific patient factors that may preclude outpatient TAA surgery, there is currently limited evidence to guide treatment; however, research in foot and ankle and other joint replacement specialties has found that various patient factors are associated with perioperative complications and a longer LOS, such as elevated HbA1c level,[33] obesity, hypoalbuminemia,[21,34] age greater than 64, increased operating room time, ASA score equal or greater than 2, and presence of comorbid conditions.[33,35,36] A study looking at forefoot surgery in smokers found higher rates of perioperative pain and other complications,[37] and multiple studies have found that smoking cessation programs started as late as 4 weeks before surgery can have positive effects on outcomes.[38–40] Although further research is needed looking at TAA specifically, the ideal candidate for successful outpatient TAA should be one who is motivated and willing to undergo an accelerated perioperative pathway, well educated regarding the perioperative and postoperative course and expectations, high functioning with good mobility, and have minimal comorbidities, with a good social support network at home. At the authors' institution, patients who are deemed to be ideal candidates for TAA are screened by the surgeon and anesthesiologist for their suitability to undergo TAA as an outpatient procedure. Patients with BMI greater than 40, history of severe and/or untreated sleep apnea, significant pulmonary function compromise, congestive heart failure, chronic kidney disease, who are undergoing bilateral TAA or TAA with multiple simultaneous additional procedures or revision TAA procedures (excluding isolated polyethylene exchange, cyst grafting, and gutter debridement) are better candidates for inpatient or short stay surgery (**Fig. 1**).

PREOPERATIVE PATIENT EDUCATION PROGRAMS

Preoperative patient education is widely used in most surgical specialties and is often included in the consent process. Studies have suggested that by managing patient expectations and making patients active participants in their own recovery, they can expect an earlier discharge from hospital.[41] Interestingly, a recent Cochrane Review failed to find significant improvements in outcome for patients undergoing preoperative education before total joint arthroplasty (TJA).[42] That same study, as well as others, however has suggested a potential role of preoperative education before total joint surgery to decrease anxiety postoperatively.[42–44] With respect to patient expectations relating to hospital discharge, it is important to discuss the planned LOS beforehand because many patients may not know what to expect following their surgical procedure. Studies have found that when expectations are not met, there is a higher rate of patient dissatisfaction.[45] A study looking at THA and TKA admission expectation found that less than 1% of patients knew that a same day discharge was possible, and only 15% of patients thought that only a one night stay would be possible; the rest assumed a lengthier hospital admission would be necessary.[46] The

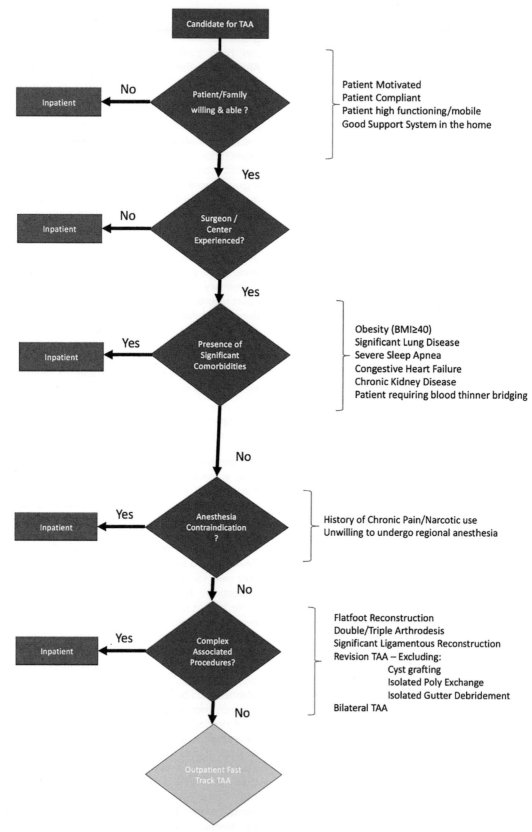

Fig. 1. Decision-making algorithm for outpatient TAA.

same study also found that half of men and a third of women were uncomfortable with the idea of being discharged home the same day.[46] These findings highlight the importance of discussing perioperative and postoperative expectations and protocols with patients before their surgery.

There is evidence to suggest that when properly administered, preoperative patient education can lead to decreased LOS.[47–49] It is important to provide appropriate and adequate information to the patient regarding the diagnosis, procedure, and postoperative course because a significant percentage of patients will access the Internet, which may not offer reliable or accurate information.[50,51] A study looking at the quality of available information on the Internet regarding TAA found that 50% of the available information was either of poor or unacceptable quality.[50] Although the most cost-effective preoperative education program has yet to be determined,[52] such a program may prove to be a valuable tool in decreasing LOS, decreasing patient anxiety, and improving patient satisfaction following TAA. At the authors' institution, every patient who is scheduled for a TAA is fully informed about the procedure, technical steps, implants being used, and length of expected recovery. The patient will then meet with the surgical coordinator, who will spend a considerable amount of time discussing the procedure, the preoperative anesthesia consult, the perioperative course, the expected LOS, and the immediate perioperative and postoperative period. In order to provide access to successful outpatient TAA, the authors believe this approach is necessary.

PREANESTHETIC ASSESSMENT, OPTIMIZATION, AND MEDICATIONS

Most osseous foot and ankle procedures are considered minor surgery, but procedures such as TAA are considered major orthopedic surgery.[53] In order to ensure a successful surgical outcome following major orthopedic procedures, preoperative optimization of medical comorbidities is extremely important and has consistently been shown to be an important step toward maximizing patient outcomes following surgery.[19,21,54] Although there is a dearth of information when it comes to TAA specifically, one can draw from other joint replacement and major surgical procedures. Emphasizing excellent glycemic control in the diabetic patient is of the utmost importance as it has been shown to have a significant impact on LOS while also decreasing local and systemic complications.[55] At the authors' institution, all patients undergo medical clearance within 4 weeks of surgery by an internal medicine specialist with experience in the assessment of TJA patients in a clinic dedicated exclusively to preoperative TJA patients. Additional issues that are managed at this point include home medications that need to be held preoperatively, postoperative deep vein thrombosis (DVT) protocols, and anesthesia modalities and postoperative pain management protocols.

ANESTHESIA MODALITY AND PAIN CONTROL

Although underappreciated, a multimodal approach to perioperative and postoperative pain management with an experienced anesthesiologist is likely one of the most important factors in ensuring a timely discharge from hospital following foot and ankle surgery. Inadequate pain control can lead to increased narcotic consumption and associated complications, such as respiratory distress, urinary retention, and delirium, among others.[56–58] Orthopedic procedures, especially lower limb reconstructive procedures including TAA, have consistently been shown to be among the most painful surgeries.[59–61] This reality has caused a shift in the choice of pain management protocols away from the oral and intravenous administration of narcotics to peripheral nerve blocks and indwelling catheters as a way to better control postoperative pain.[62] Several studies in the TAA, THA, and TKA literature have shown significant benefits to using regional anesthetic blocks, including single nerve sciatic blocks, femoral nerve blocks, and double blocks.[63–67] Continuous infusion nerve block techniques are being used more frequently and have been associated with longer-lasting and effective pain control as well as low rates of perioperative and postoperative complications.[64,65,68] A systematic review of randomized control trials found that regional anesthesia when compared with general anesthesia was associated with lower pain scores and decreased morphine consumption following TKA.[69] Regional anesthesia has also been associated with shortened LOS for major lower extremity surgery.[70] Although their overall safety has been well established, continuous popliteal sciatic nerve blocks have been associated with neuropathic complications[71] and pose a potential risk of infection,[15] which is important to keep in mind when discussing the surgical procedure and anesthetic options with the patients. A relatively new local anesthetic alternative is periarticular injection of liposomal bupivacaine (Exparel; Pacira Pharmaceuticals, Parsippany, NJ, USA), which has been approved by the US Food and Drug Administration for FDA local injection into surgical wounds. It contains DepoFoam (Pacira Pharmaceuticals), which allows for a slow and controlled release of bupivacaine into the surgical wound providing up to 72 hours of postoperative analgesia. Multiple studies looking at liposomal bupivacaine injections for total shoulder, hip, knee, and ankle replacements have shown significant benefits with respect to postoperative pain control.[72,73] A study by Mulligan and colleagues[15] found that single-shot popliteal sciatic nerve block with 0.2% ropivacaine followed by an intraoperative liposomal bupivacaine injection was as effective as a continuous popliteal sciatic nerve block in TAA with regards to total complications, emergency room visits, readmissions, reoperations, VAS pain score, and narcotic refills. At the authors' institution, following preoperative assessment and a thorough discussion between the anesthesia and surgical teams, the authors typically use either general anesthesia with a single-shot popliteal block with ropivacaine followed by periarticular liposomal bupivacaine or a continuous popliteal catheter, which is inserted preoperatively with ropivacaine infusion and intraoperative conscious sedation as required. If a catheter is used, the patient is typically discharged home with the catheter in situ with instructions to remove the catheter on the second postoperative day and to confirm that the tip of the removed catheter is intact. By following this protocol, the authors have been able to provide their patients with excellent pain control, timely discharge from hospital, and good postoperative satisfaction without compromising patient safety.

PREPROCEDURAL PHYSICAL THERAPY

There is a paucity of research assessing the benefit of pre-habilitation with respect to foot and ankle procedures. The concept of prehabilitation having a positive effect on postsurgical outcomes has been explored in the THA and TKA literature. Although some studies have found a beneficial effect,[74–78] these outcomes have not been seen universally.[79–81] A recent systematic review and meta-analysis looking at preoperative physical therapy on recovery following THA and TKA found reduced pain scores at 4 weeks and slightly increased

WOMAC scores, toilet use, time to climb stairs, and chair use in the early postoperative period.[82] This study and others have admitted that the benefits are likely minimal and reiterated the dearth of definitive knowledge and well-designed trials when it comes to answering this question.[83] At this point, there is no evidence to recommend for or against prehabilitation preceding TAA procedures, although this would represent an interesting area of future research.

CATHETERIZATION

Urinary retention following a major orthopedic procedure is not uncommon and can lead to longer LOS or emergency department visits in the immediate postoperative period.[12] The literature has shown mixed results when it comes to routine catheterization following total joint procedures; however, more recent reports have found that routine catheterization can lead to worse patient-reported outcomes and longer LOS[84] and is generally avoided in favor of intermittent catheterization as required.[85] At our institution, we prefer intermittent, as needed, catheterization as opposed to routine and patients are required to void independently without difficulty prior to discharge.

CHOICE OF SURGICAL FACILITY

When trying to implement a "fast track" protocol for outpatient TAA, it is important to consider the hospital or surgical center in which the surgery will be performed because with respect to outpatient surgery, not all centers are created equally. In order for a patient to be discharged home in a timely manner, it requires coordination from the surgeon, anesthesiologist, nursing staff, recovery room personnel, physical therapist, occupational therapist, the administration, and obviously, the patient and his or her family. If a center is not equipped or accustomed to outpatient joint replacement procedures, the results may be less than ideal. A study looking at fast tracked same day TKA found that the most common reason for failing to discharge a patient home the same day was institutional logistical problems.[86] Whether the surgical procedure will be performed at an outpatient surgical center or in an academic center is also important to consider. A study found that primary TAA being performed at an outpatient surgical center with the capacity to admit patient had significantly shorter LOS when compared with matched patients treated at an academic center with no difference in readmission or reoperation rates[87];

these findings have also been seen in other orthopedic subspecialties.[88,89] The causes are likely multifactorial, but one of the hypotheses is the presence of nurse navigators, who can help manage the patients and organize discharge planning.[87] Nurse navigator programs have been well documented to decrease LOS and increase patient satisfaction in the oncologic, medical, and surgical literature.[90–92] When considering LOS and outcomes data comparing outpatient surgical centers and academic hospitals, it is important to remember that patients who typically meet the diagnostic criteria for surgery at an outpatient surgical center are usually younger and healthier with less comorbidities, making direct comparisons difficult.[87,93–96]

OPERATIVE TECHNIQUE

Although there is currently a dearth of evidence when it comes to surgical techniques and procedures that may decrease LOS in TAA, there are several in other orthopedic subspecialties that are worth considering. The use of coagulation modifiers, such as epsilon-aminocaproic acid and tranexamic acid, has been shown to reduce blood loss and LOS following TKA.[97,98] The use of tourniquets in foot and ankle surgery is an important strategy to control operative bleeding and is used by most foot and ankle surgeons.[99] Although there is a lack of evidence in the foot and ankle literature, the use of a tourniquet has led to lower rates of transfusion and shorter LOS following TKA[100,101] but has also been associated with increased rates of DVTs,[101] although this has not been consistently found.[102] Surgeon experience and yearly procedure-specific volumes have been correlated with higher patient satisfaction in various orthopedic procedures.[103,104] A study found that surgeon experience was directly related to the risk of perioperative complications in TAA. Surgeons with less experience performing TAA were 3.1 times more likely to have a perioperative adverse event and 3.2 times more likely to have a perioperative wound complication.[105] Studies have found that surgeons who perform more yearly TAAs have decreased LOS by an average of 1 day per patient.[14,106] At the authors' institution, all surgeons participating in outpatient short stay TAA are high-volume surgeons who perform more than 50 TAA per year; the authors do not routinely administer intraoperative coagulation modifiers and they use a thigh tourniquet, which is deflated before skin closure or at 120 minutes to minimize the risk of ischemic and neurologic complications.

POSTOPERATIVE PROTOCOL

The final decision regarding whether to discharge a patient home is multifactorial and must take into consideration the patient's level of independence, discharge disposition, social support, pain control, mental status, medical comorbidities, gastrointestinal and genitourinary function, and dietary intake. Following the procedure, patients are transferred to a short stay postanesthesia care unit. In addition to the regional anesthetic, the authors' postoperative pain medication protocol includes an oral immediate-release opioid for moderate pain and an intravenously or subcutaneously delivered opioid for severe breakthrough pain. Every patient is also started on a 2-week course of gabapentin and a 3-day course of meloxicam, and alternative medications are substituted in cases of patient allergies. Standard postoperative instructions for all patients include being non-weight-bearing on the operative extremity, elevation of the extremity above the level of the heart, and anticoagulation with 81 mg aspirin in patients at low risk for DVT or pulmonary embolism (PE) risk patients, and an alternative is chosen if DVT/PE risk factors are present. For those patients planned for same-day discharge, once they are able to urinate without assistance, their pain is well controlled, and the need for breakthrough medication is minimal, they are able to safely transfer and mobilize with the use of crutches, a walker, or knee scooter, discharge home is initiated.

SUMMARY

Outpatient TAA is a potentially significant source of cost savings. The ability to institute an effective outpatient TAA program depends on appropriate patient expectations, the involvement of an experienced multidisciplinary care team, including experienced anesthesiologists, nurse navigators, recovery room nursing staff, and physical therapists, and most importantly, such a program requires complete institutional logistical support.

REFERENCES

1. Saltzman CL, Zimmerman MB, O'Rourke M, et al. Impact of comorbidities on the measurement of health in patients with ankle osteoarthritis. J Bone Joint Surg Am 2006;88:2366–72.
2. Fuchs S, Sandmann C, Skwara A, et al. Quality of life 20 years after arthrodesis of the ankle. A study of adjacent joints. J Bone Joint Surg Br 2003;85: 994–8.

3. Buchner M, Sabo D. Ankle fusion attributable to posttraumatic arthrosis: a long-term followup of 48 patients. Clin Orthop Relat Res 2003;(406): 155–64.

4. Saltzman CL. Perspective on total ankle replacement. Foot Ankle Clin 2000;5:761–75.

5. Saltzman CL, McIff TE, Buckwalter JA, et al. Total ankle replacement revisited. J Orthop Sports Phys Ther 2000;30:56–67.

6. Gould JS, Alvine FG, Mann RA, et al. Total ankle replacement: a surgical discussion. Part II. The clinical and surgical experience. Am J Orthop (Belle Mead NJ) 2000;29:675–82.

7. Bolton-Maggs BG, Sudlow RA, Freeman MA. Total ankle arthroplasty. A long-term review of the London Hospital experience. J Bone Joint Surg Br 1985;67:785–90.

8. Singh JA, Ramachandran R. Time trends in total ankle arthroplasty in the USA: a study of the national inpatient sample. Clin Rheumatol 2016;35: 239–45.

9. Stull JD, Bhat SB, Kane JM, et al. Economic burden of inpatient admission of ankle fractures. Foot Ankle Int 2017;38:997–1004.

10. Coventry LL, Pickles S, Sin M, et al. Impact of the orthopaedic nurse practitioner role on acute hospital length of stay and cost-savings for patients with hip fracture: a retrospective cohort study. J Adv Nurs 2017. https://doi.org/10.1111/jan. 13330.

11. Sibia US, Turcotte JJ, MacDonald JH, et al. The cost of unnecessary hospital days for medicare joint arthroplasty patients discharging to skilled nursing facilities. J Arthroplasty 2017;32:2655–7.

12. Gonzalez T, Fisk E, Chiodo C, et al. Economic analysis and patient satisfaction associated with outpatient total ankle arthroplasty. Foot Ankle Int 2017;38:507–13.

13. Jiang JJ, Schipper ON, Whyte N, et al. Comparison of perioperative complications and hospitalization outcomes after ankle arthrodesis versus total ankle arthroplasty from 2002 to 2011. Foot Ankle Int 2015;36:360–8.

14. Mulligan RP, Parekh SG. Safety of outpatient total ankle arthroplasty vs traditional inpatient admission or overnight observation. Foot Ankle Int 2017;38:825–31.

15. Mulligan RP, Morash JG, DeOrio JK, et al. Liposomal bupivacaine versus continuous popliteal sciatic nerve block in total ankle arthroplasty. Foot Ankle Int 2017. https://doi.org/10.1177/ 1071100717722366.

16. Huang A, Ryu JJ, Dervin G. Cost savings of outpatient versus standard inpatient total knee arthroplasty. Can J Surg 2017;60:57–62.

17. Aynardi M, Post Z, Ong A, et al. Outpatient surgery as a means of cost reduction in total hip arthroplasty: a case-control study. HSS J 2014;10: 252–5.

18. Leroux TS, Basques BA, Frank RM, et al. Outpatient total shoulder arthroplasty: a population-based study comparing adverse event and readmission rates to inpatient total shoulder arthroplasty. J Shoulder Elbow Surg 2016;25: 1780–6.

19. Lovald S, Ong K, Lau E, et al. Patient selection in outpatient and short-stay total knee arthroplasty. J Surg Orthop Adv 2014;23:2–8.

20. Richter DL, Diduch DR. Cost comparison of outpatient versus inpatient unicompartmental knee arthroplasty. Orthop J Sports Med 2017;5. 2325967117694352.

21. Winther SB, Foss OA, Wik TS, et al. 1-year follow-up of 920 hip and knee arthroplasty patients after implementing fast-track. Acta Orthop 2015;86:78–85.

22. Saltzman CL. Total ankle arthroplasty: state of the art. Instr Course Lect 1999;48:263–8.

23. Easley ME, Vertullo CJ, Urban WC, et al. Total ankle arthroplasty. J Am Acad Orthop Surg 2002;10:157–67.

24. Bonasia DE, Dettoni F, Femino JE, et al. Total ankle replacement: why, when and how? Iowa Orthop J 2010;30:119–30.

25. Rodrigues-Pinto R, Muras J, Martin Oliva X, et al. Total ankle replacement in patients under the age of 50. Should the indications be revised? Foot Ankle Surg 2013;19:229–33.

26. Dripps RD, Lamont A, Eckenhoff JE. The role of anesthesia in surgical mortality. JAMA 1961;178: 261–6.

27. Charlson ME, Pompei P, Ales KL, et al. A new method of classifying prognostic comorbidity in longitudinal studies: development and validation. J Chronic Dis 1987;40:373–83.

28. Gromov K, Kjaersgaard-Andersen P, Revald P, et al. Feasibility of outpatient total hip and knee arthroplasty in unselected patients. Acta Orthop 2017;88:516–21.

29. Storesund A, Krukhaug Y, Olsen MV, et al. Females report higher postoperative pain scores than males after ankle surgery. Scand J Pain 2016;12:85–93.

30. Schneider M, Kawahara I, Ballantyne G, et al. Predictive factors influencing fast track rehabilitation following primary total hip and knee arthroplasty. Arch Orthop Trauma Surg 2009;129:1585–91.

31. Stark AJ, Salantera S, Sigurdardottir AK, et al. Spouse-related factors associated with quality of recovery of patients after hip or knee replacement - a Nordic perspective. Int J Orthop Trauma Nurs 2016;23:32–46.

32. Meneghini RM, Ziemba-Davis M, Ishmael MK, et al. Safe selection of outpatient joint

arthroplasty patients with medical risk stratification: the "outpatient arthroplasty risk assessment score". J Arthroplasty 2017;32:2325–31.

33. Tarabichi M, Shohat N, Kheir MM, et al. Determining the threshold for hba1c as a predictor for adverse outcomes after total joint arthroplasty: a multicenter, retrospective study. J Arthroplasty 2017;32:S263–7.e1.

34. Fu MC, McLawhorn AS, Padgett DE, et al. Hypoalbuminemia is a better predictor than obesity of complications after total knee arthroplasty: a propensity score-adjusted observational analysis. HSS J 2017;13:66–74.

35. Inneh IA. The combined influence of sociodemographic, preoperative comorbid and intraoperative factors on longer length of stay after elective primary total knee arthroplasty. J Arthroplasty 2015;30:1883–6.

36. Inneh IA, Iorio R, Slover JD, et al. Role of sociodemographic, co-morbid and intraoperative factors in length of stay following primary total hip arthroplasty. J Arthroplasty 2015;30:2092–7.

37. Bettin CC, Gower K, McCormick K, et al. Cigarette smoking increases complication rate in forefoot surgery. Foot Ankle Int 2015;36:488–93.

38. Lindstrom D, Sadr Azodi O, Wladis A, et al. Effects of a perioperative smoking cessation intervention on postoperative complications: a randomized trial. Ann Surg 2008;248:739–45.

39. Moller AM, Villebro N, Pedersen T, et al. Effect of preoperative smoking intervention on postoperative complications: a randomised clinical trial. Lancet 2002;359:114–7.

40. Sorensen LT. Wound healing and infection in surgery. The clinical impact of smoking and smoking cessation: a systematic review and meta-analysis. Arch Surg 2012;147:373–83.

41. Yoon RS, Nellans KW, Geller JA, et al. Patient education before hip or knee arthroplasty lowers length of stay. J Arthroplasty 2010;25:547–51.

42. McDonald S, Page MJ, Beringer K, et al. Preoperative education for hip or knee replacement. Cochrane Database Syst Rev 2014;(5):CD003526.

43. O'Connor MI, Brennan K, Kazmerchak S, et al. Youtube videos to create a "virtual hospital experience" for hip and knee replacement patients to decrease preoperative anxiety: a randomized trial. Interact J Med Res 2016;5:e10.

44. Giraudet-Le Quintrec JS, Coste J, Vastel L, et al. Positive effect of patient education for hip surgery: a randomized trial. Clin Orthop Relat Res 2003;(414):112–20.

45. Jourdan C, Poiraudeau S, Descamps S, et al. Comparison of patient and surgeon expectations of total hip arthroplasty. PLoS One 2012;7:e30195.

46. Meneghini RM, Ziemba-Davis M. Patient perceptions regarding outpatient hip and knee arthroplasties. J Arthroplasty 2017;32:2701–5.e1.

47. Tait MA, Dredge C, Barnes CL. Preoperative patient education for hip and knee arthroplasty: financial benefit? J Surg Orthop Adv 2015;24:246–51.

48. Daltroy LH, Morlino CI, Eaton HM, et al. Preoperative education for total hip and knee replacement patients. Arthritis Care Res 1998;11:469–78.

49. Dawson J, Fitzpatrick R, Carr A, et al. Questionnaire on the perceptions of patients about total hip replacement. J Bone Joint Surg Br 1996;78:185–90.

50. Elliott AD, Bartel AF, Simonson D, et al. Is the internet a reliable source of information for patients seeking total ankle replacement? J Foot Ankle Surg 2015;54:378–81.

51. Kelly MJ, Feeley IH, O'Byrne JM. A qualitative and quantitative comparative analysis of commercial and independent online information for hip surgery: a bias in online information targeting patients? J Arthroplasty 2016;31:2124–9.

52. Pour AE, Parvizi J, Sharkey PF, et al. Minimally invasive hip arthroplasty: what role does patient preconditioning play? J Bone Joint Surg Am 2007;89:1920–7.

53. Meyr AJ, Mirmiran R, Naldo J, et al. American college of foot and ankle surgeons(r) clinical consensus statement: perioperative management. J Foot Ankle Surg 2017;56:336–56.

54. Kolisek FR, McGrath MS, Jessup NM, et al. Comparison of outpatient versus inpatient total knee arthroplasty. Clin Orthop Relat Res 2009;467:1438–42.

55. Marchant MH Jr, Viens NA, Cook C, et al. The impact of glycemic control and diabetes mellitus on perioperative outcomes after total joint arthroplasty. J Bone Joint Surg Am 2009;91:1621–9.

56. Gehling MH, Luesebrink T, Kulka PJ, et al. The effective duration of analgesia after intrathecal morphine in patients without additional opioid analgesia: a randomized double-blind multicentre study on orthopaedic patients. Eur J Anaesthesiol 2009;26:683–8.

57. Tomaszewski D, Balkota M, Truszczynski A, et al. Intrathecal morphine increases the incidence of urinary retention in orthopaedic patients under spinal anaesthesia. Anaesthesiol Intensive Ther 2014;46:29–33.

58. Nandi S, Harvey WF, Saillant J, et al. Pharmacologic risk factors for post-operative delirium in total joint arthroplasty patients: a case-control study. J Arthroplasty 2014;29:268–71.

59. Dadure C, Bringuier S, Nicolas F, et al. Continuous epidural block versus continuous popliteal nerve block for postoperative pain relief after major podiatric surgery in children: a prospective,

comparative randomized study. Anesth Analg 2006;102:744–9.

60. Chou LB, Wagner D, Witten DM, et al. Postoperative pain following foot and ankle surgery: a prospective study. Foot Ankle Int 2008;29:1063–8.

61. Bonica JJ. The management of pain. 2nd edition. Philadelphia: Lea & Febiger; 1990.

62. Elliot R, Pearce CJ, Seifert C, et al. Continuous infusion versus single bolus popliteal block following major ankle and hindfoot surgery: a prospective, randomized trial. Foot Ankle Int 2010;31: 1043–7.

63. Young DS, Cota A, Chaytor R. Continuous infra-gluteal sciatic nerve block for postoperative pain control after total ankle arthroplasty. Foot Ankle Spec 2014;7:271–6.

64. Pearce CJ, Hamilton PD. Current concepts review: regional anesthesia for foot and ankle surgery. Foot Ankle Int 2010;31:732–9.

65. Singelyn FJ, Aye F, Gouverneur JM. Continuous popliteal sciatic nerve block: an original technique to provide postoperative analgesia after foot surgery. Anesth Analg 1997;84:383–6.

66. Jamison RN, Ross MJ, Hoopman P, et al. Assessment of postoperative pain management: patient satisfaction and perceived helpfulness. Clin J Pain 1997;13:229–36.

67. Lee KT, Park YU, Jegal H, et al. Femoral and sciatic nerve block for hindfoot and ankle surgery. J Orthop Sci 2014;19:546–51.

68. Capdevila X, Pirat P, Bringuier S, et al. Continuous peripheral nerve blocks in hospital wards after orthopedic surgery: a multicenter prospective analysis of the quality of postoperative analgesia and complications in 1,416 patients. Anesthesiology 2005;103:1035–45.

69. Macfarlane AJ, Prasad GA, Chan VW, et al. Does regional anesthesia improve outcome after total knee arthroplasty? Clin Orthop Relat Res 2009; 467:2379–402.

70. Stein BE, Srikumaran U, Tan EW, et al. Lower-extremity peripheral nerve blocks in the perioperative pain management of orthopaedic patients: AAOS exhibit selection. J Bone Joint Surg Am 2012;94:e167.

71. Anderson JG, Bohay DR, Maskill JD, et al. Complications after popliteal block for foot and ankle surgery. Foot Ankle Int 2015;36:1138–43.

72. Bramlett K, Onel E, Viscusi ER, et al. A randomized, double-blind, dose-ranging study comparing wound infiltration of DepoFoam bupivacaine, an extended-release liposomal bupivacaine, to bupivacaine HCl for postsurgical analgesia in total knee arthroplasty. Knee 2012; 19:530–6.

73. Cherian JJ, Barrington J, Elmallah RK, et al. Liposomal bupivacaine suspension, can reduce length of stay and improve discharge status of patients undergoing total hip arthroplasty. Surg Technol Int 2015;27:235–9.

74. Desmeules F, Hall J, Woodhouse LJ. Prehabilitation improves physical function of individuals with severe disability from hip or knee osteoarthritis. Physiother Can 2013;65:116–24.

75. Brown K, Loprinzi PD, Brosky JA, et al. Prehabilitation influences exercise-related psychological constructs such as self-efficacy and outcome expectations to exercise. J Strength Cond Res 2014;28:201–9.

76. Walls RJ, McHugh G, O'Gorman DJ, et al. Effects of preoperative neuromuscular electrical stimulation on quadriceps strength and functional recovery in total knee arthroplasty. A pilot study. BMC Musculoskelet Disord 2010;11:119.

77. Saleh KJ, Lee LW, Gandhi R, et al. Quadriceps strength in relation to total knee arthroplasty outcomes. Instr Course Lect 2010;59:119–30.

78. Calatayud J, Casana J, Ezzatvar Y, et al. High-intensity preoperative training improves physical and functional recovery in the early postoperative periods after total knee arthroplasty: a randomized controlled trial. Knee Surg Sports Traumatol Arthrosc 2017. https://doi.org/10.1007/s00167-016-3985-5.

79. Cavill S, McKenzie K, Munro A, et al. The effect of prehabilitation on the range of motion and functional outcomes in patients following the total knee or hip arthroplasty: a pilot randomized trial. Physiother Theory Pract 2016;32: 262–70.

80. Mat Eil Ismail MS, Sharifudin MA, Shokri AA, et al. Preoperative physiotherapy and short-term functional outcomes of primary total knee arthroplasty. Singapore Med J 2016;57:138–43.

81. Cabilan CJ, Hines S, Munday J. The impact of prehabilitation on postoperative functional status, healthcare utilization, pain, and quality of life: a systematic review. Orthop Nurs 2016;35: 224–37.

82. Wang L, Lee M, Zhang Z, et al. Does preoperative rehabilitation for patients planning to undergo joint replacement surgery improve outcomes? A systematic review and meta-analysis of randomised controlled trials. BMJ Open 2016;6: e009857.

83. Peer MA, Rush R, Gallacher PD, et al. Pre-surgery exercise and post-operative physical function of people undergoing knee replacement surgery: a systematic review and meta-analysis of randomized controlled trials. J Rehabil Med 2017;49: 304–15.

84. Loftus T, Agee C, Jaffe R, et al. A simplified pathway for total knee arthroplasty improves outcomes. J Knee Surg 2014;27:221–8.

85. Walters M, Chambers MC, Sayeed Z, et al. Reducing length of stay in total joint arthroplasty care. Orthop Clin North Am 2016;47:653–60.

86. Bradley B, Middleton S, Davis N, et al. Discharge on the day of surgery following unicompartmental knee arthroplasty within the United Kingdom NHS. Bone Joint J 2017;99-B:788–92.

87. Beck DM, Padegimas EM, Pedowitz DI, et al. Total ankle arthroplasty: comparing perioperative outcomes when performed at an orthopaedic specialty hospital versus an academic teaching hospital. Foot Ankle Spec 2017;10:441–8.

88. Toy PC, Fournier MN, Throckmorton TW, et al. Low rates of adverse events following ambulatory outpatient total hip arthroplasty at a free-standing surgery center. J Arthroplasty 2017. https://doi.org/10.1016/j.arth.2017.08.026.

89. Padegimas EM, Zmistowski BM, Clyde CT, et al. Length of stay after shoulder arthroplasty-the effect of an orthopedic specialty hospital. J Shoulder Elbow Surg 2016;25:1404–11.

90. Lee T, Ko I, Lee I, et al. Effects of nurse navigators on health outcomes of cancer patients. Cancer Nurs 2011;34:376–84.

91. Seldon LE, McDonough K, Turner B, et al. Evaluation of a hospital-based pneumonia nurse navigator program. J Nurs Adm 2016;46:654–61.

92. Goodson AS, DeGuzman PB, Honeycutt A, et al. Total joint replacement discharge brunch: meeting patient education needs and a hospital initiative of discharge by noon. Orthop Nurs 2014;33:159–62.

93. Pugely AJ, Martin CT, Gao Y, et al. Comorbidities in patients undergoing total knee arthroplasty: do they influence hospital costs and length of stay? Clin Orthop Relat Res 2014;472:3943–50.

94. Menendez ME, Baker DK, Fryberger CT, et al. Predictors of extended length of stay after elective shoulder arthroplasty. J Shoulder Elbow Surg 2015;24:1527–33.

95. Husted H, Hansen HC, Holm G, et al. What determines length of stay after total hip and knee arthroplasty? A nationwide study in Denmark. Arch Orthop Trauma Surg 2010;130:263–8.

96. Pakzad H, Thevendran G, Penner MJ, et al. Factors associated with longer length of hospital stay after primary elective ankle surgery for end-stage ankle arthritis. J Bone Joint Surg Am 2014;96:32–9.

97. Harper RA, Sucher MG, Giordani M, et al. Topically applied epsilon-aminocaproic acid reduces blood loss and length of hospital stay after total knee arthroplasty. Orthopedics 2017;40:1–6.

98. Zhu M, Chen JY, Yew AK, et al. Intra-articular tranexamic acid wash during bilateral total knee arthroplasty. J Orthop Surg (Hong Kong) 2015;23:290–3.

99. Gruetter F, Rudkin G, Stavrou P, et al. Use of peripheral blocks and tourniquets in foot surgery: a survey of Australian orthopaedic foot and ankle surgeons. Foot Ankle Surg 2015;21:282–5.

100. Parvizi J, Diaz-Ledezma C. Total knee replacement with the use of a tourniquet: more pros than cons. Bone Joint J 2013;95-B:133–4.

101. Tai TW, Lin CJ, Jou IM, et al. Tourniquet use in total knee arthroplasty: a meta-analysis. Knee Surg Sports Traumatol Arthrosc 2011;19:1121–30.

102. Alcelik I, Pollock RD, Sukeik M, et al. A comparison of outcomes with and without a tourniquet in total knee arthroplasty: a systematic review and meta-analysis of randomized controlled trials. J Arthroplasty 2012;27:331–40.

103. Bozic KJ, Maselli J, Pekow PS, et al. The influence of procedure volumes and standardization of care on quality and efficiency in total joint replacement surgery. J Bone Joint Surg Am 2010;92:2643 52.

104. Jain NB, Kuye I, Higgins LD, et al. Surgeon volume is associated with cost and variation in surgical treatment of proximal humeral fractures. Clin Orthop Relat Res 2013;471:655–64.

105. Haskell A, Mann RA. Perioperative complication rate of total ankle replacement is reduced by surgeon experience. Foot Ankle Int 2004;25:283–9.

106. Basques BA, Bitterman A, Campbell KJ, et al. Influence of surgeon volume on inpatient complications, cost, and length of stay following total ankle arthroplasty. Foot Ankle Int 2016;37:1046–51.

Printed and bound by CPI Group (UK) Ltd, Croydon, CR0 4YY

08/05/2025

01864728-0002